AF443580

Update on Hepatobiliary Diseases
1996

FALK SYMPOSIUM 90

Update on Hepatobiliary Diseases 1996

Edited by

S.-K. Lam
Department of Medicine
The University of Hong Kong
Queen Mary Hospital
Hong Kong

G. Paumgartner
Department of Medicine II
Klinikum Grosshadern
University of Munich
D-81377 Munich
Germany

B. Wang
Beijing Friendship Hospital
Capital University of Medical Sciences
Beijing
People's Republic of China

Proceedings of the Falk Symposium No. 90 held in Hong Kong,
February 29 – March 1 1996

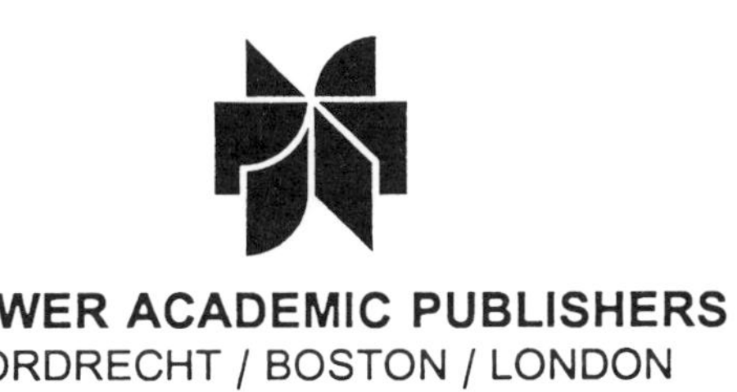

KLUWER ACADEMIC PUBLISHERS
DORDRECHT / BOSTON / LONDON

Distributors

---

for the United States and Canada: Kluwer Academic Publishers, PO Box 358, Accord Station, Hingham, MA 02018-0358, USA

for all other countries: Kluwer Academic Publishers Group, Distribution Center, PO Box 322, 3300 AH Dordrecht, The Netherlands

A catalogue record for this book is available from the British Library

ISBN 0–7923–8715–5

Copyright

Published in the United Kingdom by Kluwer Academic Publishers, PO Box 55, Lancaster, UK.

Kluwer Academic Publishers BV incorporates the publishing programmes of D. Reidel, Martinus Nijhoff, Dr W. Junk and MTP Press.

Typeset by EXPO Holdings, Malaysia

Printed and bound in Great Britain by Hartnolls Ltd., Bodmin, Cornwall.

Contents

List of principal contributors

H. E. Blum
Medizinische Klinik und Poliklinik
Universitätsklinikum
Hugstetter Str. 55
D-79106 Freiburg
Germany

J. L. Boyer
Liver Center/Section of Digestive
  Diseases
Yale University School of Medicine
333 Cedar Street
New Haven
CT 06510-8019
USA

C. E. Broelsch
Abteilung für Allgemeinchirurgie
Universitätskrankenhaus Eppendorf
Martinistr. 52
D-20253 Hamburg
Germany

M. Burdelski
Abteilung Pädiatrische
  Gastroenterologie
Universitätskrankenhaus Eppendorf
Martinistr. 52
D-20246 Hamburg
Germany

M. C. Carey
Harvard Medical School
Gastroenterology Division
Brigham and Women's Hospital
75 Francis Street
Boston
MA 02115-6195
USA

M. Colombo
Istituto di Medicina Interna
dell' Università degli Studi di Milano
University of Milan
Via Pace 9
I-20122 Milan
Italy

J. J. Fung
Division of Transplantation Surgery
Pittsburgh Transplantation Institute
3601 Fifth Avenue
Pittsburgh
PA 15213
USA

A. L. Gerbes
Medizinische Klinik II
Klinikum Grosshadern der Universität
  Munchen
Marchioninistr. 15
D-81377 München
Germany

J. L. Gollan
Harvard Medical School
Gastroenterology Division
Brigham and Women's Hospital
75 Francis Street
Boston
MA 02115-6195
USA

J. W. Halliday
Queensland Institute of Medical
  Research (Liver Unit)
The Bancroft Centre
PO Royal Brisbane Hospital
300 Herston Road
Brisbane 4029
Australia

LIST OF PRINCIPAL CONTRIBUTORS

D. Häussinger
Klinik für Gastroenterologie und
   Infektiologie
Medizinische Einrichtungen der
   Universität Dusseldorf
Moorenstr. 5
D-40225 Düsseldorf
Germany

T. Ichida
Department of Internal Medicine III
Niigata University School of Medicine
757 Asahimachi-Dori 1
Niigata City
Niigata 951
Japan

C.-L. Lai
Department of Medicine
Gastroenterology Section
Queen Mary Hospital
University of Hong Kong
Hong Kong

S.-K. Lam
Department of Medicine
The University of Hong Kong
Queen Mary Hospital
Room 419, K. Block
Hong Kong

D. Lebrec
Inserm U-24
Hôpital Beaujon
100 Blvd. du Général Leclerc
F-92118 Clichy Cedex
France

U. Leuschner
Medizinische Klinik II
Universitätsklinikum Haus 11
Theodor-Stern-Kai 7
D-60590 Frankfurt am Main
Germany

Y.-F. Liaw
Liver Research Unit
Chang Gung Memorial Hospital and
   Medical College
199 Tung Hwa North Road
Taipei
Taiwan 105

C. S. Lieber
Alcohol Research and Treatment Center
Liver Disease and Nutrition Section
Bronx VA Medical Center
130 West Kingsbridge Road, Bronx
New York
NY 10468-3904
USA

K. P. Maier
Department of Medicine
City Hospital Esslingen
Academic Department
University of Tübingen
Tübingen
Germany

M. P. Manns
Department of Gastroenterology and
   Hepatology
Medizinische Hochschule Hannover
Konstanty-Gutschow-Str. 8
D-30625 Hannover
Germany

J. Neuberger
The Liver and Hepatobiliary Unit
3rd Floor, Nuffield House
Queen Elizabeth Hospital
University Hospital Birmingham
Birmingham B15 2TH
UK

G. Paumgartner
Department of Medicine II
Klinikum Grosshadern
University of Munich
Marchioninistr. 15
D-81377 Munich
Germany

R. Poupon
Service d'Hepato-Gastro-Enterologie
Hôpital Saint Antoine
184 rue du Fbg. Saint-Antoine
F-75571 Paris Cedex 12
France

T. Sauerbruch
Klinik für Allgemeine Innere
   Medizin
Klinikum der Universität
Sigmund-Freud-Str. 25
D-53105 Bonn
Germany

N. Soehendra
Department of Endoscopic
   Surgery
University Hospital
   Hamburg-Eppendorf
Martinistr. 52
D-20246 Hamburg
Germany

LIST OF PRINCIPAL CONTRIBUTORS

S. M. Strasberg
Washington University School of
  Medicine
Section of Hepatobiliary, Pancreatic and
  Gastrointestinal Surgery
One Barnes Hospital Plaza, Box 8109
St Louis
MO 63110
USA

Z.-Y. Tang
Liver Cancer Institute
Zhong Shan Hospital
Shanghai Medical University
136 Yi Xue Yuan Road
Shanghai 200032
P.R. of China

D. H. van Thiel
C349 Transplant Center
Chandler Medical Center
University of Kentucky
800 Rose St
Lexington
KY 40536–0084
USA

B.-E. Wang
Honorary President
Beijing Friendship Hospital
Capital University of Medical Sciences
Beijing
P.R. of China

Section I
Viral Hepatitis

1
Pathogenesis and immunology of hepatitis C

M. P. MANNS

INTRODUCTION

Since the discovery of the hepatitis C virus in 1989[1] numerous investigators have concentrated on evaluating the pathogenetic mechanisms leading to liver cell destruction in hepatitis C. Closely related to this is the phenomenon that the majority of patients, at least 80%, develop a chronic infection after contact with the hepatitis C virus. This chapter reviews the present knowledge of the B- and T-cell response against hepatitis C virus proteins, the involvement of hepatitis C virus in the induction of autoimmunity and its involvement as an aetiological agent for extrahepatic diseases which may have an immune-mediated pathogenesis.

B-CELL RESPONSE AGAINST HEPATITIS C

The hepatitis C virus (HCV) was discovered by screening cDNA libraries prepared from a chimpanzee which had been inoculated with serum from a patient with post-transfusion hepatitis. First a clone was identified which expressed an epitope of the NS3 region[1]. The structure of the HCV has been well characterized and several B-cell epitopes have been identified in the structural and non-structural regions of the virus. Diagnostic tests for the detection of HCV antibodies by ELISA and RIBA techniques at present use three or four recombinant HCV proteins.

Recently human monoclonal antibodies were used to identify immunodominant B-cell epitopes of HCV[2,3]. In this context it is interesting that immunodominant conformational B-cell epitopes on NS3 spanning between amino acids 1363 and 1454 discriminate between viraemic and non-viraemic HCV sera. These B-cell epitopes characterized by human monoclonal antibodies may be used as prognostic parameters, as well as reagents, to elucidate pathogenetic mechanisms.

Different approaches are currently used to develop vaccines against HCV. So far they have all been unsuccessful. The hypervariable region 1 (HVR 1) of the E2 envelope protein is of particular interest[4]. HCV isolates were pre-incubated with human anti-HCV antibody positive sera. It was shown that incubation of HCV isolates with serum containing antibodies to HVR 1 epitopes may become non-infectious for chimpanzees. However, these obviously protecting and neutralizing epitopes on the HVR 1 region are isolate-specific. These experiments, carried out by Farci *et al.*[4], support the theory that the HCV population in serum consists of a variety of quasi-species which develop during the course of infection (Fig. 1).

A further interesting aspect of the B-cell response to HCV is that an epitope of the HCV core region obviously cross-reacts with a poorly defined self-antigen. This antigen has been named GOR. Mishiro *et al.*[5] first found that antibodies to this GOR epitope (anti-GOR) occur very early in HCV infection[5]. They found that these antibodies cross-react with a self-antigen presumably expressed in the nuclei of hepatocytes. The antibodies also react with a sequence of the HCV core antigen. Anti-GOR antibody titres are closely associated with HCV infection. LKM 1 antibodies are markers of autoimmune hepatitis type II and occur in 0–10% of patients with chronic hepatitis C[6]. When sera were tested for anti-GOR, hepatitis C antibodies, and hepatitis C RNA at the same time, it became obvious that antibodies to GOR antigen occur only in patients with replicating hepatitis C infection[7]. Further studies indicated that in hepatitis D

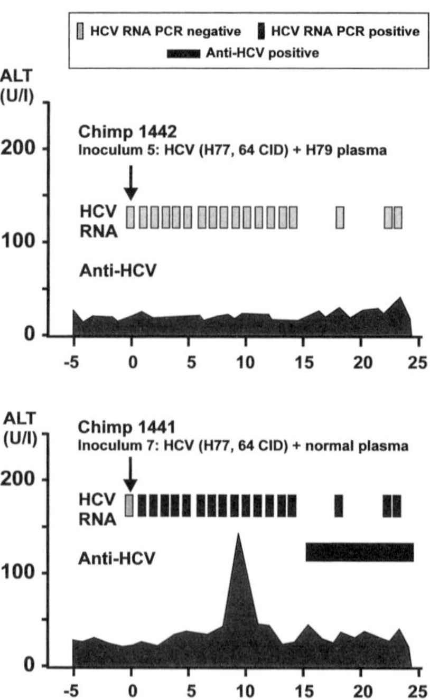

Fig. 1 Course of HCV infection in chimpanzees after antibody-mediated *in-vitro* neutralization (according to ref. 4)

Table 1 Anti-GOR: a hepatitis C antibody cross-reacting between HCV core protein and a nuclear protein

Anti-GOR antibodies occur early in acute hepatitis C infection
Anti-GOR antibodies are closely associated with hepatitis C replication
Anti-GOR titres decline if interferon treatment is effective
Anti-GOR antigen in hepatitis D indicates co-infection with hepatitis C
Anti-GOR in LKM-1 antibody-positive liver disease indicates HCV infection
Anti-GOR antibodies cross-react between a hepatitis C virus core protein sequence and a poorly defined nuclear self antigen
GOR antigen expression seems to be up-regulated in hepatocellular carcinoma tissue

virus infection GOR antibodies are detected only if there is superinfection with hepatitis C[8]. Anti-GOR never occur in hepatitis D virus infection or hepatitis B virus infection alone[8]. Anti-GOR are not only early markers of acute HCV infection, their titres also decline if interferon therapy is effective. Therefore anti-GOR antibodies seem to reflect cross-reactivity between HCV core protein and a self structure expressed in the nucleus of liver cells, and presumably other organs. Thus anti-GOR antibodies react with cross-reactive epitopes and do not represent self-perpetuating genuine autoimmunity (Table 1).

T-CELL RESPONSE AGAINST HCV

Before discussing in detail available data concerning the T-cell response in hepatitis C it is interesting to briefly summarize the data available regarding hepatitis B. It has become clear that the T-cell response in hepatitis B is poly-clonal and multispecific[9]. It is targeted at all viral proteins. The T-cell response in patients with acute hepatitis is very strong, whereas it is frequently mild or absent in chronic hepatitis B (Table 2). The T-cell response contributes to viral clearance, it suppresses viral gene expression and replication in the liver. Latest data show that the intrahepatic T-helper cell profile is mainly T-helper 2[10]. It finally became evident that natural variants of cytotoxic T-cell epitopes of the

Table 2 The cellular immune response in hepatitis B and C

Hepatitis B
The cellular immune response is polyclonal and multispecific
It is targeted against all viral proteins
It is detectable in the peripheral blood in acute hepatitis but less frequently and weaker in chronic hepatitis
It contributes to viral clearance
It suppresses viral gene expression and replication
The intrahepatic T helper cell profile is mainly T helper 2
Hepatitis C
The cellular immune response is polyclonal and multispecific
It is targeted against all viral proteins
It is detectable in the peripheral blood in acute hepatitis and also in chronic hepatitis
Resolution of acute hepatitis is associated with a T helper cell response against an immunodominant epitope in the NS3 region
The intrahepatic T helper cell profile is mainly T helper 1

hepatitis B core protein presented by HLA A2 molecules may act as T-cell receptor antagonists[11]. This phenomenon was shown to be responsible for the development of chronic hepatitis B in a minor proportion of patients. However, this mechanism is not the cause of chronicity in the majority of hepatitis B carriers[12].

Data concerning the T-cell response in hepatitis C are limited. Cellular immune response against HCV is also polyclonal and multispecific[13–18] (Table 2); it is also targeted against all viral proteins. In contrast to hepatitis B the evaluation of peripheral blood lymphocytes in hepatitis C reveals that a strong polyclonal and multispecific T-cell response against various HCV proteins is found not only in acute hepatitis but also in chronic hepatitis C patients[17]. Thus the chronic carrier rate develops despite a strong cellular immune response against various proteins of the HCV. However, it is of interest that acute hepatitis C is associated with a T-helper cell response against immunodominant epitopes in the NS3 region[19]. This epitope has been further defined on a 72 amino acid sequence of the NS3 region between amino acids 1207 and 1278[20]. Apart from the characterization of the CD4 positive T-helper cell response in hepatitis C several papers have characterized and analysed the cytotoxic T-cell response in hepatitis C. One group used recombinant virus to introduce hepatitis C viral proteins in an *in-vitro* assay for the evaluation of cytotoxic T lymphocytes against hepatitis C. This CTL response was characterized to be HLA class I restricted, and in particular relevant epitopes were expressed on HLA 2.1 molecules. The list of T-cell epitopes is continuously growing. Furthermore, transgenic mice have been used to identify T-cell epitopes[18]. Transgenic mice expressing human HLA A2 molecules were shown to recognize HCV-T-cell epitopes which were later confirmed in the human system[21,22]. This seems to be a particularly attractive experimental model. Finally CTL escape mutants were identified in a chimpanzee model for chronic hepatitis C[23].

HEPATITIS C AND EXTRAHEPATIC SYNDROMES

Hepatitis is associated with a number of extrahepatic syndromes (Table 3). Several of these syndromes are thought to be immune-mediated. Although the pathogenesis is unclear, the aetiological role of HCV for mixed cryoglobulinaemia and a proportion of patients with membranoproliferative glomerulonephritis is evident[24]. Furthermore, an association with immune thyroiditis, a Sicca syndrome (different from Sjögren syndrome) and lymphoma is probable. The relationship of other syndromes to hepatitis C virus still has to be proven.

Table 3 Extrahepatic syndromes associated with hepatitis C

Mixed cryoglobulinaemia
Membranoproliferative glomerulonephritis
Thyroiditis
Sicca syndrome (different from Sjögren syndrome)
Porphyria cutanea tarda
Panarteritis nodosa
Lymphoma

Table 4 Heterogeneity of microsomal antigens

Antibody	kDa	Target antigen	Disease association
LKM 1	50	Cytochrome P450 II D6	Autoimmune hepatitis type 2 (hepatitis C)
LKM 2	50	Cytochrome P450 II C9	Ticrynafen-induced hepatitis
LKM 3	55	Family 1 UGT / Family 2 UGT	Chronic hepatitis D, autoimmune hepatitis type 2
LM	52	Cytochrome P450 I A2	Dihydralazine-induced hepatitis Autoimmune polyendocrine syndrome type 1 (APS-1)
	57	Disulphide isomerase	Halothane hepatitis
	59	Carboxylesterase	Halothane hepatitis
	59	?	Chronic hepatitis C
	64	?	Autoimmune hepatitis
	70	?	Chronic hepatitis C

kDa = molecular weight in kilodaltons; LKM = liver–kidney microsomal antibodies; LM = anti-liver microsomal antibodies; UGT = UDP-glucuronosyltransferase.

Concerning treatment, it is accepted that interferon should be recommended for the treatment of essential mixed cryoglobulinaemia and cases of membrano-proliferative glomerulonephritis if replicating HCV infection is the cause. Concerning other syndromes the reader is referred to several review articles[24–26].

HEPATITIS C AND AUTOIMMUNITY

HCV is associated with the induction of several autoantibodies. In Asia and Africa hepatitis C infection is frequently associated with high-titre antinuclear antibodies. The induction of antinuclear antibodies by HCV in the European population is relatively rare. Antithyroid antibodies may be detected in hepatitis C before the start of interferon treatment. Clinically overt immune thyroiditis may manifest during treatment. Of particular interest is the association of HCV infection with liver/kidney microsomal antibodies in a proportion of patients. This proportion varies between 0% and 7% depending on the geographical origin of the patients (Table 5). In southern Europe up to 10% of patients show LKM 1 antibodies while this is very rare in Northern America[7,27–32], LKM 1 antibodies in hepatitis C may not be distinguished by immunofluorescence from LKM 1 antibodies in autoimmune hepatitis type II. In autoimmune hepatitis type II LKM 1 antibodies are directed against the core epitope of eight amino acids on cytochrome P450 II D6[33], these LKM 1 antibodies are very heterogeneous in hepatitis C[8]. A proportion recognizes cytochrome P450 II D6[8] (Table 4). Usually they recognize a larger epitope or different epitopes on cytochrome P450 II D6[8,33–35]. Additional LKM 1 antibodies react with other microsomal proteins[8] at 59 kDa and 70 kDa. Half of the sera reacting in fluorescence with an LKM 1-like pattern do not react with recognized proteins in Western blot[8]. This may be due to conformational epitopes[8,34]. Preliminary data suggest that patients with hepatitis C and LKM 1 antibodies show a specific genetic background as

Table 5 HCV-associated autoimmunity: association of HCV infection with liver–kidney microsomal antibodies (LKM 1)

(a) HCV prevalence among LKM-1 positive patients
Todros *et al.* 1991[29]: 73% (*n* = 33) Italian
Lenzi *et al.* 1991[27]: 88% (*n* = 33) Italian
                        0% (*n* = 10) UK
Lunel *et al.* 1992[28]: 49% (*n* = 83) French
Michel *et al.* 1992[7]: 48% (*n* = 29) German
Miyakawa *et al.* 1995[a]: 100% (*n* = 24) Japanese

(b) LKM-1 prevalence among HCV-positive patients
Reddy *et al.* 1993[30]: 3.7% (*n* = 428) French
                        0% (*n* = 204) US
Czaja *et al.* 1993[31]: 3% (*n* = 29) US
Abuaf *et al.* 1993[32]: 5% (*n* = 272) French
Pawlotsky *et al.* 1994[48]: 5% (*n* = 61) French

LKM 1 = anti liver–kidney microsomal antibodies; HCV = hepatitis C virus.
[a] Personal communication

determined by HLA phenotypes[36,37]. In addition these patients may experience increased risks under treatment with interferon[37–39]. Single-case reports demonstrate an elevation of transaminases under interferon treatment in patients with hepatitis C and LKM 1 antibodies[37–39]. Three out of six patients from Italy showed a deterioration of disease under interferon treatment; all shared the HLA haplotype B51, DR2 and DQ1[37]. A larger series from Torino showed that one out of 18 patients with chronic hepatitis C and LKM 1 antibodies treated with interferon showed deterioration, while none out of 90 patients with chronic hepatitis C developed an increase in transaminases when LKM 1 antibodies were missing[39]. Preliminary data suggest that reactivity with the microsomal antigens at 70 kDa may have a more favourable response to interferon than patients with LKM 1 antibodies reacting against the other microsomal antigens (Durazzo *et al.*, unpublished). Overall the development of serological markers of autoimmunity may be influenced by the host rather than by the virus[40]. Transmission of hepatitis C via the donor liver demonstrates that autoimmunity is induced by HCV infection[41]. However, genotypes in patients with or without LKM 1 antibodies do not seem to be significantly different[40].

There is another example of an RNA hepatitis virus inducing autoimmunity: hepatitis D. A number of autoantibodies are associated with hepatitis D virus infection[42]. LKM 3 antibodies occur in up to 13% of patients with chronic hepatitis D[43]. These LKM 3 antibodies react with a 55 kDa microsomal protein[8]. The antigen was cloned and identified on proteins of the family 1-UDP glucuronosyltransferases[44]. A minor epitope was recognized on family 2-UGT[44]. Recently a recombinant bacculovirus-expressed protein was used to establish an ELISA technique[45]. LKM 3 antibodies against UGT are restricted to patients with chronic hepatitis D and autoimmune hepatitis type 2. The application of this ELISA based on recombinant bacculovirus expressed UGT-1 protein showed that LKM 3 antibodies in autoimmune hepatitis show significantly higher titres[45]. Even in patients with chronic hepatitis D and LKM 3 antibodies titres of Italian patients are higher than those of German patients[45]. The evaluation of the B-cell epitope has shown that the length of sequence is rather large for patients with chronic hepatitis D compared to patients with autoimmune hepatitis[46]. Interestingly, again there seems to be a difference between patients with viral hepatitis and those suffering from autoimmune hepatitis. The minimum sequence seems to be larger in patients with chronic viral hepatitis, and conformational epitopes are most important.

LKM 1 antibodies in hepatitis C and LKM 3 antibodies in hepatitis D share a number of characteristics (Table 5). In genuine autoimmune liver disease LKM 1 and LKM 3 antibodies are of high titre, the autoepitopes are linear and small and in general the B-cell response is more homogeneous. In contrast, in virus-induced autoimmunity caused by hepatitis C or hepatitis D, autoantibody titres are low, autoepitopes are heterogeneous, and there are multiple linear and conformational autoepitopes. In general the B-cell response is more heterogeneous.

It is interesting that microsomal autoantigens are localized in the endoplasmic reticulum and belong to the cytochrome P450 supergene family or to another superfamily of drug-metabolizing enzymes, i.e. UDP glucuronosyltransferases. It is interesting that autoimmunity in genuine autoimmune liver disease and virus-induced liver disease may be distinguished based on B-cell epitope characterization. However, the mechanisms leading to the induction of autoantibodies in viral hepatitis are not clear. It is of interest than all the hepatitis viruses inducing autoimmunity are RNA viruses. They may be packaged in the membranes of the endoplasmic reticulum. A specific HLA background may be necessary to present these autoepitopes to the immune system. Furthermore, it is known that several of the cytochrome P450 molecules, or parts of them, are expressed on the surface of the liver cell membrane. However, this has to be proven for autoepitopes expressed on UGT proteins. Until now we do not know whether and how this type of autoimmunity contributes to the tissue damage seen in chronic viral hepatitis, in particular hepatitis C. However, the molecular characterization of hepatocellular autoantigens in autoimmune liver disease, viral liver disease and drug-induced liver disease (Table 5) will certainly aid study of the pathogenesis of those liver diseases[7,8]. In this sense members of the cytochrome P450 supergene family and the UDP-glucuronosyltransferases are good models to study autoimmune liver disease, drug-induced immune-mediated liver disease and virus-induced autoimmunity in humans.

References

1. Choo QL, Kuo G, Weiner AJ *et al.* Isolation of a cDNA clone derived from a blood-borne non-A, non-B viral hepatitis genome. Science. 1989;244:359–62.
2. Cerino A, Boender P, La Monica N, Rosa C, Habets W, Mondelli M. A human monoclonal antibody specific for the N terminus of the hepatitis C virus nucleocapsid protein. J Immunol. 1993;151:7005–15.
3. Mondelli M, Cerino A, Boender P *et al.* Significance of the immune response to a major conformational B-cell epitope on the hepatitis C virus NS3 region defined by a human monoclonal antibody. J Virol. 1994;68:4829–36.
4. Farci P, Alter HJ, Wong DC *et al.* Prevention of hepatitis C virus infection in chimpanzees after antibody-mediated *in vitro* neutralization. Proc Natl Acad Sci USA. 1994;91:7792–6.
5. Mishiro S, Hoshi Y, Takeda K. Non-A, non-B hepatitis specific antibodies directed at host derived epitope: implication for an autoimmune process. Lancet. 1990;2:1400–3.
6. Strassburg C, Manns MP. Viral hepatitis and autoimmunity: chicken or egg? Viral Hepatitis Rev. 1995;1:97–109.

7. Michel G, Ritter A, Gerken G, Meyer zum Büschenfelde K-H, Decker R, Manns M. Anti-GOR and hepatitis C virus in autoimmune liver disease. Lancet. 1992;339:267–9.
8. Durazzo M, Philipp T, van Pelt FNAM *et al.* Heterogeneity of microsomal autoantibodies (LKM) in chronic hepatitis C and D virus infection. Gastroenterology. 1995;108:455–62.
9. Rehermann B. Immunopathogenesis of viral hepatitis. In: Manns MP, editor. Bailliére's Clinical Gastroenterology. In press.
10. Bertolotti A, Del Prete G, D'Elios M *et al.* Different cytokine profiles of liver-derived T-cell clones in chronic hepatitis B and hepatitis C virus infections. IX Triennial International Symposium on Viral Hepatitis and Liver Diseases, Rome 21–25 April 1996, Abstract D36.
11. Bertoletti A, Sette A, Chisari FV *et al.* Natural variants of cytotoxic epitopes are T-cell receptor antagonists for antiviral cytotoxic T-cells. Natural (Lond.). 1994;369:407–10.
12. Rehermann B, Pasquinelli C, Mosier SM, Chisari FV. Hepatitis B virus (HBV) sequence variation in cytotoxic T lymphocyte epitopes is not common in patients with chronic HBV infection. J Clin Invest. 1995;96:1527–34.
13. Weiner AJ, Geysen HM, Christopherson C *et al.* Evidence for immune selection of hepatitis C virus (HCV) putative envelope glycoprotein variants: Potential role in chronic HCV infections. Proc Natl Acad Sci USA. 1992;89:3468–72.
14. Koziel MJ, Dudley D, Wong JT *et al.* Intrahepatic cytotoxic T lymphocytes specific for hepatitis C virus in persons with chronic hepatitis. J Immunol. 1992;149:3339–44.
15. Minutello MA, Pileri P, Unutmaz D *et al.* Compartmentalization of T lymphocytes to the site of disease: intrahepatic CD4+ T cells specific for the protein NS4 of hepatitis C virus in patients with chronic hepatitis C. J Exp Med. 1993;178:17–25.
16. Koziel MJ, Dudley D, Afdhal N *et al.* Hepatitis C virus (HCV)-specific cytotoxic T lymphocytes recognize epitopes in the core and envelope proteins of HCV. J Virol. 1993;67:7522–32.
17. Cerny A, McHutchinson JG, Pasquinelli C *et al.* Cytotoxic T lymphocyte response to hepatitis C virus-derived peptides containing the HLA A2.1 binding motif. J Clin Invest. 1995;95:521–30.
18. Battegay M, Fikes J, Di Bisceglie AM *et al.* Patients with chronic hepatitis C have circulating cytotoxic T cells which recognize hepatitis C virus-encoded peptides binding to HLA-A2.1 molecules. J Virol. 1995;69:2462–70.
19. Diepolder HM, Zachoval R, Hoffmann RM *et al.* Possible mechanism involving T lymphocyte response to non-structural protein 3 in viral clearance in acute hepatitis C virus infection. Lancet. 1995;346:1006–7.
20. Diepolder HM, Zachoval R, Hoffmann RM *et al.* Virus Elimination während akuter Hepatitis C: funktionelle und molekulare Analyse der NS3-spezifischen CD4+- T-Zellreaktion. Z Gastroenterologie. 1996;23:80–1.
21. Shirai M, Okada H, Nishioka M *et al.* An epitope in hepatitis C virus core region recognized by cytotoxic T cells in mice and humans. J Virol. 1994;68:3334–42.
22. Shirai M, Arichi T, Nishioka M *et al.* CTL response of HLA-A2.1 transgenic mice specific for hepatitis C viral peptides predict epitopes for CTL of humans carrying HLA-A2.1. J Immunol. 1994;154:2733–42.
23. Erickson AL, Houghton M, Choo QL *et al.* Hepatitis C virus-specific CTL response in the liver of chimpanzees with acute and chronic hepatitis C. J Immunol. 1993;151:4189–99.
24. Manns MP. Autoimmunity and hepatitis C virus. In: Miguet JP, Dhumeaux D, editors. Progress in Hepatology 93. Paris: John Libbey Eurotext; 1993:79–87.
25. Manns MP. Autoantibodies in chronic hepatitis: diagnostic reagents and scientific tools to study etiology, pathogenesis and cell biology. In: Boyer JL, Ockner RK, editors. Progress in liver diseases, Vol. XII. Philadelphia, PA: WB Saunders; 1994:137–56.
26. Vergani D, Mieli-Vergani G. Type II autoimmune hepatitis. What is the role of the hepatitis C virus? Gastroenterology. 1993;104:1870–3.
27. Lenzi M, Johnson PJ, Mcfarlane IG *et al.* Antibodies to hepatitis C virus in autoimmune liver disease: evidence for geographical heterogeneity. Lancet. 1991;338:277–80.
28. Lunel F, Abuaf N, Frangeul L *et al.* Liver/kidney microsome antibody type 1 and hepatitis C virus infection. Hepatology. 1992;16:630–6.
29. Todros T, Touscoz G, D'Urso N *et al.* Hepatitis C virus-related chronic liver disease with autoantibodies to liver–kidney microsomes (LKM). Clinical characterzation from idiopathic LKM-positive disorders. J Hepatol. 1991;13:128–31.
30. Reddy KR, Kravitt EL, Radick J *et al.* Absence of LKM-1 antibody in hepatitis C viral infection in the United States. Hepatology. 1993;18:173A.

31. Czaja AJ, Carpenter HA, Santrach PJ, Moore B, Taswell HF, Homburger HA. Evidence against hepatitis viruses as important causes of severe autoimmune hepatitis in the United States. J Hepatol. 1993;18:342–52.
32. Abuaf N, Lunel F, Giral P *et al.* Non-organic specific autoantibodies associated with chronic C virus hepatitis. J Hepatol. 1993;18:359–64.
33. Manns M, Griffin KJ, Sullivan KF, Johnson EF. LKM-1 autoantibodies recognize a short linear sequence in P450 II D6, a cytochrome P450 monooxygenase. J Clin Invest. 1991;88:1370–8.
34. Duclos-Vallee JC, Hajoui O, Yamamoto AM, Jacqz-Aigrain E, Alvarez F. Conformational epitopes on CYP2D6 are recognized by liver/kidney microsomal antibodies. Gastroenterology. 1995;108:470–6.
35. Yamamoto AM, Cresteil D, Homberg JC, Alvarez F. Characterization of anti-liver–kidney microsome antibody (anti-LKM1) from hepatitis C virus-positive and -negative sera. Gastroenterology. 1993;104:1762–7.
36. Manns M, Scheucher S, Jentzsch M *et al.* Genetics in autoimmune hepatitis type 2. Hepatology. 1991;14:60A.
37. Muratori L, Lenzi M, Cataleta M *et al.* Interferon therapy in liver/kidney microsomal antibody type 1-positive patients with chronic hepatitis C. J Hepatol. 1994;21:199–203.
38. Ruiz-Moreno M, Rua MJ, Carreno V *et al.* Autoimmune chronic active hepatitis type 2 manifested during interferon therapy in children. J Hepatol. 1991;12:265–6.
39. Todros L, Saracco G, Durazzo M *et al.* Efficacy and safety of interferon alfa therapy in chronic hepatitis C with autoantibodies to liver–kidney microsomes. Hepatology. 1995;22:1374–8.
40. Michitaka K, Durazzo M, Tillmann HL, Walker D, Phillipp T, Manns MP. Analysis of hepatitis C virus genome in patients with autoimmune hepatitis type 2. Gastroenterology. 1994;106:1603–10.
41. Mackie FD, Peakman M, Yun M *et al.* Primary and secondary liver/kidney microsomal autoantibody response following infection with hepatitis C virus. Gastroenterology. 1994;106:1672–5.
42. Philipp T, Straub P, Durazzo M, Tukey RH, Manns MP. Molecular analysis of autoantigens in hepatitis D. J Hepatol. 1995;22(Suppl. 2):132–5.
43. Crivelli O, Lavarini C, Chiaberge E *et al.* Microsomal autoantibodies in chronic infection with the HBsAg associated delta (d) agent. Clin Exp Immunol. 1983;54:232–8.
44. Philipp T, Durazzo M, Trautwein C *et al.* Recognition of uridine diphosphate glucuronosyl transferase by LKM-3 antibodies in chronic hepatitis D. Lancet. 1994;344:578–81.
45. Strassburg CP, Obermayer-Straub P, Alex B, Philipp T, Tukey RH, Manns MP. Autoepitopes on UDP-glucuronosyltransferase (LKM-3) in autoimmune hepatitis differ from those on hepatitis C. Gastroenterology. 1995;108:A1177.
46. Obermayer-Straub P, Strassburg CP, Clemente MG, Phillipp T, Tukey RH, Manns MP. Recognition of three different epitopes on UDP-glucuronosyltransferases by LKM-3 antibodies in patients with autoimmune hepatitis and hepatitis D. Gut. 1995;37(Suppl. 2):A100.
47. Van Pelt FNAM, Straub P, Manns MP. Molecular basis of drug-induced immunological liver injury. Sem Liver Dis. 1995;15:283–300.
48. Pawlotsky J-M, Ben Yahia M, Andre C *et al.* Immunological disorders in C virus chronic active hepatitis: a prospective case–control study. Hepatology. 1994;9:841.

2
The clinical course of hepatitis C

K. P. MAIER

The clinical course of hepatitis C virus (HCV) infection can be described as the interplay between the virus and the host defence, resulting in different clinical outcomes. The *acute* clinical presentation of hepatitis C has mainly been documented in transfusion-associated cases. Acute HCV infection leads to symptoms only in a minority of cases, and few patients (about 10%) become jaundiced. Therefore, the acute disease is often overlooked.

Fulminant cases of hepatitis non-A–non-B have been reported. However, most of these cases have later been shown not to be related to HCV infection (Table 1[1]). Recently, however, it was shown that HCV could be transmitted from patients with fulminant hepatitis to a chimpanzee, thus providing evidence for an aetiological role of HCV in humans[2]. Clinically, fulminant hepatitis was characterized by very high titres of HCV viraemia in each case, and by multiple genotypes (1a, 1b, 2a). In clinical practice, however, documented fulminant hepatitis C must still be regarded as an extremely rare complication of acute HCV infection.

Given the rarity of fulminant cases, and the general benign condition of the acute disease, the significance of HCV infection resides in its penchant to

Table 1 Fulminant hepatitis – the role of HCV infection

	n	*Cases*	*Serum HCV RNA positive (%)*
France			
Feray *et al.*, 1994[1]	23	HBsAg-negative ('sporadic') (1/23 HBV DNA-positive)	0
	17	HBsAg-positive (10/17 HBV DNA-positive)	45 (co-/superinfection?)
Asia			
Chu *et al.*, 1994[8]	11	HBsAg-negative ('sporadic')	45
	19	HBsAg-positive	32
USA			
Farci *et al.*, 1994[2]	3	HBV DNA (PCR)-negative	100*

* Genotype: 1a, 1b, 2a (1b was experimentally transmitted to a chimp: induction of an unusually severe acute hepatitis C (ALT 744 U/L), self-limited

Table 2 Symptoms and signs in chronic HCV infection (PTH) (percentages)

Symptoms or signs	No. of patients (n=131)	Chronic hepatitis (n=27)	Chronic active hepatitis (n=30)	Cirrhosis (n=67)	HCC (n=7)[*]
Symptom					
Fatigue	67	52	57	75	100
Abdominal pain	19	15	10	24	43
Anorexia	14	11	13	13	43
Weight loss	6	4	—	6	43
Jaundice	1	—	—	3	—
Sign					
Hepatomegaly	68	56	60	75	86
Splenomegaly	21	4	—	37	29

[*] All the patients with HCC had either clinical or histological evidence of cirrhosis
Data from ref. 3

become chronic. Indeed, progression from acute to chronic hepatitis C is extremely common, perhaps universal.

Chronic infection, usually defined as a persistently elevated alanine aminotransferase (ALT) activity of more than 2.5 times normal for 1 year, is largely a silent process[3]. Fatigue is the predominant clinical symptom. In most patients the liver is enlarged (Table 2). Spontaneous resolution beyond 12 months appears unusual (about 1% of cases). In Japan the rate of natural loss of HCV was calculated to be 0.4% per year. Male gender, old age, a large viral dose and HCV genotype 1b (?) have been found to favour the development of chronic HCV infection. Initially there was some scepticism as to whether HCV infection represented anything more than unspecific 'transaminitis' in a largely asymptomatic person. Serial liver biopsies, however, disclosed that up to 50% of patients with the initial diagnosis of mildly active hepatitis, formerly called CPH, progressed to severely active chronic hepatitis within 11 years of observation. The

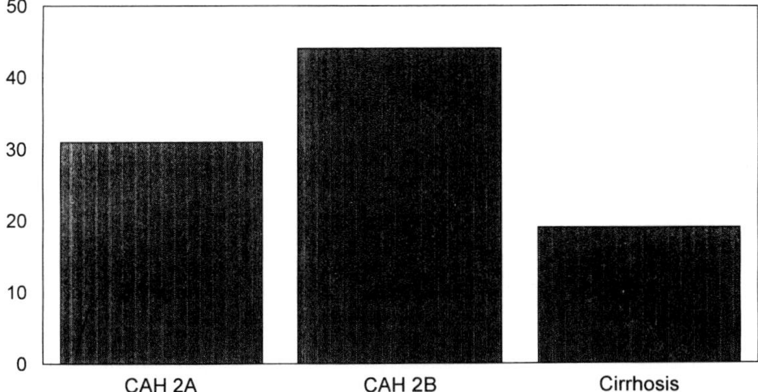

Fig. 1 Histological course of chronic hepatitis C – moderately active CH (first biopsy). Time interval to second biopsy: 9 ± 6 years. Histologically improved: 6%. Data from ref. 4

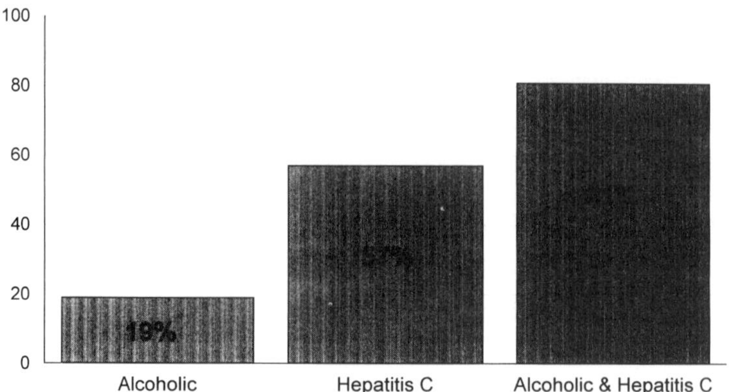

Fig. 2   Cumulative rate (10 years) of HCC development in cirrhosis. Data from ref. 5

sequelae of severe chronic hepatitis C are potentially substantial: within 5–8 years up to 20% (perhaps more) of patients develop cirrhosis (Fig. 1[4]).

The annual rate of developing cirrhosis in Italy is about 8% of chronically infected patients. Additional factors (co-infection with HBV and HIV, alcohol) may accelerate this process[5]. Moreover, alcohol represents a substantial risk factor for the development of liver carcinoma (HCC) in patients suffering from cirrhosis due to HCV infection (Fig. 2).

On the other hand there are some patients who have consistently normal ALT values despite the presence of HCV RNA in serum. Histological data in this group are conflicting: although 47% of patients had significant liver pathology[6], most lesions were not very severe (Table 3). It has been speculated that the 'healthy' HCV carrier state could reflect a very early event of chronic viral infection, followed – years later – by chronic hepatitis C. At present, however, it seems fair to emphasize that the question of a truly 'healthy carrier' of HCV is still unresolved. The overall severity of chronic hepatitis C is controversial. There is no question that HCV can lead to cirrhosis and HCC, and in many centres end-stage chronic hepatitis C is today the leading indication for OLT.

Table 3   Liver histology in hepatitis C infection. Comparison of histological assessment between persistently normal and abnormal liver function

Histological assessment	Normal AST[*]	Abnormal AST	Total
Normal	2	0	2
Minimal	8	5	13
Chronic persistent hepatitis	6	6	12
Chronic active hepatitis	3	10	3
Cirrhosis	0	2	2

[*] Significant liver pathology in 47% of cases (nine of 19 patients)
Data from ref. 6

How often do these serious consequences occur, and how soon? A controlled study has shown that, after a mean of 18 years follow-up, mortality rates in patients with hepatitis C (post-transfusion hepatitis; PTH); were identical as compared to controls (transfused patients without hepatitis). While overall mortality was the same, a small but statistically significant excess of liver-related mortality was noted[7]. Recently, patients with proven chronic hepatitis C (PTH) were followed for a mean of 3.9 (1–15) years. Alcoholics were excluded. Fifty-one per cent had cirrhosis, 5% HCC. During follow-up, 20 patients (15%) died from complications of cirrhosis and from HCC. Mean intervals from blood transfusion to the diagnosis of HCV-induced liver disease could be calculated: 13.9 years for chronic hepatitis, 18.4 years for chronic active hepatitis, 20.6 years for cirrhosis and 28.3 years for HCC[3]. Therefore, the paradox between the relatively benign mortality figures up to 18 years and the observed fatal outcome resides in the indolent nature of progressive HCV infection. In this particular situation progression of the disease should be measured not in years but in decades.

In summary, prognostication is difficult in the case of chronic HCV infection. ALT activity fluctuates and can be normal for weeks or months. Serial liver biopsies are prognostically important, especially in patients with persistently abnormal ALT activity. However, even with established cirrhosis, some patients do very well over a period of years, while others progress to a fatal outcome in less than 5–10 years (viral load? virulent strain? different immune response?).

References

1. Féray C, Gigou M, Samuel D *et al*. Hepatitis C virus RNA and hepatitis B virus DNA in serum and liver of patients with fulminant hepatitis. Gastroenterology. 1993;104:549–55.
2. Farci P, Munez S, Alter H *et al*. Hepatitis C virus (HCV) associated fulminant hepatitis and its transmission to a chimpanzee. Hepatology. 1994;20:265A.
3. Tong MJ, El-Farra NS, Reikes AR, Co RL. Clinical outcomes after transfusion-associated hepatitis C. N Engl J Med. 1995;332:1463–6.
4. Takahashi M, Yamada G, Miyamoto R, Doi T, Endo H, Tsuji T. Natural course of chronic hepatitis C. Am J Gastroenterol. 1993;88:240–3.
5. Yamauchi M, Nakahara M, Maezawa S. Prevalence of hepatocellular carcinoma in patients with alcoholic cirrhosis and prior exposure to hepatitis C. Am J Gastroenterol. 1993;88:39–43.
6. Healey CJ, Chapmann RWG, Fleming KA. Liver histology in hepatitis C infection: a comparison between patients with persistently normal or abnormal transaminases. Gut. 1995;37:274–8.
7. Seeff LB, Buskel-Bales Z, Wright EC *et al*. Long-term mortality after transfusion-associated non-A, non-B hepatitis. N Engl J Med. 1992;327:1906–11.
8. Chu CM, Sheen IS, Liaw YF. The role of hepatitis C virus in fulminant viral hepatitis in an area with endemic hepatitis A and B. Gastroenterology. 1994; 107:189–95.

3
Concurrent hepatitis B virus and hepatitis C virus infection

Y.-F. LIAW

INTRODUCTION

Hepatitis C virus (HCV), hepatitis B virus (HBV) and hepatitis delta virus (HDV) share similar transmission routes, thus concurrent infection with two or three viruses may occur in the same patient. In addition, these viral infections may persist to cause chronic hepatitis or chronic carrier state[1-3], superinfection of a new virus may occur and persist in patients who have been chronically infected with others. Earlier studies employing less sophisticated tests for hepatitis markers have already demonstrated sequential or simultaneous acute infections by two or even four hepatitis agents[4-7]. Non-A–non-B hepatitis (NANB) virus superinfections have long been suspected to play a significant role in acute exacerbations during the course of chronic HBV infection[8], or to account for acute hepatitis in previously unrecognized HBsAg carriers[9]. The advent of HCV assays has enabled investigators to examine the issues of HCV co-infection or superinfection more precisely. Several authors have recently shown that dual or triple infection involving HCV is not uncommon. There is emerging evidence to suggest that multiple hepatotropic virus infections involving HCV have significant clinical or virological implications, and this is the topic of this review.

CO-INFECTION WITH HBV AND HCV

Simultaneous acute infections with NANB and HBV were first described in an intensive-care unit nurse who developed an attenuated acute hepatitis B that was preceded by an earlier onset of NANB hepatitis[4]. Besides this single case report, an outbreak of exceptionally severe hepatitis in haemodialysis units was encountered in two Edinburgh hospitals during 1969–70, and was suspected to be the result of concurrent infection with NANB and HBV[10]. Retrospective HCV assays for the stored serum specimens of these patients have recently confirmed that they were concurrently infected with HCV and HBV[11]. Krogsgaard *et al.*[12]

re-evaluated their Copenhagen patients with acute hepatitis B seen during 1980–82, and also found that some patients had acute HCV co-infection. More recently, at least seven patients with concurrent post-transfusion acute HCV and HBV infection have been documented[13,14].

Similar to the findings in chimpanzee studies[15,16], patients with acute HBV and HCV co-infection generally have a delay in the appearance of HBsAg with shortened duration of HBsAg antigenaemia and a lower level of HBsAg and ALT as compared with patients with acute HBV infection alone[14]. These observations suggest that HCV co-infection interferes with HBV and attenuates its clinical presentation. However, acute HCV and HBV co-infection may lead to fulminant hepatitis[17]. A substantial number of HCV and HBV co-infections in HBsAg-positive fulminant hepatitis have also been observed in India[18], France[19] and the Edinburgh outbreak (B. P. Marmion, personal communication 1994). It seems that concurrent acute infection with HCV and HBV can significantly increase the risk of fulminant hepatitis on the one hand, but suppress HBV on the other. The mechanisms of these effects require further study, but seem similar to the obligatory interaction between HDV and HBV.

HCV SUPERINFECTION IN CHRONIC HBV INFECTION

Unless the onset of HBV and/or HCV infections was clearly known and delineated serologically, such as in the prospective follow-up study of patients with chronic hepatitis virus infections[20], one can rarely tell which virus comes first. The chronological sequences of seropositivity for HBsAg and anti-HCV can be prospectively documented in some patients, such as haemophiliacs, parenteral drug abusers, and those on maintenance haemodialysis[21–23], but not in most of the clinical cases. In a HBV endemic area where HBV infection usually occurs perinatally or at childhood, e.g. Taiwan or other Southeast Asian countries, most patients with both HBV and HCV markers could be chronic HBV-infected patients with HCV superinfection. In the case of clinical acute hepatitis, *de novo* seroconversion of anti-HCV in a HBsAg-positive but IgM-anti-HBc-negative patient indicates an acute HCV superinfection on chronic HBV state[9,12,21]. The presence of serum anti-HCV with a low enzyme immunoassay optical density (OD) ratio in such patients also indicates acute HCV super-infection if the OD ratios increase in the follow-up assays[11]. In contrast, acute HBV superinfection in patients with preceding or past HCV infection can be suggested by the presence of IgM anti-HBc as well as anti-HCV of high OD ratio in the acute-phase serum samples[12].

Seroprevalence studies in patients with HBsAg-positive chronic hepatitis, cirrhosis and hepatocellular carcinoma (HCC) have shown that concurrent infection with HBV and HCV is not uncommon in Asia[24–29] or in Western countries[30–36]. The prevalence is around 10–15% in patients with chronic HBV infection, although it may vary from country to country (Table 1). This is possibly due to different assay methods used, and the size of the studies. The prevalence tends to be higher in studies involving less than 100 patients[26,32,33,36] or in studies using first-generation anti-HCV assays[30,35].

Table 1 Prevalence of serum anti-HCV in patients with chronic HBV infection

Country	Year	Reference	No. of cases	Anti-HCV	
				No.	Percentage
East					
China	1994	Tao *et al.*[24]	1345	119	9
India	1994	Panigrahi *et al.* [25]	91	11	12
Japan	1994	Ohkawa *et al.*[27]	156	20	13
Korea	1993	Kim and Park[28]	185	16	9
Taiwan	1994	Liaw *et al.*[29]	1498	173	12
West					
Germany	1995	Jilg *et al.*[35]	518	139	27
Italy	1991	Fattovich *et al.*[30]	184	27	15
Niger	1995	Cénac *et al.*[36]	65	13	20
Spain	1994	Crespo *et al.*[34]	132	17	13
UK	1992	Brown *et al.*[32]	26	6	23
USA	1991	Fong *et al.*[31]	148	16	11
USSR	1992	Favorov *et al.*[33]	76	15	20

Anti-HCV: antibodies against hepatitis C virus. HBV: hepatitis B virus

HBV SUPERINFECTION IN CHRONIC HCV INFECTION

To the best of our knowledge, acute HBV infection during the follow-up course of patients with chronic HCV infection has not been reported. Although the data are limited, the Copenhagen study showed that 22 of 69 patients who developed typical acute hepatitis B had evidence of antecedent or past HCV infection[12]. The finding that two of 10 Taiwanese patients with fulminant/subfulminant hepatitis were seropositive for IgM anti-HBc as well as anti-HCV of high OD during the acute phase also suggested HBV superinfection in pre-existing chronic HCV infection[37,38].

CONCURRENT HBV, HCV AND HDV TRIPLE INFECTION

Several seroprevalence studies have shown that triple infections with HBV, HCV and HDV are not rare. The prevalence of serum anti-HCV in patients with HDV infection ranged between 9% and 32%[29,30,33,36,39–41], or around 10% in studies involving more than 100 patients (Table 2). Clinical studies have shown that there are patients with acute HBV, HCV and HDV co-infection, or acute HBV and HDV co-superinfection in pre-existing chronic HCV infection[12]. As expected, acute HDV superinfection can occur in pre-existing dual infection with HCV and HBV. Likewise, acute HCV and HDV co-superinfection is seen in pre-existing chronic HBV infection[41]. Successive or sequential HCV and HDV superinfections in patients with chronic HBV infection are also seen in our liver unit.

Acute HCV superinfection in previously unrecognized asymptomatic HBsAg carriers with HDV markers (acute or chronic) presents much more severe liver injury than in those without the HDV markers. For instance, 100% of 11 HDV-

Table 2 Prevalence of serum anti-HCV in patients with HDV infection

Country	Year	Reference	No. of cases	Anti-HCV	
				No.	*Percentage*
Italy	1991	Fattovich *et al.*[30]	28	9	32
Niger	1995	Cénac *et al.*[36]	41	10	24
Taiwan	1994	Liaw[29]	194	19	10
USA	1992	Ackerman *et al.*[39]	46	10	22
USSR	1992	Favorov *et al.*[33]	101	9	9

Anti-HCV: antibodies against hepatitis C virus. HDV: hepatitis delta virus

positive patients developed hepatic decompensation and 45% died of failure (Liaw *et al.*, unpublished data, 1996). Acute HCV and HDV co-superinfection as the aetiology of fulminant/subfulminant hepatitis in previously unrecognized HBsAg carriers is well documented in two Taiwanese studies[37,38]. In the Greek study the parenteral drug abusers showing fulminant/subfulminant hepatitis were exclusively those having triple viral infection[42]. These findings indicate that triple viral infection increases the risk of severe hepatitis.

EFFECT OF CONCURRENT INFECTION WITH HBV AND HCV

Suppressive effect of HCV

Similar to the findings in chimpanzees[15,16] and in humans[14] that acute HCV co-infection interferes with HBV, earlier studies in chimpanzees have also illustrated that NANB (HCV) superinfection exerts a suppressive or inhibitory effect on the replication of the pre-existing HBV[43,44]. Clinical studies in patients with chronic HBV infection have also demonstrated that anti-HCV-positive patients are mostly hepatitis B e antibody (anti-HBe) seropositive[26,27,30,31,34,45,46], generally have a low HBV-DNA polymerase activity[26,31] or weak HBV-DNA positivity[30,34,40,45]. In fact, gradual loss of HBV-DNA with subsequent HBeAg seroconversion, and even HBsAg clearance, has been observed in acute HCV superinfection[20,40,47]. A study on patients with concurrent HCV and HBV infection has shown that HCV-RNA-positive patients rarely had detectable IgA anti-HBc, suggesting a decrease of active immune response against HBV[26]. An immunological study assessing the proliferative response of peripheral blood mononuclear cells to viral antigens also demonstrated that such patients responded primarily to HCV antigens, and this suggests that HCV prevails in causing liver damage, and was a suppressive effect on HBV in humans[48].

A recent case–control study showed that patients with chronic HBV infection undergoing HBsAg seroclearance had a significantly higher (5–6 times) prevalence of anti-HCV than their age/sex-matched controls[49]. Another study showed that anti-HCV was found significantly more often in patients with antibody against HBV core (anti-HBc) alone than in chronic HBsAg carriers[35]. These observations provide indirect evidence to support the concept that HCV superinfection exerts a viral interference effect that can suppress or terminate the chronic HBsAg carrier state. The longitudinal follow-up study and multivariate analysis in a large series of patients further indicates that the annual incidence of HBsAg seroclearance increased strikingly from < 0.5% in patients with HBV infection alone to > 2% in patients with concurrent HCV infection, and that the HCV is the sole hepatotropic virus accountable for enhanced HBsAg seroclearance in chronic HBV infection[50].

In addition, HCV infection may somehow influence the replication of HDV, as the serum marker(s) for HDV replication were generally undetectable in patients seropositive for both anti-HDV and anti-HCV[33]. Further evidence that HCV tends to suppress HDV comes from the immunohistological finding that HDAg was detected much less frequently in patients with concurrent HCV infection[41].

Usurpation of HBV by HCV as the agent in continuing chronic hepatitis

Serum ALT levels usually returned to normal after HBsAg seroclearance in patients with chronic HBV infection. However, abnormal ALT and hepatitis activity may persist in some patients. Clinicopathological and molecular biological studies in such patients have provided evidence to suggest that HCV superinfection may not only have terminated chronic HBsAg antigenaemia but may also take over the role of HBV in causing continuing chronic hepatitis[47]. It is noteworthy that such patients usually remain anti-HBc-positive but anti-HBs-negative after HBsAg seroclearance[47]. Therefore, anti-HCV-seropositive patients with anti-HBc as the sole HBV marker might be originally chronic HBsAg carriers who had cleared their serum HBsAg following clinical or subclinical HCV superinfection[35,47].

Suppression of HCV by other viruses

Interestingly, a reciprocal suppression of HCV replication by HBV or HDV resulting in a state of latent HCV infection has been noted in patients with concurrent infection[26,40,46]. A recent study in human immunodeficiency virus (HIV) infected patients showed that HBV may have taken advantage of a severe immunodeficiency state, and effectively suppresses HCV expression[51]. Patients showing an alternating appearance of serum HBV-DNA or HCV-RNA with concomitant disappearance of the other virus have also been documented[11,46]. The finding of coexistence or alternating appearance of HDV-RNA or HCV-RNA[11], and the finding that HCV-RNA was frequently absent in the serum and liver of patients seropositive for both anti-HDV and anti-HCV[40] also suggest that HDV may suppress HCV.

Aggravation of disease by HCV

Paradoxically, HCV superinfection can cause a much more severe liver disease in patients with chronic HBV infection. In fact, acute HCV superinfection in HBsAg carriers, as well as acute HCV and HBV co-infection, may be the major cause of fulminant/subfulminant hepatitis[17-19]. Two independent studies from Taiwan have also demonstrated that a significant proportion (10–20%) of fulminant/subfulminant hepatitis in chronic HBsAg carriers could be attributed to

HCV superinfection[37,38]. These studies lend support to the suggestion that HCV superinfection in HBV carriers may enhance the risk of fulminant hepatitis[19]. However, whether HBV superinfection in patients with pre-existing chronic HCV infection may also aggravate the disease severity or increase the risk of fulminant hepatitis remains to be investigated.

Besides such a catastrophic effect of acute HCV superinfection, liver disease may progress (Fig. 1), and appears to be more severe in terms of histology and clinical decompensation in patients seropositive for both HBsAg and anti-HCV than in patients seropositive for HBsAg alone[31,34], or HCV alone[52]. This has been well documented in the follow-up study of renal allograft recipients who have concurrent HCV and HBV infection[53], and in severely immunodeficient HIV-infected patients with both HBV and HCV viraemia[51]. Furthermore, case–control studies have indicated that concurrent infection with HCV and

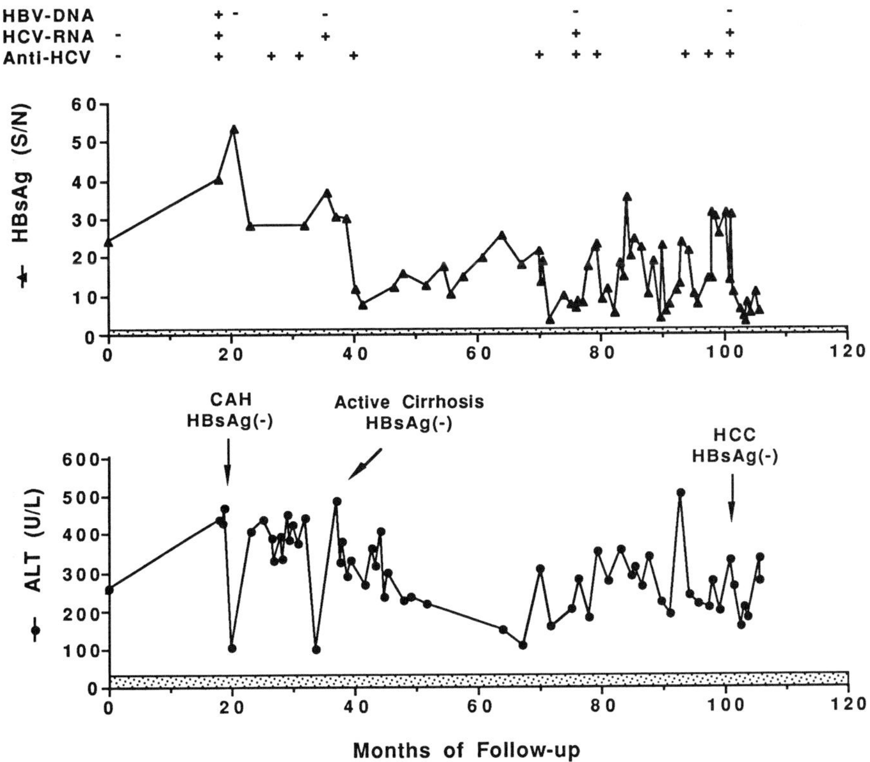

Fig. 1 Clinical course after acute hepatitis C virus (HCV) superinfection in a patient with chronic hepatitis B virus (HBV) infection. Along with persistent serum alanine aminotransferase (ALT) elevation and seropositivity of HCV-RNA, the liver disease progressed from chronic active hepatitis (CAH) to cirrhosis within 20 months, and to hepatocellular carcinoma (HCC) within 80 months. Note seroclearance of HBV-DNA with a trend of decreasing serum to negative count ratio (S/N) of hepatitis B surface antigen (HBsAg) and absence of HBsAg immunopathologically throughout the course. Shaded areas represent normal ranges; arrows indicate timing of liver biopsy

HBV has a much higher relative risk for the development of HCC[54–56]. A prospective follow-up study in Italy suggests that concurrent HBsAg and anti-HCV positivity in patients with cirrhosis is an independent and significant determinant for the development of HCC[57], although this trend is not so obvious in a similar study from Japan[58]. Several studies on HBsAg-negative patients with HCC have demonstrated that a significant number of patients seropositive for anti-HCV have both HBV and HCV genomic sequences in tumorous and non-tumorous liver tissue[59–61]. These findings provide the evidence implicating the importance of persistent concurrent infection with HCV and HBV in hepato-carcinogenesis. However, it is possible that HCV infection is related to HCC development indirectly through the cirrhotic process[62].

Viral interference

Evidence form both animal experiments and human clinical studies clearly indicates that chronic HBV infection with HCV co-infection or superinfection are associated with viral interference[4,15,16,43,44]. The precise mechanism is unknown. Possible alterations in the mechanism(s) responsible for virus absorption, penetration and/or replication and induction of interferon (IFN), IFN-like substance, or other soluble mediator(s) were considered[43]. However, IFN was not detected in the serial serum samples in NANB infection in chimpanzees[15]. Cytokines, including tumour necrosis factor alpha (TNF-α) and interleukin-6 may also be candidates, as they may activate certain intracellular pathways that can negatively regulate HBV expression, as shown in a transgenic mouse model[63]. In addition, the hepatocyte-derived TNF-α may exert its actions, leading to cytotoxic effect in the same cell that produced it, as well as to neighbouring cells[64]. Since the subcellular localization of HBV core protein can be regulated by the cell cycle[65], it is possible that HCV-induced liver injury and the accompanying cell renewal may increase the expression of HBV epitopes on the hepatocyte surface. This may lead to cytotoxic T-cell-effected elimination of HBV-infected hepatocytes, thus lowering HBV levels in liver and blood. A recent cotransfection study in a human hepatoma cell line demonstrated that HCV suppresses the HBV replication involving the process of transcription and encapsidation of HBV pregenomic RNA. This suppressive effect may be mediated by the HCV core protein, which can also function as a gene-regulatory protein[66].

In essence, many of the variabilities encountered in HCV-associated multiple virus infection cannot be simply explained. The information gathered so far implicates a complex interplay of humoral and cellular immune networks, as well as the virus-specific replicating process.

ANTIVIRAL THERAPY IN PATIENTS WITH CONCURRENT HCV AND HBV INFECTION

IFN-α is currently the most effective antiviral agent that has been used worldwide in the treatment of chronic HBV or HCV infection. However, little is known about the effect of IFN in patients seropositive for both HBsAg and anti-

HCV. Limited experience showed that such patients responded poorly to IFN therapy[11,26,67]. This is analogous to the therapeutic effect of IFN in HBV patients with HDV superinfection. It is noteworthy that IFN therapy in patients seropositive for HBsAg and anti-HCV may occasionally result in HBV hepatitis following seroclearance of HCV-RNA or HCV hepatitis following seroclearance of HBV-DNA[11,68]. It appears that the interactions between HCV and HBV could influence the effect of IFN therapy in such patients. However, we have noted that patients with continuing chronic hepatitis C following seroclearance of HBsAg respond to IFN as well as do patients with HCV infection alone.

CONCLUSIONS AND OUTLOOK

This review concludes that the prevalence of concurrent HBV and HCV infection covers more than 10% of patients with chronic HBV or HDV infection worldwide. Concurrent infection involving HCV tends to aggravate the severity and progression of the liver disease which appears to be resistant to antiviral therapy. On the other hand, HCV has been shown to increase the HBsAg clearance rate, to suppress HDV, and even to usurp the role of HBV to cause continuing chronic hepatitis. It seems clear that serum HCV markers, at least anti-HCV, should be tested in all patients with chronic HBV and HDV infection, particularly those who develop an acute hepatitis-like episode, or in those who undergo spontaneous HBsAg clearance, as well as in individuals seropositive for anti-HBc alone. The recognition of concurrent infection is essential for adequate follow-up and monitoring of patients with chronic HBV infection.

At present, antiviral therapy outside clinical trials is not recommended for patients with concurrent infections until more information is available. The understanding of the mechanisms by which hepatotropic viruses interact is also incomplete. Several important issues remain to be answered, namely: (1) What are the viral factors, such as genotype/strain and concentration of each virus, that may determine the impact of HCV on the outcome of dual or triple hepatitis virus infection? (2) What are the molecular mechanism(s) regulating these changes? (3) What are the immune responses of the host and other host factor(s) that may be involved in dual or triple virus infection? It is hoped that future research will clarify these issues and, in particular, the molecular mechanism(s) of the suppressive effect of HCV on HBV or HDV. Such knowledge may help in designing new therapeutic approaches in the treatment of chronic HBV and HDV infections.

Acknowledgements

The author acknowledges grant support from the National Science Council, National Health Research Institutes, Chang Gung Medical Research Fund and the Prosporus Foundation, Taipei, Taiwan, and the excellent secretarial assistance of Ms M. H. Tsai.

References

1. Liaw YF. Natural history of chronic hepatitis B virus infection. In: Liaw YF, Chronic hepatitis. Amsterdam: Elsevier, editor. 1986:9–18.

2. Rizzetto M, Bonino F, Verme G. Hepatitis delta virus infection of the liver: progress in virology, pathology and diagnosis. Semin Liver Dis. 1988;8:350–60.

3. Genesca, J, Esteban, JI, Alter HJ. Blood borne non-A, non-B hepatitis: hepatitis C. Semin Liver Dis. 1991;11:147–64.

4. Liaw YF, Chu CM, ChangChien CS, Wu CS. Simultaneous acute infections with hepatitis non-A, non-B and B viruses. Dig Dis Sci. 1982;27:762–4.

5. Mosley JW, Redeker AG, Feinstone SM, Purcell RH. Multiple hepatitis viruses in multiple attacks of acute viral hepatitis. N Engl J Med. 1977;296:75–8.

6. Norkrans G, Frösner G, Hermodsson S, Iwarson S. Multiple hepatitis attacks in drug addicts. J Am Med Assoc. 1980;243:1056–8.

7. Mathiesen LR, Hardt SF, Nielson JO et al. and the Copenhagen Hepatitis Acute Programme. Epidemiology and clinical characteristics of acute hepatitis types A, B, and non-A, non-B. Scand J Gastroenterol. 1979;14:849–56.

8. Liaw YF, Tai DI, Chu CM, Pao CC, Chen TJ. Acute exacerbation of chronic type B hepatitis: comparison between HBeAg and antibody-positive patients. Hepatology. 1987;7:20–3.

9. Chu CM, Liaw YF, Pao CC, Huang MJ. The etiology of acute hepatitis superimposed upon previously unrecognized HBsAg carriers. Hepatology. 1989;9:452–6.

10. Marmion BP, Burrell CJ, Tonkin RW, Dickson J. Dialysis-associated hepatitis in Edinburgh; 1969–1978. Rev Infect Dis. 1982;4:619–37.

11. Liaw YF. Role of hepatitis C virus in dual and triple hepatitis virus infection. Hepatology. 1995;22:1101–8.

12. Krogsgaard K, Wantzin P, Mathisen L, Ring Larsen H and the Copenhagen Hepatitis Acute Programme. Chronic evolution of acute hepatitis B: the significance of simultaneous infections with hepatitis C and D. Scand J Gastroenterol. 1991;26:275–80.

13. Baginski I, Chemin I, Hantz O et al. Transmission of serologically silent hepatitis B virus along with hepatitis C virus in two cases of posttransfusion hepatitis. Transfusion. 1992;32:215–20.

14. Mimms LT, Mosley JW, Hollinger FB et al. Effect of concurrent acute infection with hepatitis C virus on acute hepatitis B virus infection. Br Med J. 1993;307:1095–7.

15. Brotman B, Prince AM, Huima T, Richardson L, van den Ende MC, Pfeifer U. Interference between non-A, non-B and hepatitis B virus infection in chimpanzees. J Med Virol. 1983;11:191–205.

16. Hollinger FB, Dolana G, Thomas W, Gyorkey F. Reduction in risk of hepatitis transmission by heat-treatment of a human factor VIII concentrate. J Infect Dis. 1984;150:250–62.

17. Chu CM, Liaw YF. Simultaneous acute hepatitis B virus and hepatitis C virus infection leading to fulminant hepatitis and subsequent chronic hepatitis C. Clin Infect Dis. 1995;20:703–5.

18. Tandon BN, Irshad M, Acharya SK, Joshi YK. Hepatitis C virus infection is the major cause of severe liver disease in India. Gastroenterol Jpn. 1991;26:S192–5.

19. Feray C, Gigou M, Samuel D et al. Hepatitis C virus RNA and hepatitis B virus DNA in serum and liver of patients with fulminant hepatitis. Gastroenterology. 1993;104:549–55.

20. Liaw YF, Lin SM, Sheen IS, Chu CM. Acute hepatitis C virus superinfection followed by spontaneous HBeAg seroconversion and HBsAg elimination. Infection. 1991;19:250–1.

21. Alter HJ, Purcell RH, Shih WJ et al. Detection of antibody to hepatitis C virus in prospectively followed transfusion recipients with acute and chronic non-A, non-B hepatitis. N Engl J Med. 1989;321:1494–500.

22. Estaban JI, Estaban R, Viladomiu L et al. Hepatitis C virus antibodies among risk groups in Spain. Lancet. 1989;2:294–7.

23. Lin HH, Huang CC, Sheen IS, Lin DY, Liaw YF. Prevalence of antibodies to hepatitis C virus in hemodialysis unit. Am J Nephrol. 1991;11:192–4.

24. Tao QM, Wang Y, Du SC, Guo JP. Epidemiology of hepatitis B and C in China. In: Nishioka K, Suzuki H, Mishiro S, Oda T, editors. Viral hepatitis and liver disease. Tokyo: Springer-Verlag, 1994:412–15.

25. Panigrahi AK, Nanda SK, Dixit RK, Acharya SK, Zuckerman AJ, Panda SK. Diagnosis of hepatitis C virus-associated chronic liver disease in India: comparison of HCV antibody assay with a polymerase chain reaction for the 5′ noncoding region. J Med Virol. 1994;44:176–9.

26. Sato S, Fujiyama S, Tanaka M et al. Coinfection of hepatitis C virus in patients with chronic hepatitis B infection. J Hepatol. 1994;21:159–66.

27. Ohkawa K, Hayashi N, Yuki N et al. Hepatitis C virus antibody and hepatitis C virus replication in chronic hepatitis B patients. J Hepatol. 1994;21:509–14.

28. Kim BS, Park YM. Prevalence of hepatitis C virus related to liver disease in Korea. Gastroenterol Jpn. 1993;28:S17–22.
29. Liaw YF. Viral hepatitis in Taiwan: Status in the 1990s. In: Nishioka K, Suzuki H, Mishiro S, Oda T, editors. Viral hepatitis and liver disease. Tokyo: Springer-Verlag, 1994;419–21.
30. Fattovich G, Tagger A, Brollo L et al. Hepatitis C virus infection in chronic hepatitis B virus carriers. J Infect Dis. 1991;163:400–2.
31. Fong TL, Di Bisceglie AM, Waggoner JG, Banks SM, Hoofnagle JH. The significance of antibody to hepatitis C virus in patients with chronic hepatitis B. Hepatology. 1991;13:64–7.
32. Brown J, Dourakis S, Karayiannis P et al. Seroprevalence of hepatitis C virus nucleocapsid antibodies in patients with cryptogenic chronic liver disease. Hepatology. 1992;15:175–9.
33. Favorov MO, Fields HA, Yashina TL et al. Hepatitis C virus in the etiology of chronic hepatitis and liver cirrhosis: possibility of mixed viral infections due to parenteral transmission. J Med Virol. 1992;36:184–7.
34. Crespo J, Lozano JL, de la Cruz F et al. Prevalence and significance of hepatitis C viremia in chronic active hepatitis B. Am J Gastroenterol. 1994;89:1147–51.
35. Jilg W, Sieger E, Zachoval R, Schätzl H. Individuals with antibodies against hepatitis B core antigen as the only serological marker for hepatitis B infection: high percentage of carriers of hepatitis B and C virus. J Hepatol. 1995;23:14–20.
36. Cénac A, Pedroso ML, Djibo A et al. Hepatitis B, C and D virus infections in patients with chronic hepatitis, cirrhosis and hepatocellular carcinoma: a comparative study in Niger. Am J Trop Med Hyg. 1995;52:293–6.
37. Wu JC, Chen CL, Hou MC, Chen TZ, Lee SD, Lo KJ. Multiple viral infection as the most common cause of fulminant and subfulminant viral hepatitis in an area endemic for hepatitis B: application and limitation of the polymerase chain reaction. Hepatology. 1994;19:836–40.
38. Chu CM, Sheen IS, Liaw YF. The role of hepatitis C virus in fulminant viral hepatitis in an endemic area of hepatitis A and B. Gastroenterology. 1994;107:189–95.
39. Ackerman Z, Valinluck B, McHutchison JG, Redeker AG, Goviadarajan S. Spontaneous exacerbation of disease activity in patients with chronic delta hepatitis infection: the role of hepatitis B, C or D? Hepatology. 1992;16:625–9.
40. Pontisso P, Ruvoletto MG, Fattovich G et al. Clinical and virological profiles in patients with multiple hepatitis virus infections. Gastroenterology. 1993;105:1529–33.
41. Liaw YF, Chien RN, Chen TJ, Sheen JS, Chu CM. Concurrent hepatitis C virus and hepatitis delta virus superinfection in patients with chronic hepatitis B virus infection.. J Med Virol. 1992;37:294–7.
42. Tassopoulos NC, Koutelou MG, Papatheodoridis GV, Kalantzakis YS, Hatzakis AE. Acute delta hepatitis in Greek parenteral drug abusers. Prog Clin Biol Res. 1993;382:221–7.
43. Bradley DW, Maynard JE, McCaustland KA, Murphy BL, Cook EH, Ebert JW. Non-A, non-B hepatitis in chimpanzees: interference with acute hepatitis A virus and chronic hepatitis virus infection. J Med Virol. 1983;11:207–13.
44. Tsiquaye KN, Portmann B, Tovey G et al. Non-A, non-B hepatitis in persistent carriers of hepatitis B virus. J Med Virol. 1983;11:179–83.
45. Yeh CT, Chiu CT, Tsai SL, Hong ST, Chu CM, Liaw YF. Absence of precore stop mutant in chronic dual (B and C) and triple (B, C and D) hepatitis viruses infection. J Infect Dis. 1994;170:1582–5.
46. Koike K, Yasuda K, Yotzuyanagi H et al. Dominant replication of either virus in dual infection with hepatitis viruses B and C. J Med Virol. 1995;45:236–9.
47. Liaw YF, Tsai SL, Chang JJ et al. Displacement of hepatitis B virus by hepatitis C virus as the cause of continuing chronic hepatitis. Gastroenterology. 1994;106:1048–53.
48. Tsai SL, Liaw YF, Yeh CT, Chu CM, Kuo G. Cellular immune responses in patients with dual infections of hepatitis B and C viruses: dominant role of hepatitis C virus. Hepatology. 1995;21:908–12.
49. Sheen IS, Liaw YF, Chu CM, Pao CC. Role of hepatitis C virus infection in spontaneous hepatitis B surface antigen clearance during chronic hepatitis B virus infection. J Infect Dis. 1992;165:831–4.
50. Sheen IS, Liaw YF, Lin DY, Chu CM. Role of hepatitis C and delta viruses in the termination of chronic HBsAg carrier state: A multivariate analysis in a longitudinal follow-up study. J Infect Dis. 1994;170:358–61.
51. Garcia-Samaniego J, Sariano V, Bravo R, González-Lahoz J, Múnoz F. Viral replication in patients with multiple hepatitis virus infections. Gastroenterology. 1994;107:322–3.

52. Villa E, Grottola A, Buttafoco P *et al*. Evidence for hepatitis B virus infection in patients with chronic hepatitis C with and without serological markers of hepatitis B. Dig Dis Sci. 1995;40:8–13.

53. Huang CC, Liaw YF, Lai MK, Chu SH, Chuang CK, Huang JY. Clinical outcome of hepatitis C virus antibody-positive renal allograft recipients. Transplantation. 1992;53:763–5.

54. Yu MW, You SL, Chang AS, Lu SN, Liaw YF, Chen CJ. Association between hepatitis C virus antibodies and hepatocellular carcinoma in Taiwan. Cancer Res. 1991;51:5621–5.

55. Kaklamani E, Trichopoulous D, Tzonou A *et al*. Hepatitis B and C viruses and their interaction in the origin of hepatocellular carcinoma. J Am Med Assoc. 1991;15:1974–6.

56. Simonetti RG, Camma C, Fiorello F *et al*. Hepatitis C virus infection as a risk factor for hepatocellular carcinoma in patients with cirrhosis. A case control study. Ann Intern Med. 1992;116:97–102.

57. Benvegnu L, Fottovich G, Noventa F *et al*. Concurrent hepatitis B and C virus infection and risk of hepatocellular carcinoma. A prospective study. Cancer. 1994;74:2442–8.

58. Kato Y, Nakata K, Omagari K *et al*. Risk of hepatocellular carcinoma in patients with cirrhosis in Japan. Cancer. 1994;74:2234–8.

59. Sheu JC, Huang GT, Shih LN *et al*. Hepatitis C and B viruses in hepatitis B surface antigen-negative hepatocellular carcinoma. Gastroenterology. 1992;103:1322–7.

60. Paterlini P, Driss F, Nalpas B *et al*. Persistence of hepatitis B and C viral genomes in primary liver cancers from HBsAg-negative patients: A study of a low endemic area. Hepatology. 1993;17:20–9.

61. Diamantis ID, McGandy CE, Chen TJ, Liaw YF, Gudat F, Bianchi L. Detection of hepatitis B and C viruses in liver tissue with hepatocellular carcinoma. J Hepatol. 1994;20:405–9.

62. Goritsas CP, Athanasiadou A, Arvaniti A, Lampropoulou-Karatza C. The leading role of hepatitis B and C viruses as risk factors for the development of hepatocellular carcinoma. A case control study. J Clin Gastroenterol. 1995;20:220–4.

63. Gilles PN, Fey G, Chisari FV. Tumor necrosis factor alpha negatively regulates hepatitis B virus gene expression in transgenic mice. J Virol. 1992;66:3955–60.

64. González-Amaro R, Garcia-Monzón C, Garcia-Buey L *et al*. Induction of tumor necrosis factor α production by human hepatocytes in chronic viral hepatitis. J Exp Med. 1994;179:841–8.

65. Yeh CT, Wong SW, Fung YK, Ou JH. Cell cycle regulation of nuclear localization of hepatitis B virus core protein. Proc Natl Acad Sci USA. 1993;90:6459–63.

66. Shih CM, Lo SJ, Miyamura T, Chen SY, Wu Lee YH. Suppression of hepatitis B virus expression and replication by hepatitis C virus core protein in Huh-7 cells. J Virol. 1993;5823–32.

67. Weltman WD, Brotodihardjo A, Crewe EB *et al*. Coinfection with hepatitis B and C or B, C and D viruses results in severe chronic liver disease and responds poorly to interferon-α treatment. J Virol Hepatol. 1995;2:39–45.

68. Villa E, Grottola A, Trande P *et al*. Reactivation of hepatitis B virus infection induced by interferon in HBsAg-positive, anti-HCV positive patients (letter). Lancet. 1993;341:1413.

4
Treatment of viral hepatitis

M. COLOMBO, P. LAMPERTICO and M. G. RUMI

INTRODUCTION

Chronic hepatitis B is progressive, although there are patients who have long-lasting spontaneous remissions and healthy carriers of HBsAg. Advanced age, histological features of chronic active hepatitis with bridging necrosis and persistence of serum HBV-DNA are the most important factors that predict progression to cirrhosis[1]. The calculated annual probability of developing cirrhosis for patients with HBeAg chronic hepatitis B was approximately 6%. Chronic hepatitis C is also progressive, since approximately 30% of all chronically infected patients will develop cirrhosis in 10–30 years[2].

Thus, treatment of virus infection is the only approach available for halting the progression of chronic viral hepatitis and preventing the development of devastating sequelae, such as cirrhosis and liver cancer. Interferon alpha (IFN-α) has been shown to be active against hepatitis B virus (HBV), hepatitis C virus (HCV) and hepatitis D virus (HDV), for all of which it is now considered to be the standard therapy.

HBeAg–POSITIVE CHRONIC HEPATITIS B

Choice of patients

HBsAg, HBeAg-positive patients with detectable serum HBV-DNA, abnormal alanine aminotransferase (ALT) and histological diagnosis of chronic hepatitis B are candidates for IFN therapy.

Standard therapy and assessment of response

Standard therapy is 5 MU IFN daily or 10 MU three times weekly for 12–24 months. Response is defined as clearance of serum HBV-DNA by dot–blot, normalization of ALT levels and HBe seroconversion. Clearance of serum HBV-DNA usually occurs during treatment, but loss of HBeAg and development of anti-HBe may be delayed. About 30–50% of the patients may have flare-ups of ALT during IFN treatment, but discontinuation of treatment is

Table 1 Efficacy of IFN-α in chronic hepatitis B

Outcomes	Difference in proportion	95% confidence interval	p-Value
Loss of HBsAg	0.06	0.02–0.09	0.001
Loss of HBeAg	0.21	0.15–0.26	0.0001
Loss of HBV-DNA	0.20	0.14–0.26	0.001
Normal ALT	0.23	0.13–0.33	0.0001

generally unnecessary. In a recently reported meta-analysis all the randomized controlled trials analysed showed that IFN-α was beneficial[3]; 6% more IFN-treated patients had lost HBsAg and 20% more IFN-treated patients had lost HBV-DNA than controls. Treated patients were also significantly more likely to have normalized ALT levels (Table 1). In most studies a successful antiviral response was accompanied by histological improvement of the liver disease, but complete eradication of HBV was seldom achieved. As for the long-term outcome of patients treated with IFN, loss of HBsAg was reported for 65% of US patients who had sustained loss of HBeAg, but for only 24% of Spanish and none of the Chinese responders[4–6]. Clearance of HBV-DNA by polymerase chain reaction (PCR) was frequently achieved in those patients who cleared HBeAg and HBsAg, but not in those who cleared HBeAg only. Although it is widely held that sustained resolution of necroinflammatory activity will reduce the risk of developing cirrhosis and hepatocellular carcinoma, such data are not yet available.

Factors associated with a sustained response

IFN therapy is most likely to benefit those patients with replicating infections and an ongoing immune reaction against infected liver cells (active disease). The most important factors that predict a favourable response to IFN-α therapy are elevated ALT and low serum HBV-DNA levels[7–9]. Patients who have persistently normal ALT levels despite active virus replication are unlikely to benefit from IFN therapy, even with prednisone priming. These patients should be monitored regularly, because immune tolerance may break down later in life, rendering them more responsive to IFN treatment.

ANTI-HBe POSITIVE CHRONIC HEPATITIS B

Following spontaneous or IFN-induced HBe seroconversion, some patients will have inactive liver disease and no evidence of HBV replication, while others will continue to have replicating infections and chronic active hepatitis. Anti-HBe-positive chronic hepatitis B is the most frequent chronic hepatitis B in Mediterranean countries and the Far East[10]: it is sustained by HBV strains with mutations in the pre-core region that prevent the synthesis of HBeAg, and characterized by spontaneous reactivation and severe hepatitis. Six months administration of high doses of IFN therapy can suppress HBV replication and induce remission of liver disease in these patients, but the relapse rate is very high[11–13].

The sustained response rate may be improved by long-term administration of IFN to these patients[14].

Treatment of problematic patients

Children

IFN therapy with or without prednisone priming gave disappointing results in Chinese children[15,16], but this is related to the fact that most of the children in those studies were still in the immune tolerant phase. The responses in European children who had elevated alanine aminotransferase (ALT) levels were similar to those in adults[17–21].

Cirrhotic patients

In cirrhotic patients with active HBV replication, IFN can inhibit HBV replication, resulting in improvement of liver disease, but there is a high risk of precipitating liver failure and infectious complications[22]. Low-dose (0.15–3 MU) titratable IFN therapy is safer than previously described regimens, and induced sustained virological and clinical responses in 5/5 patients in Child's A status, and 5/15 Child's B, but was ineffective in 6 Child's C patients. This treatment should be given to patients with mild-to-moderate hepatic decompensation only, preferably in Child's A[22,23].

Future strategies

New therapeutic strategies include new antiviral agents and immunomodulatory therapy. Pilot studies have shown promising results for new orally administered nucleoside analogues, such as famciclovir and lamivudine[24,25]. In a preliminary trial, 100–300 mg of lamivudine administered for 12 weeks was well tolerated and reduced HBV-DNA to undetectable levels in HBeAg-positive patients. Other antiviral agents were ineffective (acyclovir) or too toxic (adenine arabinoside).

As for immunomodulatory therapy, large-scale studies failed to confirm the therapeutic efficacy of prednisone priming, interleukin-2 or thymosin[8,26,27]. The effect of granulocyte–macrophage colony-stimulating factor (GM-CSF) on HBV replication awaits further studies.

Although vaccines are considered to be preventive and not therapeutic, several recent studies have shown that vaccine therapy may boost natural immunity in several conditions, such as HIV, herpes, leprosy, tuberculosis, and leishmaniasis. Recent data from France have shown that standard doses of anti-HBV vaccine may clear HBV-DNA in some patients, suggesting that large-scale, randomized controlled studies should be done[28].

Other approaches to stimulate host immune response to hepatitis B antigens are also under investigation. Patients with chronic HBV infection have been demonstrated to have impaired cytotoxic T cell responses to HBcAg, resulting in ineffective removal of infected hepatocytes. A phase II study is under way to see if vaccinating chronic hepatitis B patients with a synthetic peptide that contains the corresponding HLA-restricted HBcAg epitope will stimulate the cytotoxic T cell response to HBcAg.

CHRONIC HEPATITIS DELTA

Preliminary reports suggested that a 3–4-month course of IFN-α suppressed HDV replication and improved liver disease in some patients, but in almost all cases discontinuation of therapy was followed by a relapse. IFN-α (9 MU), administered for 48 weeks, was generally well tolerated and resulted in normal ALT values, clearance of serum HDV-RNA and histological improvement in 50% of patients[29]. Normal ALT persisted up to 4 years in half of the patients who had normal ALT at the end of therapy, but the effects on viral replication were not sustained. Further studies will be necessary to determine whether long-term treatment with higher doses of IFN can prolong the duration of the response, with changes in the natural history of the disease.

HEPATITIS C

Choice of patients

Priority patients for treatment are immunocompetent adults 18–65 years of age who have serum antibodies to HCV (anti-HCV), AST/ALT levels at least 1.5 times the upper normal limit, and chronic hepatitis by liver biopsy.

Standard therapy and assessment of response

Standard treatment for chronic hepatitis C is 3×10^6 units (MU) of recombinant IFN-α three times a week for 6 months. This is the regimen that was adopted in three randomized controlled trials[30–32] in which treatment normalized serum ALT and histology in 30–50% of the patients. Subsequent virological analysis of these cohorts revealed that in approximately 15–20% of the patients as a whole serum HCV-RNA was no longer detectable by PCR at 1–5 years after IFN was stopped.

Lymphoblastoid IFN-α has also been recommended for treating patients with chronic hepatitis C, on the assumption that a mixture of 22 IFN should be more effective than a single IFN therapy. In a randomized study of 250 such patients assigned to either recombinant or lymphoblastoid IFN, sustained complete responses were achieved in 18% of the patients in both groups, negating any advantage of treating these patients with more than one IFN.

A primary response is defined as normalization of ALT within 3 months after starting IFN, and it is currently acknowledged that treatment should be stopped for patients who fail to respond within this time. A complete response consists of normal ALT/AST and negative serum HCV-RNA (detected by PCR) at the end of treatment. Approximately 10% of all patients responding to IFN have transient elevations of serum transminases (breakthrough) while on treatment[33]. Breakthroughs are thought to be due to development of neutralizing antibodies to IFN-α[34] or to multiplication of genetic variants of HCV, escaping most of the immune response[35]. Hepatitis relapses are indicated by persistent elevations of serum ALT above the upper limit of normal after cessation of treatment. Approximately two-thirds of patients with primary responses to IFN have had hepatitis relapses. In non-selected patients with chronic hepatitis C, approximately 50% of the patients will not respond to treatment, 30% will have transient responses, and only 20% will show long-lasting biochemical and virological (complete) responses[30,36,37].

The high-dose regimens

To increase the rates of sustained responses in patients with hepatitis C, high doses and long treatment periods[33] have been attempted. The superiority of high doses and long-duration treatments was prospectively demonstrated in 171 Italian patients[38]; 54 were given 6 MU for 6 months (group 1), 61 were given 3 MU for 12 months (group 2) and 54 were given 6 MU for 6 months followed by 3 MU for 6 months (group 3). While the response rates at the end of therapy did not differ in the groups, the prolonged response rates 4 years after IFN was stopped were higher in group 3 than in the other two groups (Table 2). High doses and prolonged treatment are unlikely to increase the number of patients with primary responses, but they do seem to increase the durability of the response.

Table 2 Long-term responses to INF-α 2a in patients with chronic hepatitis C treated with different schedules

Group	No.	Treatment	IFN (MU)	Normal ALT and negative HCV-RNA	
				12 months	48 months
1	54	6 MU × 6 months	468	76%	26%
2	61	3 MU × 12 months	468	65%	25%
3	54	6 MU × 6 months+ 3 MU × 6 months	702	74%	42%*

* $p<0.01$.

Factors associated with a sustained response

There was significant correlation between patient age and treatment outcome: patients younger than 45 years responded better than older patients[39,40]. In one study of 61 long-term responders out of 361 patients treated with IFN, multistep regression analysis revealed that duration of disease and severity of disease, but not patient age, were the independent variables associated with treatment outcome (Table 3)[41]. These studies could not ascertain whether patients with more protracted infections were also those at increased risk of cirrhosis, which is itself an important predictor of a poor response. A clear-cut correlation between cirrhosis and low rates of long-term biochemical and virological response to IFN had already emerged from analyses of previous trials[39,42]. In one study the rate of sustained virological response to IFN in patients with HCV-related cirrhosis was zero[43].

Table 3 Predictors of a sustained response to recombinant and lymphoblastoid IFN-α in patients with chronic hepatitis C

Pretreatment	Univariate analysis			Multivariate analysis
	LTR	NR	p	p
Age (years)	44	48	<0.01	n.s.
Duration (<24 months)	34	82	<0.0002	<0.001
Cirrhosis (%)	16	47	<0.00002	<0.0001

LTR = sustained responders; NR = non-sustained responders.

Important virological features, such as levels of viraemia and HCV genotypes, have also been shown to be associated with treatment outcome. Quantitative assays of serum HCV-RNA based on dilutional PCR, competitive PCR or branched DNA assay have shown that long-term responders have 2 or 3 log lesser amounts of HCV-RNA than non-responders or relapsers[40,44]. By multivariate analysis, pretreatment viraemia was an independent predictor of treatment outcome even for patients with cirrhosis[45–47].

Other studies have also shown a clear-cut correlation between HCV genotype and treatment outcome, with type 1b being more often associated with poor responses[40,48–50]. In general, infection with HCV 1b was found to be associated with long-duration infections, cirrhosis and high levels of HCV-RNA, whereas patients infected with genotype 2a had less aggressive disease and less HCV-RNA. In more than one study it was not clear which factor, viraemia or genotype, predicts treatment outcome better[48].

Treatment of problematic patients

Since treatment outcome is inversely related to disease duration, treatment of patients during acute infection might prevent development of chronic disease. In a multicentre trial of patients with acute post-transfusion hepatitis there was long-term eradication of HCV infection for 39% of the patients treated with 3 MU of IFN for 3 months, a figure twice that achieved in the same centre for patients with chronic hepatitis C (Table 4).[51] Studies with intravenous administration of IFN-β have clearly shown that up to 90% of the patients with acute

Table 4 Multicentre randomized controlled study of effects of IFN-α 2b in patients with acute post-transfusion hepatitis C

Period	Month	Complete response	
		Treated (n = 22)	Controls (n = 16)
Prior to therapy	0	0	0
End of therapy	3	53%[*]	0
End of follow-up	18	39%[**]	0

[*] p = 0.0087; [**] p = 0.035.

hepatitis (community-acquired + post-transfusion) were permanently cured with high cumulative doses (336 MU)[52].

Another controversial issue is whether or not HCV carriers who are also HIV-positive should be treated with IFN. These patients, in fact, have higher HCV-RNA levels, and are at higher risk for severe liver disease, than HIV-negative patients with chronic hepatitis C[53], though with similar life expectancy[54]. Half of haemophiliacs and intravenous drug users have had transient normalization of serum ALT and HCV-RNA suppression following IFN therapy[55,56]. Treatment of post-transplantation hepatitis is another debated issue. HCV recurs in 77–100% of patients after liver transplantation for which HCV-related cirrhosis was the primary indication, and 36% of them developed chronic active hepatitis or cirrhosis within 3 years[57]. IFN treatment of post-transplantation hepatitis C patients has had conflicting results. A controlled study of 42 patients in whom hyperbilirubinaemia was the primary indication for IFN therapy showed no differences between treated and untreated patients in terms of number of rejection episodes or improvement of liver function[58]. In another study[59], irreversible chronic rejection occurred in five of 14 treated patients in the face of poor virological and biochemical responses. Immunosuppression might account for the poor response rates of patients with post-transplantation hepatitis C, as suggested by the 10–20-fold higher levels of HCV-RNA after transplantation than before transplantation[60]. In one study[61] the amount of viral antigens in the liver was correlated directly with the severity of liver damage. In more than one study HCV subtype lb was the predominant genotype (41%) in the transplant population: since patients infected with this genotype were twice as likely to resist IFN than those infected with other genotypes, many feel that genotype lb may be an important predictor of the outcome of treatment of post-transplantation hepatitis[62].

Another strategy against post-transplantation HCV was attempting to clear viraemia before transplantation. Limited experience with IFN therapy of patients with decompensated cirrhosis due to HCV indicates that IFN can be administered to most of these patients with good results, and with no risk of further decompensation. Van Thiel and associates[63] have randomly assigned 40 such patients to daily doses of 5 MU IFN with G-CSF for 3 months or nothing, and demonstrated clearance of viraemia in 12 of 14 treated patients versus none of the controls.

HCV may also contribute to mortality in patients treated with kidney grafts. In two studies IFN treatment resulted in 30% rates of responses in the face of high rates of kidney rejection, sepsis or IgA nephropathy[64,65]; for OLT, also, a strategy against recurring HCV could be to attempt to clear viraemia during the phase of renal dialysis prior to transplantation. However, treatment of the patients has yielded unsatisfactory results in terms of long-term virus suppression and of compliance to therapy[66].

Patients with mixed cryoglobulinaemia are a heterogeneous group, but only a minority of them develop clinically important complications[67]. IFN has been successfully administered to patients with mixed cryoglobulinaemia who were unresponsive to cytotoxic drugs before HCV was recognized as an important factor[68]. More recently a randomized controlled study[69] showed transient improvement of renal, hepatic and cutaneous lesions in half of the patients treated with IFN.

Asymptomatic individuals who are actively replicating HCV but have normal aminotransferase levels may occasionally develop severe liver disease. The general opinion is that, until more information about the natural history of these patients has been obtained, they should not be treated with IFN. One study showed that IFN therapy caused ALT elevation in 60% of such asymptomatic carriers without eliminating serum HCV-RNA[70].

Side-effects

Side-effects are usually dose-dependent, mild and reversible after treatment is stopped. The most frequent short-term side-effect is the so-called 'flu-like syndrome', which occurs in virtually all patients and can easily be controlled with paracetamol. Fewer than 5% of the patients require stopping of treatment or reduction of dose. Mild and transient myelosuppression and hair loss are common long-term side-effects of therapy. Loss of libido, psychological depression, anxiety, fatigue, increasing titres of serum autoantibodies and thyroid disfunction can also occur during IFN therapy[71].

Conclusion and future strategies

IFN is the only treatment available for chronic HCV infection, but it is far from satisfactory in terms of effectiveness, tolerability or cost. To enhance the cost-effectiveness of hepatitis C treatment, one might elect to give priority to young patients, patients without cirrhosis or those with low levels of viraemia. However, by doing so a number of patients will not be treated who might develop progressive liver disease, and might have responded to therapy. Therefore, prospective studies are needed to determine which criteria are the more cost-effective for patient selection. Controlled trials assessing IFN efficacy in patients selected on the basis of virus genotypes or pretreatment levels of viraemia, or based on HCV-RNA as an 'early' end-point for stopping or continuing treatment, are under way. The potential of the nucleoside analogue ribavirin as a single agent, or in combination with IFN, is being investigated in many centres. Preliminary data indicate that combination therapy is better than ribavirin alone, and that patients who relapse after IFN therapy are those most likely to benefit from combination therapy. The future of antiviral therapy will probably depend on the development of newer antiviral agents, such as antisense oligomers and virus-specific enzyme inhibitors, as well as on immunotherapy with recombinant virus proteins.

References

1. Fattovich G, Brollo L, Giustina G *et al*. Natural history and prognostic factors for chronic hepatitis type B. Gut. 1991;32:294–8.
2. Di Bisceglie AM, Goodman ZD, Ishak KG, Hoofnagle JH, Melpolder JJ, Alter HJ. Long-term clinical and histopathological follow-up of chronic posttransfusion hepatitis. Hepatology. 1991;14:969–74.
3. Wong DKH, Cheung AM, O'Rourke K, Naylor CD, Detsky AS, Heathcote J. Effect of alpha-interferon treatment in patients with hepatitis B e antigen-positive chronic hepatitis B. Ann Intern Med. 1993;119:312–23.

4. Korenman J, Baker B, Waggoner J, Everhart JE, Di Bisceglie AM, Hoofnagle JH. Long-term remission of chronic hepatitis after alpha-interferon therapy. Ann Intern Med. 1991;114:629–34.
5. Carreno V, Castillo I, Moina J, Porres JC, Bartolome J. Long-term follow-up of hepatitis B chronic carriers who responded to interferon therapy. J Hepatol. 1992;15:102–6.
6. Lok ASF, Chung HT, Liu VWS, Ma OCK. Long-term follow-up of chronic hepatitis B patients treated with interferon alfa. Gastroenterology. 1993;105:1833–8.
7. Lok ASF, Wu PC, Lai CL *et al*. A controlled trial of interferon with or without prednisone priming for chronic hepatitis B. Gastroenterology. 1992;102:2091–7.
8. Perrillo RP, Schiff ER, Davis GL *et al*. and the Hepatitis Interventional Therapy Group. A randomized, controlled trial of interferon alfa-2b alone and after prednisone withdrawal for the treatment of chronic hepatitis B. N Engl J Med. 1990;323:295–301.
9. Brook MG, Karayannis P, Thomas HC. Which patients with chronic hepatitis B virus infection will response to alpha-interferon therapy. A statistical analysis of predictive factors. Hepatology. 1989;10:761–3.
10. Carman W, Thomas H, Domingo E. Viral genetic variation: hepatitis B virus as a clinical example. Lancet. 1993;341:349–53.
11. Brunetto MR, Oliveri F, Rocca G *et al*. Natural course and response to interferon of chronic hepatitis B accompanied by antibody to hepatitis B e antigen. Hepatology. 1989;10:198–202.
12. Pastore G, Santantonio T, Milella M *et al*. Anti-HBe positive chronic hepatitis B with HBV-DNA in the serum: response to a 6-month course of lymphoblastoid interferon. J Hepatol. 1992;14:221–5.
13. Fattovich G, Farci P, Rugges M *et al*. A randomized controlled trial of lymphoblastoid interferon-alpha in patients with chronic hepatitis B lacking HBeAg. Hepatology. 1992;15:585–9.
14. Lampertico P, Rumi MG, Donato MF *et al*. Long-term treatment with recombinant interferon (IFN) alpha-2b of anti-HBe positive chronic hepatitis B: a randomized controlled trial. Hepatology. 1995;22 (Suppl.): abstract 874.
15. Lai CL, Lok ASF, Lin HJ, Wu PC, Yeoh EK, Yeung CY. Placebo-controlled trial of recombinant alpha 2 interferon in Chinese HBsAg-carrier children. Lancet. 1987;2:877–80.
16. Lai CL, Lin HJ, Lau JKN *et al*. Effect of recombinant alpha 2 interferon with or without prednisone in Chinese HBsAg carrier children. Q J Med. 1991;78:155–63.
17. Ruiz-Moreno M, Jimenez J, Porres JC, Bartolome J, Moreno A, Carreno V. A controlled trial of recombinant interferon-alpha in Caucasian children with chronic hepatitis B. Digestion. 1990;45:26–33.
18. Moreno MR, Rua MJ, Molina J *et al*. Prospective, randomized controlled trial of interferon-alpha in children with chronic hepatitis B. Hepatology. 1991;13:1035–9.
19. Sokal EM, Wirth S, Goyens P, Depreterre A, Cornu C. Interferon alpha-2b therapy in children with chronic hepatitis B. Gut. 1993(Suppl.):S87–90.
20. Utili R, Sagnelli E, Gaeta GB *et al*. Treatment of chronic hepatitis B in children with prednisone followed by alfa-interferon: a controlled randomized study. J Hepatol. 1994;20:163–7.
21. Barbera C, Bortolotti F, Crivellaro C *et al*. Recombinant interferon alpha-2a hastens the rate of HBeAg clearance in children with chronic hepatitis B. Hepatology. 1994;20:287–90.
22. Hoofnagle JH, Di Bisceglie AM, Waggoner JG, Park Y. Interferon alfa for patients with clinically apparent cirrhosis due to chronic hepatitis B. Gastroenterology. 1993;104:1116–21.
23. Perrillo R, Tamburro C, Regenstein F *et al*. Low-dose, titratable interferon alfa in decompensated liver disease caused by chronic infection with hepatitis B virus. Gastroenterology. 1995;109:908–16.
24. Kruger M, Tillmann HL, Trautwein C *et al*. Famciclovir treatment of hepatitis B virus recurrence after orthotopic liver transplantation: a pilot study. Hepatology. 1995;22(Suppl.):abstract 449.
25. Dienstag JL, Perrillo RP, Schiff ER, Bartholomew M, Vicary C, Rubin M. A preliminary trial of lamivudine for chronic hepatitis B infection. N Engl J Med. 1995;333:1657–61.
26. Reichen J, Bianchi L, Frei PC, Male PJ, Lavanchy D, Schmid M. Efficacy of steroid withdrawal and low-dose interferon treatment in chronic active hepatitis B. Results of a randomized multicenter trial. J Hepatol. 1994;20:168–74.
27. Liaw YF, Lin SM, Chen TJ, Chien RN, Sheen IS, Chu CM. Beneficial effect of prednisolone withdrawal followed by human lymphoblastoid interferon on the treatment of chronic type B hepatitis in Asians: a randomized controlled trial. J Hepatol. 1994;20:175–80.

28. Pol S, Driss F, Carnot F, Michel ML, Berthelot P, Brechot C. Efficacie d'une immunotherapie par vaccination contre le virus de l'hepatite B sur la multiplication virale B. CR Acad Sci Paris. 1993;316:668–91.
29. Farci P, Mandas A, Coiana A *et al.* Treatment of chronic hepatitis D with interferon alfa-2a. Results of a randomized, controlled trial of high doses of alpha interferon given for prolonged periods. N Engl J Med. 1994;330:88–94.
30. Davis GL, Balart LA, Schiff ER *et al.* Treatment of chronic hepatitis C with recombinant interferon alfa. A multicenter randomized, controlled trial. N Engl J Med. 1989;321:1501–6.
31. Di Bisceglie AM, Martin P, Kassianides C *et al.* Recombinant interferon alfa therapy for chronic hepatitis C. A randomized, double-blind, placebo-controlled trial. N Engl J Med. 1989;321:1506–10.
32. Marcellin P, Boyer N, Giostra E *et al.* Recombinant human alpha-interferon in patients with chronic non-A, non-B hepatitis: a multicenter randomized controlled trial from France. Hepatology. 1991;13:393–7.
33. Negro F, Baldi M, Mondardini A *et al.* Continuous versus intermittent therapy for chronic hepatitis C with recombinant interferon alfa-2a. Gastroenterology. 1994;107:479–85.
34. Giannelli G, Antonelli G, Fera G *et al.* Biological and clinical significance of neutralizing and binding antibodies to interferon alpha (IFN-α) during therapy for chronic hepatitis C. Clin Exp Immunol. 1994;97:4–9.
35. Enomoto N, Sato C, Kurosaki M, Marumo F. Hepatitis C virus after interferon treatment has the variation in the hypervariable region of envelope 2 gene. J Hepatol. 1994;20:252–61.
36. Rumi MG, Del Ninno E, Parravicini ML *et al.* Long-term titrated recombinant interferon alfa-2a in chronic hepatitis C: a randomized controlled trial. J Viral Hepatitis. 1995;2:73–6.
37. Saracco G, Rosina F, Abate ML *et al.* Long-term follow-up of patients with chronic hepatitis C treated with different doses of interferon-alfa 2b. Hepatology. 1993;18:1300–5.
38. Alberti A, Chemello L, Bonetti P *et al.* Treatment with interferon(s) of community-acquired chronic hepatitis and cirrhosis type C. J Hepatol. 1993;17:S123–6.
39. Causse X, Godinot H, Chevalier M *et al.* Comparison of 1 or 3 MU of interferon alfa-2b and placebo in patients with chronic non-A, non-B hepatitis. Gastroenterology. 1991;101:497–502.
40. Yoshioka K, Kakumu S, Wakita T *et al.* Detection of hepatitis C virus by polymerase chain reaction and response to interferon-alfa therapy: relationship to genotypes of hepatitis C virus. Hepatology. 1992;16:293–9.
41. Pagliaro L, Craxì A, Cammaa C *et al.* Interferon-alpha for chronic hepatitis C. An analysis of pretreatment clinical predictors of response. Hepatology. 1994;19:820–8.
42. Jouet P, Roudot-Thoraval F, Dhumeaux D, Metreau JM, and Le group Française pour l'etude du traitement des hepatites croniques NANB/C. Comparative efficacy of interferon alfa in cirrhotic and noncirrhotic patients with non-A, non-B, C hepatitis. Gastroenterology. 1994;106:686–90.
43. Sieck JO, Ellis ME, Alfurayh O *et al.* Histologically advanced chronic hepatitis C treated with recombinant alpha-interferon: a randomized placebo-controlled double-blind cross-over study. J Hepatol. 1993;19:418–23.
44. Kobayashi Y, Watanabe S, Konishi M *et al.* Detection of hepatitis C virus RNA by nested polymerase chain reaction in sera of patients with chronic non-A, non-B hepatitis treated with interferon. J Hepatol. 1992;16:138–44.
45. Marcellin P, Pouteau M, Martinot-Peignoux M *et al.* Lack of benefit of escalating dosage of interferon alfa in patients with chronic hepatitis C. Gastroenterology. 1995;109:156–65.
46. Kasahara A, Hayashi N, Hiramatsu N *et al.* Ability of prolonged interferon treatment to suppress relapse after cessation of therapy in patients with chronic hepatitis C: a multicenter randomized controlled trial. Hepatology. 1995;21:291–7.
47. Yamada G, Takatani M, Kishi F *et al.* Efficacy of interferon alfa therapy in chronic hepatitis C patients depends primarily on hepatitis C virus RNA level. Hepatology. 1995;22:1351–4.
48. Hino K, Sainokami S, Shimoda K *et al.* Genotypes and titers of hepatitis C virus for predicting response to interferon in patients with chronic hepatitis C. J Med Virol. 1994;42:299–305.
49. Tsubota A, Chayama K, Ikeda K *et al.* Factors predictive of response to interferon-α therapy in hepatitis C virus infection. Hepatology. 1994;12:1088–94.
50. Chemello L, Bonetti P, Cavalletto L *et al.* Randomized trial comparing three different regimens of alpha-2a-interferon in chronic hepatitis C. Hepatology. 1995;22:700–6.
51. Lampertico P, Rumi MG, Romeo R *et al.* A multicenter randomized controlled trial of recombinant interferon alpha-2b in patients with acute transfusion-associated non-A, non-B hepatitis. Hepatology. 1994;19:19–22.

52. Takano S, Satomura Y, Omata M, and the Japan Acute Hepatitis Cooperative Study Group. Effects of interferon beta on non-A, non-B acute hepatitis: a prospective, randomized, controlled-dose study. Gastroenterology. 1994;107:805–11.
53. Eyster ME, Fried MW, Di Bisceglie AM, Goedert JJ, for the Multicenter Hemophilia Cohort Study. Increasing hepatitis C virus RNA levels in hemophiliacs: relationship to human immunodeficiency virus infection and liver disease. Blood. 1994;84:1020–3.
54. Wright TL, Hollander H, Pu X et al. Hepatitis C in HIV-infected patients with and without AIDS: prevalence and relationship to patient survival. Hepatology. 1994;20:1152–5.
55. Makris M, Preston FE, Triger DR, Underwood JC, Westlake L, Adelman MI. Interferon alfa for chronic hepatitis C in haemophiliacs. Gut. 1993;34(Suppl. 2):S121–3.
56. Telfer P, Devereux H, Colvin B, Hayden S, Dusheiko G, Lee C. Alpha interferon for hepatitis C virus infection in haemophilic patients. Haemophilia. 1995;1:54–8.
57. Feray C, Gigoun M, Samuel D et al. The course of hepatitis C infection after liver transplantation. Hepatology. 1994;20:1127–43.
58. Sheiner PA, Fisher A, Schluger LK et al. Treatment with α-interferon does not alter the course of recurrent hepatitis C. Hepatology. 1994;20:abstract 147.
59. Feray C, Samuel D, Gigou M, Paradis V, Reynès M, Bismuth H. Effects of interferon in liver recipients with post-transplantation chronic hepatitis C. J Hepatol. 1994;abstract GS 5/28.
60. Chazouillers O, Kim M, Combs C et al. Quantitation of hepatitis C virus RNA in liver transplant recipients. Gastroenterology. 1994;106:994–9.
61. Gretch DR, Bacchi CE, Corey L et al. Persistent hepatitis C virus infection following liver transplantation: clinical and virologic features. Hepatology. 1995;21:1–9.
62. Feray C, Gigou N, Samuel D et al. Influence of genotypes of hepatitis C virus on the severity of recurrent liver disease after liver transplantation. Gastroenterology. 1995;108:1088–96.
63. Van Thiel DH, Faruki H, Fagiuoli S et al. Successful treatment of end stage liver disease due to hepatitis C prior to liver transplantation. Hepatology. 1994;20:abstract 161.
64. Hanafusa T, Ichikawa Y, Kyo M et al. Long-term impact of hepatitis virus infection on kidney transplant recipients and a pilot study of effects of interferon alpha on chronic hepatitis C. Transplant Proc. 1995;27:956–7.
65. Durlikn M. Gaciong Z, Rancewicz Z et al. Renal allograft function in patients with chronic viral hepatitis B and C treated with interferon alpha. Transplant Proc. 1995;27:958–9.
66. Koenig P, Vogel W, Umlauft F et al. Interferon treatment for chronic hepatitis C virus in uremic patients. Kidney Int. 1994;45:1507–9.
67. Gumber SC, Chopra S. Hepatitis C: A multifaceted disease. Review of extrahepatic manifestation. Ann Intern Med. 1995;123:615–20.
68. Casato M, Lagan B, Antonelli G, Dianzani F, Bonomo L. Long-term results of therapy with interferon-α for type II essential mixed cryoglobulinemia. Blood. 1991;78:3142–7.
69. Misiani R, Bellavita P, Fenili D et al. Interferon alfa-2a therapy in cryoglobulinemia associated with hepatitis C virus. N Engl J Med. 1994;330:751–6.
70. Sangiovanni A, Spinzi GC, Ceriani R et al. Randomized controlled trial of HCV healthy carriers treatment with interferon (IFN). Hepatology. 1995;22(Suppl.):abstract 734.
71. Balkwill FR. Interferons. Lancet. 1989;2:1060–3.

5
Ursodeoxycholic acid for chronic viral hepatitis

R. POUPON, P. PODEVIN and R. E. POUPON

INTRODUCTION

Recombinant interferon (IFN)-α is the base treatment for chronic hepatitis C but its efficacy remains unsatisfactory. Many patients either relapse after cessation of IFN or do not normalize their serum alanine aminotransferase (ALT) activities while receiving IFN, irrespective of the dose and duration of IFN. Therefore, there is a need for more effective and sustained forms of therapy. The factors predictive of response to IFN treatment are listed in Table 1. In addition to viral load, genotype, quasi-species diversity, the state of the liver – and in particular, the presence or absence of cholestasis – has also been found to be predictive of response to IFN therapy[1]. This might suggest that metabolic liver events could modulate antiviral defences.

The three following points will be addressed: (a) ursodeoxycholic acid (UDCA) as monotherapy for chronic viral hepatitis; (b) UDCA as an adjunct to IFN therapy; and (c) the putative mechanisms of action of UDCA in chronic viral hepatitis. As such, we will propose a hypothesis which might account for the specific therapeutic effect of UDCA in this setting.

UDCA AS MONOTHERAPY

Japanese investigators were first to report an improvement in liver function tests during UDCA treatment in patients with chronic active hepatitis[2]. In Europe,

Table 1 Factors associated with complete response to interferon treatment

Body weight (<86 kg)
Absence of cirrhosis
Low serum ferritin
Normal γ-glutamyltransferase
Low serum bile acids
Not genotype 1b
Low serum HCV-RNA levels

Data from ref. 1.

Leuschner *et al.*[3] reported a decrease in serum transaminases in six patients with chronic active hepatitis and gallstones while they were being treated with UDCA. Subsequent to these reports, seven controlled trials have been carried out[2,4–9]. Endpoints were enzyme activities. In two of the seven trials, endpoints were enzyme activities and liver histology[4,5]. The viral load was not assessed in any of these studies. All these trials confirmed the favourable effect of UDCA administration on serum liver enzymes with constant relapses after UDCA withdrawal. The improvement size was more pronounced for serum γ-glutamyl-transpeptidase activity than for serum ALT activity. Interestingly, the effect size of UDCA treatment was markedly different in the presence or absence of cirrhosis; the improvement in serum γ-glutamyltranspeptidase and ALT activities was significantly more important in patients with cirrhosis than in those without[5]. The mechanism by which UDCA is more efficient in the presence of cirrhosis is probably related to the degree of cholestasis and hepatic accumulation of bile acids in the liver in cases of liver cirrhosis. Supporting this hypothesis is the significant inverse relationship between the degree of changes in serum enzyme activities and the rate of changes in the hydrophilic–hydrophobic balance of the circulating bile acids under UDCA treatment[10]. In two studies[4,5] liver histology was evaluated before and at 12 months of UDCA therapy. In these two studies there was no significant change in Knodell's score. In one study[4] a biliary score, including bile duct damage and ductular changes, was assessed. A significant improvement in this score was noted after 1 year of UDCA therapy. The degrees of changes in the biliary score and in serum γ-glutamyltranspeptidase activity were significantly correlated.

UDCA AS AN ADJUVANT THERAPY

Two randomized controlled studies of the efficacy of UDCA plus IFN-α versus IFN-α alone in the treatment of chronic hepatitis C have recently been published[11,12]. Patients who had never previously received antiviral treatment were enrolled; less than 20% of the included patients had cirrhosis. Results of these two studies can be summarized as follows: (1) the primary response during IFN-α treatment did not differ between the two groups; (2) the relapse rate and its severity were significantly lower in the combination group; (3) the post-treatment histology was similar in the two groups with the exception of the degree of portal inflammation, which was improved only in the UDCA plus IFN group; and (4) there was no difference between therapies regarding sustained clearance of HCV-RNA after 24 months of follow-up.

The efficacy of adjuvant UDCA in IFN-resistant patients was assessed in a pilot study. Twenty-one patients with chronic hepatitis C resistant to a first course of IFN received a second course (3 MU three times a week) combined with UDCA (10 mg/kg per day) for 6 months. At the end of the treatment with UDCA plus IFN, ALT activity had returned to normal in six patients and PCR amplification of viral RNA was negative in three of these cases, suggesting that chronic administration could partially reverse resistance to IFN in chronic hepatitis C. A multicentre double-blind controlled trial aimed at assessing

UDCA as an adjuvant therapy in resistant patients to IFN has been carried out in France. The results of this trial will be available soon.

PUTATIVE MECHANISMS OF ACTION OF UDCA: A HYPOTHESIS

UDCA protects against the toxicity of endogenous bile acids and corrects cholestasis through, at least in part, an effect on hepatobiliary transport pathways and membrane stability. To explain the effects of UDCA in chronic viral hepatitis we hypothesize that: (a) cholestasis promotes viraemia, and (b) UDCA therapy may reduce viraemia by correcting cholestasis (Fig. 1). What is the clinical and experimental evidence supporting this hypothesis?

Clinical evidence

There is circumstantial evidence supporting a link between cholestasis and viraemia. Indices of cholestasis (serum γ-glutamyltranspeptidase activity and serum bile acid levels) have been shown to be predictive of resistance to IFN in chronic hepatitis C[13]. After liver transplantation, HCV-RNA levels increase and peak at the time of acute graft dysfunction and cholestasis. A syndrome defined by the association of severe cholestasis and very high levels of viraemia has been described in recurrent hepatitis B and C after liver transplantation. Rapid clinical deterioration generally occurs in this setting. It is possible that cholestasis, whatever its cause, (graft dysfunction, rejection, cyclosporin- or drug-induced intrahepatic cholestasis or extrahepatic cholestasis) by promoting immunosuppression and impairing antiviral defences might induce high virus replication, which in turn may aggravate cholestasis through a cytopathic effect.

Experimental evidence

Cell-mediated immunity is impaired during cholestasis of various origins. Experimentally, bile duct ligation results in suppressing *in-vitro* cell-mediated immune response, in delaying cardiac allograft rejection and in reducing incidence of graft-versus-host disease. This is illustrated by our studies aimed at assessing the respective influence of cholestasis, chenodeoxycholic acid and

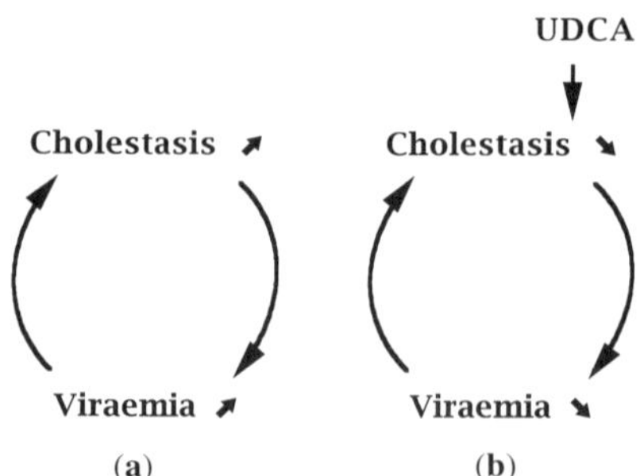

Fig. 1 This hypothesis is proposed in order to explain the effects of ursodeoxycholic acid (UDCA) in chronic viral hepatitis: (a) cholestasis by decreasing cell-mediated immunity and antiviral defences promotes viraemia; (b) UDCA therapy, by correcting cholestasis, may reduce viraemia

UDCA on the mixed lymphocyte culture (MLC), a model of cellular immune response[14,15]. MLC was profoundly depressed when responder cells, or both stimulator and responder cells, were obtained from bile duct-ligated animals. Chenodeoxycholic acid induced a dose-dependent inhibition of MLC response with 50% inhibition at 25 μmol/L and almost complete inhibition at 50 μmol/L. In comparison, cyclosporin induced 50% inhibition at concentrations between 10 μg/L and 30 μg/L in the same conditions. UDCA had no significant effect at concentrations ranging from 12.5 to 50 μmol/L.

Interferon and natural killer cells (NK) are involved in the eradication of virus-infected cells. When a cell is infected by a virus, IFN is produced, and binds to receptors on nearby cells, inducing these cells to make antiviral proteins which then limit the spread of viral infection. NK activity is increased, allowing the eradication of virus-infected cells. In a first series of experiments we studied the effects of cholestasis on oligoadenylate synthetase (OAS) activity in liver and spleen from common bile duct-ligated rats: cholestasis induced a time-dependent inhibition of both spleen and liver OAS activities. Twenty-four hour cholestasis reduced enzyme activities by 86% and 70% relative to baseline in spleen and liver, respectively. *In vitro*, chenodeoxycholic acid and its conjugated forms had a concentration-dependent inhibitory effect on IFN-induced OAS and NK activities in fresh human mononuclear cells. The inhibitory effect correlates with the surface activity index of bile acids. UDCA and its conjugated forms had little if any effect. In sum, cholestasis and chenodeoxycholic acid both decrease cell-mediated immunity and diminish the biological activity of IFN and NK cell activity. These properties are not shared by UDCA or tauro-UDCA[16].

Finally, it is also possible that UDCA may have a direct effect on viral replication by inducing cell swelling[17]. Tauro-UDCA at micromolar concentrations has been shown to induce hepatocyte swelling. Hypo-osmotic cell swelling inhibits viral replication and the synthesis of viral protein, as shown in primary cultured hepatocytes from ducks infected *in vivo* with the duck hepatitis B virus[17].

CONCLUSION

Circumstantial evidence strongly suggests that cholestasis and chenodeoxycholic acid, the major human bile acid, might promote viral replication. The correction of cholestasis provided by UDCA might restore, at least in part, cell-mediated immunity and antiviral defences, and thus might lead to reduced viral replication. This hypothesis merits testing with appropriate therapeutic controlled trials.

References

1. Davis GL. Prediction of response to interferon treatment of chronic hepatitis C. J Hepatol. 1994;21:1–3.
2. Yamanaka M. Study of curative effect of ursodeoxycholic acid for chronic hepatitis by double-blind trial. Diagn Treat. 1976;64:2150.
3. Leuschner U, Leuschner M, Sieratzki J, Kurtz W, Hübner K. Gallstone dissolution with ursodeoxycholic acid in patients with chronic active hepatitis and two years follow-up. A pilot study. Dig Dis Sci. 1985;30:642–9.

4. Attili AF, Rusticali A, Varriale M, Carli L, Repice AM, Callea F. The effect of ursodeoxycholic acid on serum enzymes and liver histology in patients with chronic active hepatitis. A 12-month double-blind, placebo-controlled trial. J Hepatol. 1994;20:315–20.

5. Bellentani S, Tabarroni G, Barchi T *et al*. Effect of ursodeoxycholic acid treatment on alanine aminotransferase and γ-glutamyltranspeptidase serum levels in patients with hyper-transaminasemia. Results from a double-blind controlled-trial. J Hepatol. 1989;8:7–12.

6. Floreani A, Chiaramonte M, Fabris P, Ngatchu T, Naccarato R. Poor effect of ursodeoxycholic acid in anti-hepatitis C virus-positive chronic liver disease. Curr Ther Res. 1991;50:635–42.

7. Portincasa P, Palmieri V, Doronzo F *et al*. Effect of tauroursodeoxycholic acid on serum liver enzymes and dyspeptic symptoms in patients with chronic active hepatitis. Curr Ther Res. 1993;53:521–31.

8. Puoti C, Magrini A, Filippi T, Annovazzi G, Pannullo A. Effects of ursodeoxycholic acid on serum liver enzymes in patients with hepatitis C virus-related chronic liver disease. Eur J Gastroenterol Hepatol. 1995;7:151–4.

9. Rolandi E, Franceschini R, Cataldi A, Cicchetti V, Carati L, Barreca T. Effects of urso-deoxycholic acid (UDCA) on serum liver damage indices in patients with chronic active hepati-tis. A double-blind controlled study. Eur J Clin Pharmacol. 1991;40:473–6.

10. Takano S, Ito Y, Yokosuka O *et al*. A multicenter randomized controlled dose study of ursodeoxycholic acid for chronic hepatitis C. Hepatology. 1994;20:558–64.

11. Boucher E, Jouanolle H, André P *et al*. Interferon and ursodeoxycholic acid combined therapy in the treatment of chronic viral C hepatitis: results from a controlled randomized trial in 80 patients. Hepatology. 1995;21:322–7.

12. Angelico M, Gandin C, Pescarmona E *et al*. Recombinant interferon-α and ursodeoxycholic acid versus interferon-α alone in the treatment of chronic hepatitis C: a randomized clinical trial with long-term follow-up. Am J Gastroenterol. 1995;90:263–9.

13. Serfaty L, Giral P, Loria A, Andréani T, Lengendre C, Poupon R. Factors predictive of the response to interferon in patients with chronic hepatitis C. J Hepatol. 1994;21:12–17.

14. Calmus Y, Weill B, Ozier Y, Chéreau C, Houssin D, Poupon R. Immunosuppressive pro-perties of chenodeoxycholic and ursodeoxycholic acid in the mouse. Gastroenterology. 1992;103:617–21.

15. Calmus Y, Guéchot J, Podevin P, Bonnefis MT, Giboudeau J, Poupon R. Differential effects of chenodeoxycholic and ursodeoxycholic acid on interleukin 1, interleukin 6 and tumor necrosis factor α production by monocytes. Hepatology. 1992;16:719–23.

16. Podevin P, Calmus Y, Bonnefis M-T, Veyrunes C, Chéreau C, Poupon R. Effect of cholestasis and bile acids on interferon-induced 2′,5′-adenylate synthetase and natural killer activities. Gastroenterology 1995;108:1192–8.

17. Offenspereger WB, Offensperger S, Stoll B, Gerok W, Haussinger D. Effects of anisotonic exposure on duck hepatitis B virus replication. Hepatology. 1994;20:1–7.

6
Experimental therapies in viral hepatitis

H. E. BLUM, S. WIELAND, F. V. WEIZSÄCKER,
W.-B. OFFENSPERGER, S. OFFENSPERGER,
D. MORADPOUR, I. CHEMIN and E. WALTER

INTRODUCTION

Chronic liver disease is caused by a wide spectrum of aetiologies, including viral infections which are among the most important causes worldwide. The viruses leading to chronic hepatitis are the hepatitis B virus (HBV), hepatitis C virus (HCV), hepatitis D virus (HDV) and possibly the newly discovered hepatitis G virus (HGV)[1,2]. The natural course of these chronic infections is characterized by frequent progression to liver cirrhosis. Thus, chronic hepatitis and its sequelae are major health problems worldwide, and are associated with significant morbidity and mortality from liver cirrhosis and hepatocellular carcinoma (HCC)[3].

The prevention of chronic hepatitis and its progression to more severe forms of liver diseases is, therefore, of major clinical importance. Preventive and therapeutic strategies depend on the aetiology of the liver disease and are aimed at three different levels: (1) prevention of acute hepatitis; (2) prevention of progression of acute to chronic liver disease; and (3) prevention of progression of chronic liver disease to liver cirrhosis. In clinical practice the prevention of the progression of chronic hepatitis to liver cirrhosis and HCC through therapy of the underlying viral infection is a major challenge. Since currently available therapies are of limited efficacy in chronic viral hepatitis, novel therapeutic strategies are being experimentally explored. These strategies fall into two main categories, as will be discussed below: antiviral strategies and elimination of infected cells.

CURRENT THERAPEUTIC STRATEGIES IN CHRONIC VIRAL HEPATITIS

Antiviral strategies

Antiviral strategies in principle attempt to interfere with one or several aspects of the viral life cycle: attachment of the virus to the cell membrane,

Table 1 Steps in viral life cycle and antiviral targets

Viral life cycle	Targets
Attachment	Receptor
Internalization and uncoating	Lysosomal pathway
Replication	DNA polymerase, RNA polymerase, reverse transcriptase, chain elongation
Gene expression	DNA, RNA, proteins
Virus assembly	Packaging
Export	Envelope protein

internalization, uncoating, viral replication and gene expression, virus assembly and finally virion export (Table 1). To date, interference with viral replication by various antiviral agents has been explored most extensively. These agents include inhibitors of viral DNA polymerase or RNA polymerase, viral reverse transcriptase or protease, chain-terminating nucleoside analogues and others. Examples are aciclovir, ganciclovir[4], famciclovir, penciclovir, didanosine, zidovudine, zalcitabine, lamivudine[5], and ribavirin[6]. As monotherapies these agents are, in general, either non-effective or only transiently effective, with reappearance of viral replication after cessation of therapy. Thus, it is likely that these agents may be most useful in combination with other therapeutic strategies, such as interferon-alpha or -beta (see below).

Elimination of infected cells

The elimination of infected cells can be achieved, in principle, by immune mechanisms, such as cytotoxic T cells, by introduction into infected cells of a 'suicide gene', such as a gene coding for herpes simplex thymidine kinase (HSVtk), followed by the administration of aciclovir or ganciclovir, or by the introduction of directly cytotoxic agents, such as diphtheria toxin A or ricin. All these strategies result in direct cytotoxicity with elimination of the infected cells. To date the clinically best established therapeutic strategy is interferon-alpha or -beta, which acts, among others, via immunomodulation, resulting in the immune-mediated elimination of infected hepatocytes.

In selected patients with chronic HBV, HCV or HDV infection, interferon-alpha (IFN-α) results in a long-term response in 30–40% of HBV-infected patients[7], about 20% of HCV-infected patients[8] and about 10% of HDV-infected patients[9,10]. Predictors of response in patients with chronic HBV infection are high transaminases, low HBV DNA, absence of HIV or HDV infection and short duration of disease. Predictors of response in patients with chronic HCV infection are: age younger than 50 years, absence of cirrhosis, normal γ-glutamyltranspeptidase activity, low HCV-RNA levels and absence of HCV genotype 1b[11]. Prolonged treatment of patients with chronic HCV infection appears to improve the long-term response to IFN-α to some degree[12,13]. Given the limited efficacy, the long-term economic benefit of treatment of chronic hepatitis B and C with IFN-α is less than certain[14,15].

Clearly, these therapeutic results with IFN-α or IFN-β are not yet satisfactory, and led to the exploration of alternative strategies. Therefore, a number of non-interferon therapies have been evaluated in clinical studies, none of which appears to be highly effective. Combination therapies of ribavirin[6] or urso-deoxycholic acid with IFN-α[16] may be more effective than either drug alone. To date, no combination therapy has been sufficiently established, however, to justify routine clinical use. IFN-α or IFN-β, therefore, are the only drugs currently available for clinical use in selected patients, despite their limited efficacy.

EXPERIMENTAL THERAPEUTIC STRATEGIES IN CHRONIC VIRAL HEPATITIS

Antiviral strategies

Given the limited efficacy of currently available drugs, newer antiviral strategies are being explored. These strategies are based on the concept that, from a genetic point of view, infections are acquired genetic diseases. Blocking viral gene expression, therefore, may be a molecular or genetic approach to treat viral infections efficiently. Conceptually, molecular or genetic interventions can block viral gene expression at five different levels (Fig. 1), as will be discussed below.

Sense strategy (RNA decoys)

The sense strategy involves the introduction into cells of oligonucleotides or vectors synthesizing RNA fragments which are designed to specifically bind to transcription factors. The binding of the transcription factors then results in a block of transcription viral genes. The interaction with cellular transcription factors, controlling the expression of cellular and viral genes, may limit this therapeutic approach, however.

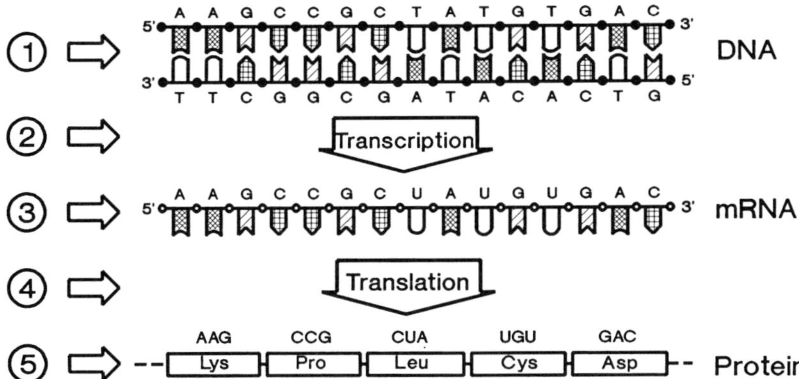

Fig. 1 Antiviral strategies by block of gene expression: (1) sense strategy; (2) anti-gene strategy (triple helix formation); (3) ribozymes; (4) antisense strategy; (5) interfering peptides or proteins

Anti-gene strategy

The anti-gene strategy involves the introduction into cells of oligonucleotides which are designed to bind to double-stranded DNA, resulting in triple-helix formation and reduction of messenger RNA (mRNA) synthesis[17–19].

Ribozymes

Ribozymes are naturally occurring RNA enzymes that catalyse RNA cleavage and RNA splicing reactions[20,21]. Ribozymes that catalyse RNA cleavage are being developed for gene therapeutic applications as inhibitors of gene expression and viral replication. *In-vitro* studies have demonstrated that ribozymes can specifically cleave HBV-RNA[22]. *In-vivo* analyses of this strategy, however, have not been successful to date.

Antisense oligonucleotides

Antisense oligonucleotides are designed to specifically bind to mRNA, resulting in a translational arrest[23]. This strategy has been successfully applied to a number of malignant and viral diseases *in vitro*, including HBV[24–26] or HCV infections[27–29], as well as to the duck hepatitis B virus (DHBV) model of HBV infection *in vivo*[30].

As shown for HBV *in vitro*, cotransfection of the human hepatoma cell line HuH-7 with a replication-competent HBV-DNA construct and a 40-mer antisense oligonucleotide (ATC-40) results in a very strong sequence- and polarity-specific inhibition of HBsAg and HBeAg synthesis (Fig. 2), as well as of intracellular viral replication and export of virions into the culture medium (Fig. 3)[25]. Similarly, experimental studies in the DHBV model demonstrate a specific and dose-dependent inhibition of DHBV replication in primary duck hepatocytes *in vitro* (Fig. 4), as well as infected duct livers *in vivo* (Fig. 5)[30].

Interfering peptides or proteins

The intracellular synthesis of interfering peptides or proteins, including antibodies, is aimed at the specific interference with the assembly or function of viral structural or non-structural proteins, and represents a type of intracellular immunization. This approach is being explored, among others, for the inhibition of HBV core particle production using modified viral core proteins[31–33].

Cytokine-mediated antiviral mechanisms

Recent evidence suggests that virus-specific cytotoxic T cells (CTL) can abolish HBV gene expression and replication in liver cells without hepatocyte killing[34]. This antiviral effect is mediated through IFN-γ and tumour necrosis factor (TNF)-α secreted by the CTL or by the antigen-non-specific macrophages and T cells that they activate following antigen recognition[34,35]. These cytokines appear to act via elimination of nucleocapsid particles and replicating viral genomes, as well as through destabilization of viral RNA[34]. IFN-α and IFN-β, as well as interleukin (IL)-2 appear to act, at least in part, via the same pathways[36,37]. Gene therapy aimed at the local expression of IFN-γ or IFN-α,

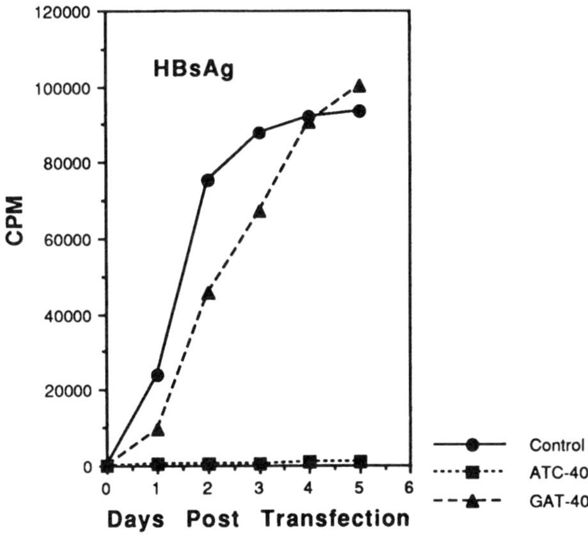

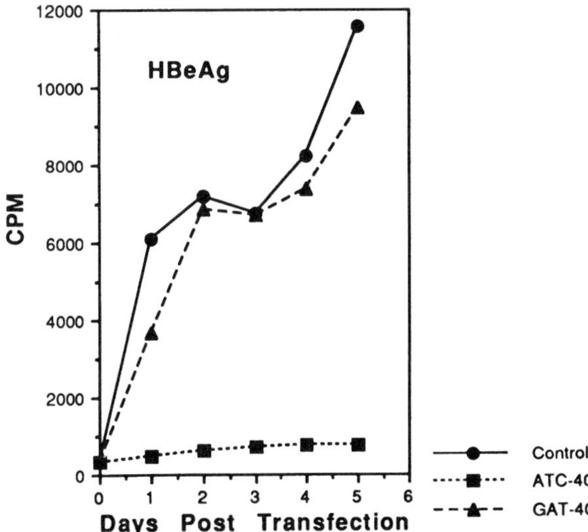

Fig. 2 Inhibition of HBsAg and HBeAg synthesis *in vitro* by cotransfection of a replication-competent HBV-DNA construct with a 40-mer antisense oligonucleotide (ATC-40). Controls include phosphate-buffered saline (control) and a 40-mer sense oligonucleotide (GAT-40)[25]

therefore, may prove to be an effective antiviral strategy. Therapeutic DNA vaccination (see below) possibly also acts via cytokine-mediated intracellular inactivation of viral replication and gene expression[34].

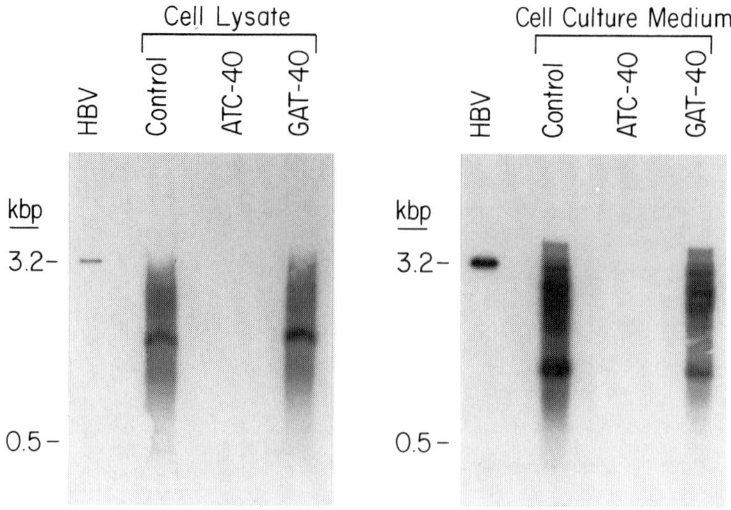

Fig. 3 Inhibition of HBV-DNA replication and virion export *in vitro* by cotransfection of a replication-competent HBV-DNA construct with a 40-mer antisense oligonucleotide (ATC-40). Controls include phosphate-buffered saline (control) and a 40-mer sense oligonucleotide (GAT-40)[25]

The molecular strategies presently being explored to block viral gene expression at different levels still face a number of problems. Apart from the optimal design of oligonucleotides or DNA constructs, a major problem is the stability of these therapeutic nucleic acids or proteins *in vivo*, as well as their specific cellular and intracellular targeting. Viral and non-viral vectors, including liposomes[38] or immunoliposomes[39] and recombinant cylomicrons[40], are being investigated, and should allow the specific delivery of antiviral molecules to infected cells, thereby improving therapeutic efficacy and reducing extrahepatic side-effects.

Elimination of infected cells

The elimination of infected cells can be achieved, in principle, by immune mechanisms, such as cytotoxic T cells, by introduction of a 'suicide gene', such as a gene encoding for herpes simplex thymidine kinase (HSVtk), followed by the administration of aciclovir or ganciclovir[41,42], or by the introduction of inducible cytotoxic agents, such as diphtheria toxin A or ricin. All these strategies result in a direct cytotoxic effect with elimination of the infected cells. To date the most commonly and successfully used therapeutic strategies are IFN-α or IFN-β which act, among other methods, via immunomodulation, resulting in the immune-mediated elimination of infected hepatocytes.

Most exciting new developments are muscle-mediated gene transfer[43] and the naked-DNA vaccine strategy, both of which represent most elegant applications of gene therapy[44].

DNA-based prophylactic vaccination against HBV infection, for example, is possible by intramuscular introduction of a plasmid expressing HBsAg. HBsAg

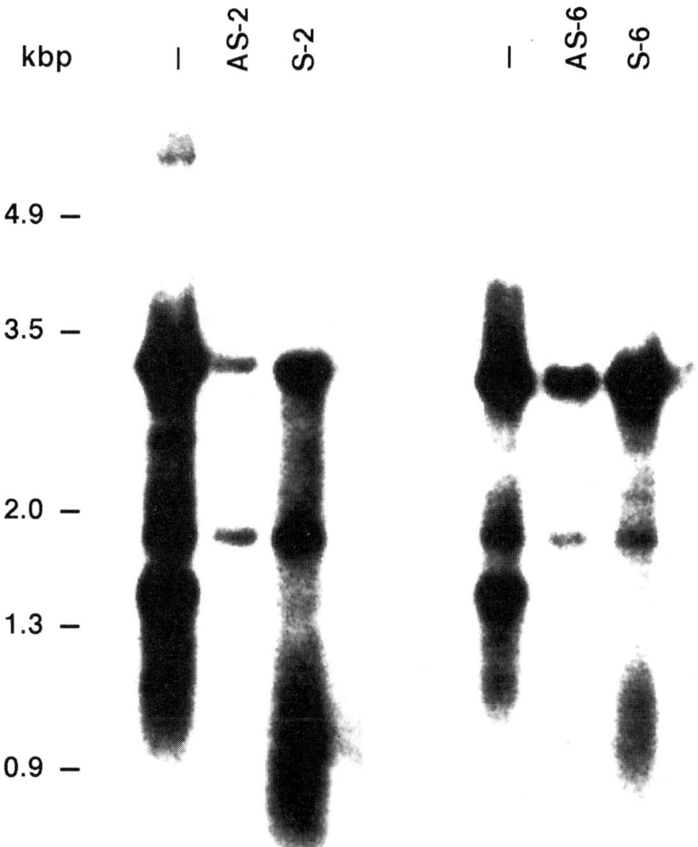

Fig. 4 Inhibition of DHBV replication in duck liver *in vitro* by antisense oligonucleotide 2 or antisense oligonucleotide 6, as compared to untreated primary duck hepatocytes and the corresponding sense oligonucleotides[30]

is secreted from the muscle cells and taken up by cells via phagocytosis or endocytosis. It is processed through the major histocompatibility complex (MHC) class II system, and primarily stimulates an antibody response through CD4+ helper T cells with the production of anti-HBs[44,45]. These antibodies are most important for the neutralization of extracellular virus, especially for viruses released from infected cells during the viral life cycle, or after cell death due to viral infection or destruction by cytotoxic T cells.

By contrast, the therapeutic DNA vaccine acts by the intracellular plasmid-derived synthesis of a viral protein which enters the cell's MHC class I pathway[44]. Only proteins that originate within the cell can be processed by MHC class I molecules that carry fragments of the viral protein to the cell surface. There they stimulate CD8+ cytotoxic T cells, resulting in cell-mediated immunity and possibly in the cytokine-mediated intracellular inactivation of viral replication and gene expression described above[34]. This approach has

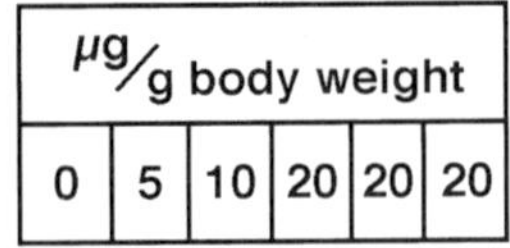

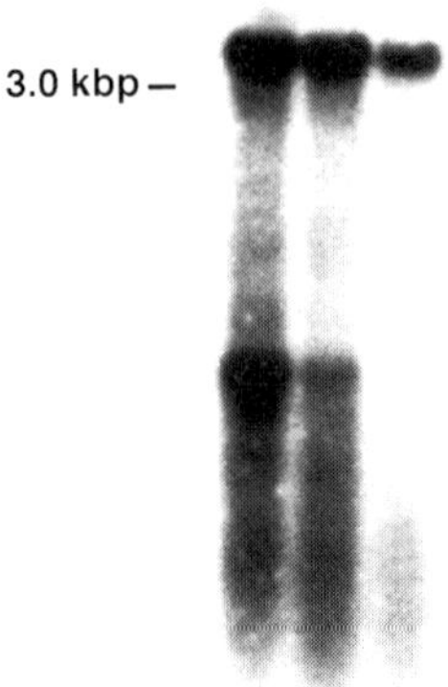

Fig. 5 Dose-dependent inhibition of DHBV replication in duck liver *in vivo* by intravenous injection of antisense oligonucleotide 2[30]

already been experimentally explored for HBV[46,47], as well as for HCV[48,49], and holds great promise as an effective molecular therapy for these viral infections.

SUMMARY AND PERSPECTIVES

Chronic viral hepatitis is caused by four distinct hepatotropic viruses: HBV, HCV, HDV and possibly HGV. Most of these viruses have been characterized in great detail and can be specifically identified by serological and molecular techniques[50]. Chronic viral hepatitis frequently progresses to liver cirrhosis and HCC. Strategies aimed at the prevention of liver cirrhosis include primary prevention of infection with HBV, HCV, HDV or HGV by various measures, as well as secondary prevention by therapy of acute or chronic hepatitis as precursors of liver cirrhosis and HCC development.

For the treatment of chronic viral hepatitis IFN-α or IFN-β are the only drugs currently available for clinical use in selected patients. Given their limited efficacy, combination therapies of IFN-α or IFN-β with synthetic antiviral agents or other drugs are presently being explored. Novel therapeutic strategies (Table 2) are aimed at the molecular nucleic acid-based intervention to block viral gene expression at different levels (sense strategy, antigene strategy, ribozymes, antisense oligonucleotides and interfering peptides or proteins), to introduce cytotoxic drugs or genes (HSVtk and ganciclovir) and to induce a specific cytotoxic immune response by therapeutic naked-DNA vaccination.

Table 2 Therapeutic strategies, targets and mechanisms in chronic viral hepatitis

Strategy	Targets and mechanisms
Antiviral	*Viral life cycle*
Current	Inhibition of viral polymerases, chain termination
Future	Molecular block of gene expression
Cytotoxic	*Infected cells*
Current	Immune modulation
Future	Direct cytotoxicity, suicide gene expression, DNA vaccination

Despite these exciting prospects of molecular nucleic acid-based therapy of viral infections, various aspects of delivery, targeting and safety need to be solved before these concepts can enter clinical practice[51,52]. Apart from further exploring and developing these novel therapeutic strategies, therefore, currently available prophylactic measures should be implemented for the primary prevention of these viral infections.

References

1. Simons JN, Leary TP, Dawson GJ *et al.* Isolation of novel virus like sequences associated with human hepatitis. Nature Med. 1995;1:564–9.
2. Linnen J, Wages Jr J, Zhang-Keck Z-Y *et al.* Molecular cloning and disease association of hepatitis G virus: a transfusion-transmissible agent. Science. 1996;271:505–8.
3. Wands JR, Blum HE. Primary hepatocellular carcinoma (editorial). N Engl J Med. 1991;325:729–31.
4. Gish RG, Lau JYN, Brooks L *et al.* Ganciclovir treatment of hepatitis B virus infection in liver transplant recipients. Hepatology. 1996;23:1–7.
5. Dienstag JL, Perrillo RP, Schiff ER, Bartholomew M, Vicary C, Rubin M. A preliminary trial of lamivudine for chronic hepatitis B infection. N Engl Med. 1995;333:1657–61.
6. Brillanti S, Garson J, Foli M *et al.* A pilot study of combination therapy with ribavirin plus interferon alfa for interferon alfa-resistant chronic hepatitis C. Gastroenterology. 1994;107:812–17.
7. Wong DK, Cheung AM, O Rourke K, Naylor CD, Detsky AS, Heathcote J. Effect of alpha-interferon treatment in patients with hepatitis B e antigen-positive chronic hepatitis B. A meta-analysis. Ann Intern Med. 1993;119:312–23.
8. Davis GL, Balart LA, Schiff ER. Group atHIT. Treatment of chronic hepatitis C with recombinant interferon alfa. N Engl J Med. 1989;321:1501–6.
9. Farci P, Mandas A, Coiana A *et al.* Treatment of chronic hepatitis D with interferon alfa-2a. N Engl J Med. 1994;330:88–94.
10. Rosina F, Cozzolongo R. Interferon in HDV infection. Antiviral Res. 1994;24:165–74.
11. Hayashi J, Ohmiya M, Kishihara Y *et al.* A statistical analysis of predictive factors of response to human lymphoblastoid interferon in patients with chronic hepatitis C. Am J Gastroenterol. 1994;89:2151–6.
12. Reichard O, Glaumann H, Norkrans G *et al.* Histological outcome in patients with chronic hepatitis C given a 60-week interferon alfa-2b treatment course. Liver. 1994;14:169–74.
13. Kasahara A, Hayashi N, Hiramatsu N *et al.* Ability of prolonged interferon treatment to suppress relapse after cessation of therapy in patients with chronic hepatitis C: a multicenter randomized controlled trial. Hepatology. 1995;21:291–7.
14. Dusheiko GM, Roberts JA. Treatment of chronic type B and C hepatitis with interferon alfa: an economic appraisal. Hepatology. 1995;22:1863–73.
15. Koff RS, Seeff LB. Economic modelling of treatment in chronic hepatitis B and chronic hepatitis C: promises and limitations. Hepatology. 1995;22:1880–2.

16. Boucher E, Jouanolle H, Andre P *et al.* Interferon and ursodeoxycholic acid combined therapy in the treatment of chronic viral C hepatitis: results from a controlled randomized trial in 80 patients. Hepatology. 1995;21:322–7.
17. Strobel SA, Dervan PB. Site specific cleavage of a yeast chromosome by oligonucleotide directed triple helix formation. Science. 1990;249:73–5.
18. Postel EH, Flint SJ, Kessler DJ, Hogan ME. Evidence that a triplex forming oligodeoxyribonucleotide binds to the c-myc promoter in HeLa cells, thereby reducing c-myc mRNA levels. Proc Natl Acad Sci USA. 1991;88:8227–31.
19. Duval VG, Thuong NT, Helene C. Specific inhibition of transcription by triple helix-forming oligonucleotides. Proc Natl Acad Sci USA. 1992;89:504–8.
20. Haseloff J, Gerlach WL. Simple RNA enzymes with new and highly specific endoribonuclease activities. Nature. 1988;334:585–91.
21. Thompson JD, Macejak D, Couture L, Stinchcomb DT. Ribozymes in gene therapy. Nature Med. 1995;1:277–8.
22. von Weizsäcker F, Blum HE, Wands JR. Cleavage of hepatitis B virus RNA by three ribozymes transcribed from a single DNA template. Biochem Biophys Res Commun. 1992;189:743–8.
23. Wagner RW. Gene inhibition using antisense oligodeoxynucleotides. Nature. 1994;372:333–5.
24. Goodarzi G, Gross SC, Tewari A, Watabe K. Antisense oligodeoxyribonucleotides inhibit the expression of the gene for hepatitis B virus surface antigen. J Gen Virol. 1990;71:3021–5.
25. Blum HE, Galun E, Weizsäcker F, Wands JR. Inhibition of hepatitis B virus by antisense oligodeoxynucleotides (letter). Lancet. 1991;337:1230.
26. Wu GY, Wu CH. Specific inhibition of hepatitis B viral gene expression *in vitro* by targeted antisense oligonucleotides. J Biol Chem. 1992;267:12436–9.
27. Wakita T, Wands JR. Specific inhibition of hepatitis C virus expression by antisense oligodeoxynucleotides. *In-vitro* model for selection of target sequence. J Biol Chem. 1994;269:14205–10.
28. Mizutani T, Kato N, Hirota M, Sugiyama K, Murakami A, Shimotohno K. Inhibition of hepatitis C virus replication by antisense oligonucleotide in culture cells. Biochem Biophys Res Commun. 1995;212:906–11.
29. Alt M, Renz R, Hofschneider PH, Paumgartner G, Caselmann WH. Specific inhibition of hepatitis C viral gene expression by antisense phosphorothioate oligodeoxynucleotides. Hepatology. 1995;22:707–17.
30. Offensperger WB, Offensperger S, Walter E, Teubner K, Igloi G, Blum HE, Gerok W. *In-vivo* inhibition of duck hepatitis B virus replication and gene expression by phosphorothioate modified antisense oligodeoxynucleotides. EMBO J. 1993;12:1257–62.
31. Delaney MA, Goyal S, Seeger C. Design of modified core genes that inhibit replication of woodchuck hepatitis virus. In: Hollinger FB, Lemon SM, Margolis H, editors. Viral hepatitis and liver disease. Baltimore, MD: Williams & Wilkins; 1991:667–8.
32. Horwich AL, Furtak K, Pugh J, Summers J. Synthesis of hepadnavirus particles that contain replication-defective duck hepatitis B virus genomes in cultured HuH7 cells. J Virol. 1990;64:642–50.
33. Scaglioni PP, Melegari M, Wands JR. Characterization of hepatitis B virus core mutants that inhibit viral replication. Virology. 1994;205:112–20.
34. Guidotti LG, Ishikawa T, Hobbs MV, Matzke B, Schreiber R, Chisari FV. Intracellular inactivation of the hepatitis B virus by cytotoxic T lymphocytes. Immunity. 1996;4:25–36.
35. Guidotti LG, Ando K, Hobbs MV *et al.* Cytotoxic T lymphocytes inhibit hepatitis B virus gene expression by a noncytolytic mechanism in transgenic mice. Proc Natl Acad Sci USA. 1994;91:3764–8.
36. Guilhot S, Guidotti LG, Chisari FV. Interleukin-2 downregulates hepatitis B virus gene expression in transgenic mice by a posttranscriptional mechanism. J Virol. 1993;67:7444–9.
37. Guidotti LG, Guilhot S, Chisari FV. Interleukin-2 and alpha/beta interferon down-regulate hepatitis B virus gene expression in vivo by tumor necrosis factor-dependent and -independent pathways. J Virol. 1994;68:1265–70.
38. Rose JK, Buonocore L, Whitt MA. A new cationic liposome reagent mediating nearly quantitative transfection of animal cells. Biotechniques. 1991;10:520–5.
39. Kalvakolanu DV, Abraham A. Preparation and characterization of immunoliposomes for targeting of antiviral agents. Biotechniques. 1991;11:218–22.

40. Rensen PCN, Vandijk MCM, Havenaar EC, Bijsterbosch MK, Krujit JK, Vanberkel TJC. Selective liver targeting of antivirals by recombinant chylomicrons: a new therapeutic approach to hepatitis B. Nature Med. 1995;1:221–5.
41. Qian C, Bilbao R, Bruna O, Prieto J. Induction of sensitivity to ganciclovir in human hepatocellular carcinoma cells by adenovirus mediated gene transfer or herpes simplex virus thymidine kinase. Hepatology. 1995;22:118–23.
42. Kuriyama S, Nakatani T, Masui K *et al.* Bystander effect caused by suicide gene expression indicates the feasibility of gene therapy for hepatocellular carcinoma. Hepatology. 1995;22:1838–46.
43. Blau HM, Springer ML. Muscle mediated gene therapy. N Engl J Med. 1995;333:1554–6.
44. McDonnell WM, Askari FK. DNA vaccines. N Engl J Med. 1996;334:42–5.
45. Davis HL, Michel ML, Whalen RG. DNA-based immunization induces continuous secretion of hepatitis B surface antigen and high levels of circulating antibody. Hum Mol Genet. 1993;2:1847–51.
46. Schirmbeck R, Bohm W, Ando K, Chisari FV, Reimann J. Nucleic acid vaccination primes hepatitis B virus surface antigen specific cytotoxic T lymphocytes in nonresponder mice. J Virol. 1995;69:5929–34.
47. Vitiello A, Ishioka G, Grey HM *et al.* Development of a lipopeptide based therapeutic vaccine to treat chronic HBV infection. I. Induction of a primary cytototix T lymphocyte response in humans. J Clin Invest. 1995;95:341–9.
48. Lagging LM, Meyer K, Hoft D, Houghton M, Belsche RB, Ray R. Immune responses to plasmid DNA encoding the hepatitis C virus core protein. J Virol. 1995;69:5859–63.
49. Major ME, Vitvitski L, Mink MA *et al.* DNA based immunization with chimeric vectors for the induction of immune responses against the hepatitis C virus nucleocapsid. J Virol. 1995;69:5798–805.
50. Purcell RH. Hepatitis viruses: changing patterns of human disease. Proc Natl Acad Sci USA. 1994;91:2401–6.
51. Crystal RG. Transfer of genes to humans: early lessons and obstacles to success. Science. 1995;270:404–10.
52. Friedmann T. Human gene therapy – an immature genie, but certainly out of the bottle. Nature Med. 1996;2:144–7.

7
New antiviral treatment for chronic hepatitis B

C.-L. LAI

INTRODUCTION

It is estimated that there are 300–350 million hepatitis B surface antigen (HBsAg) carriers in the world[1-5]. Twenty-five to forty per cent of these carriers will eventually die of liver problems; i.e. from cirrhosis and hepatocellular carcinoma (HCC)[6]. It has been suggested that, since there is a progressive increase in the incidence of HCC with age, all HBsAg carriers would eventually die from HCC and/or cirrhosis if they do not die from other causes first[7].

The ultimate aim in the treatment of HBsAg carriers is therefore to prevent, or at least to decrease, the development of cirrhosis and HCC. Since this requires the long-term follow-up of treated patients for decades, more realistic short-term objectives are usually used in clinical trials. These are as follows:

1. Viral suppression as evidenced by the disappearance of hepatitis B virus (HBV) DNA (using hybridization assay) and hepatitis B e antigen (HBeAg) with or without the appearance of antibody against HBeAg (anti-HBe).
2. Reduction in liver damage as evidenced by the normalization of serum transaminase levels (if these are elevated), and by an improvement in histological appearance on liver biopsies.
3. Complete eradication of the virus as evidenced by the loss of HBsAg and the inability to detect HBV-DNA in the serum and the liver even using polymerase chain reaction (PCR) assays. This last objective is seldom achieved with the treatment presently in use or under trial.

The agents currently used or under trial for the treatment of chronic hepatitis B can be broadly divided into two groups (Table 1). The first group is the immunomodulators. These act by modulating the immune response of the host to HBV antigens expressed on the surface of the hepatocytes[8]. Interferon-α (IFN-α) is listed under the immunodulators, even though it also has direct antiviral actions, because immunomodulation is probably its main mode of action in HBsAg carriers. Other newer immunomodulators include thymosin-α_1 (T-α_1) and therapeutic vaccines, e.g. Theradigm-HBV.

Table 1 Agents currently used or under trial for chronic hepatitis B infection

I. Immunomodulators
   Interferon-α
   Thymosin-α_1
   Therapeutic vaccines, e.g. Theradigm-HBV

II. Viral suppressors
   Famiciclovir
   Lamivudine
   (Ganciclovir)

The second group of agents used in the treatment of chronic hepatitis B comprises the viral suppressors. The most promising agents are famciclovir and lamivudine. Since exciting results have also been obtained using viral suppressors (including ganciclovir and the two agents mentioned above) in preventing or treating the recurrence of HBV infection after liver transplantation for HBsAg carriers, this topic will also be mentioned briefly at the end of this chapter.

INTERFERON-α (IFN-α)

This is the only approved agent for use in the treatment of HBsAg carriers. It is given parenterally (subcutaneously) in a 16-week course of either 5 mU daily or 10 mU three times weekly. A meta-analysis of 15 randomized placebo-controlled studies showed that IFN-α was beneficial (Table 2)[9]. However, its usefulness was limited. Loss of HBeAg and HBV-DNA occurred only 20% more often in treated patients than in the controls; and loss of HBsAg occurred 6% more often. IFN-α had significant effect on normalization of alanine aminotransferase (ALT) levels. Most studies showed that, in the patients in whom treatment was successful, there was improvement in histology.

A more recent report calculated the cost-effectiveness of IFN-α treatment[10]. Based on their own meta-analysis of nine randomized trials, and on a large set of probabilities, the authors concluded that for a 35-year-old person with chronic hepatitis B who was HBeAg-positive, IFN-α would increase life expectancy by 3.1 years or 3.4 quality-adjusted life-years. This relatively modest increase in life expectancy was based on certain assumptions that are questionable. According to the authors, patients who were HBeAg-positive and HBsAg-positive had a 12.1% probability of developing compensated cirrhosis annually; whereas patients who were HBeAg-negative and HBsAg-positive had only a

Table 2 Summary of the results of a meta-analysis of 15 randomized placebo-controlled trials of interferon-α (IFN-α) in chronic hepatitis B infection[9]

	IFN-α-treated group (%)	*Control group (%)*	*p*
Loss of HBV-DNA	37	17	0.0001
Loss of HBeAg	33	12	0.0001
Loss of HBsAg	7.8	1.8	0.001

1.0% probability of developing the same condition. It is now generally agreed that cirrhosis develops as a result of immunological injury to the liver during the phase of viral clearance when the patient is seroconverting from HBeAg positivity to anti-HBe positivity[11–13]. Therefore the assumption that HBeAg-negative patients are much less likely to develop cirrhosis compared to HBe-Ag-positive patients seems to me unjustifiable.

I would like to address four other issues concerning IFN-α in chronic hepatitis B.

Firstly, should IFN-α treatment be preceded by a short course of steroid? Steroid therapy in chronic hepatitis B causes enhanced viral replication[14], possibly acting through the glucocorticoid-responsive element that is found in the hepatitis B viral genome[15]. Following withdrawal of a short course of steroid, there is a decline in HBV-DNA and HBV-DNA polymerase, coinciding with an immunological rebound with enhancement of T lymphocyte function[16]. It is this enhancement of T lymphocyte function which may potentiate the effect of interferon. However, in a large multicentre trial[17] there was an almost identical rate of HBeAg seroconversion in patients treated with IFN-α alone and in patients treated with steroid withdrawal followed by IFN-α (though a distinct trend did exist for the patients with low pretreatment ALT levels to respond more frequently with steroid preceding IFN-α than with IFN-α alone). Moreover, steroid withdrawal is documented to precipitate hepatic decompensation, possibly fatal, in patients with marginal liver function due to hepatic necrosis superimposed on the chronic disease[18–20]. Such fatal reactivation on withdrawal of steroid can occur even in *completely asymptomatic* HBsAg carriers[21]. Steroid should therefore be used with extreme care in HBsAg carriers. Withdrawal of steroid is not recommended as a routine procedure prior to treatment of IFN-α.

Secondly, do Oriental HBsAg carriers respond less well to IFN-α when compared with Caucasian HBsAg carriers? About 75% of HBsAg carriers are Orientals. At least 50% of these Oriental carriers acquire the hepatitis B infection perinatally[22], and a large proportion of the remaining Oriental carriers acquire the infection within the first few years of life[23]. Such early infection induces immune tolerance to the hepatitis B virus, possibly through the deletion of T cells that can 'recognize' HBeAg and the hepatitis B core antigen (HBcAg).

Two large-scale trials were carried out in adult Chinese HBsAg carriers[24,25]. In the later trial the carriers were randomized into those with normal pretreatment ALT levels and those with persistently elevated pretreatment ALT levels for over 3 consecutive months. The results are summarized in Table 3. In patients with normal ALT the IFN-α had little effect. In patients with elevated ALT the response to IFN-α (with or without prednisone) was slightly better. However, the elevated ALT in these patients suggests that they were in the phase of viral clearance. The spontaneous HBe seroconversion rate in the control group was therefore as high as 19% within 1 year. Thus the authors concluded that, even in patients with elevated ALT levels, 'it is not clear whether interferon merely hastened the process of endogenous inhibition of HBV replication or provided actual benefit to some patients'[25].

Two randomized trials were also carried out in Chinese HBsAg children carriers[26,27], since it was thought that the poor response in the adult carriers

Table 3 Summary of the response to interferon-α (IFN-α) treatment in Chinese adult HBsAg carriers[25]

	Prednisone + IFN-α	IFN-α alone	Control	p
Patients with elevated ALT				
Percentage lost HBeAg	43	33	19	n.s.
Percentage lost HBsAg	0	6	0	n.s.
Patients with normal ALT				
Percentage lost HBeAg	0	10	0	n.s.
Percentage lost HBsAg	0	5	0	n.s.

n.s. = Not significant.

might be related to delayed treatment. However, the results were equally disappointing.

How effective is IFN-α in inducing viral eradication as evidenced by the loss of HBsAg and HBV-DNA as tested by PCR? As mentioned above, meta-analysis of 15 randomized trials shows that loss of HBsAg occurs 6% more often in IFN-α-treated patients than in controls 6 months after the cessation of treatment[9]. On long-term follow-up, 65% of IFN-α-treated Caucasian patients who have sustained loss of HBeAg also lose HBsAg[28]. However, only 24% of the Spanish responders, and none of the Chinese responders, lose HBsAg on long-term follow-up[29,30].

Complete disappearance of HBV-DNA, as tested by PCR assay, occurs only rarely in IFN-α-treated patients who clear HBeAg but remain positive for HBsAg. Of 272 Chinese adult and children HBsAg carriers who participated in three randomized placebo-controlled trials, 5.9% of the treated patients and 1.2% of the control patients became HBV-DNA-negative on long-term follow-up (p = n.s.)[31].

What are the adverse effects of IFN-α? The major adverse effects are listed in Table 4. These can be severe, and are dose-related. Though most adverse effects can be decreased by reduction of the dose of IFN-α, some can lead to premature cessation of therapy. The initial influenza-like syndrome can be minimized by gradual escalation of the dose during initiation of therapy. Induction of auto-antibodies, usually clinically silent, can lead to overt hypo- and hyperthyroidism and idiopathic thrombocytopenic purpura[32]. It may also induce the development

Table 4 Adverse effects of interferon-α

Influenza-like syndrome (rapid tachyphylaxis)
Myalgia
Marrow suppression (usually moderate)
Alopecia
Depression (occasionally severe)
Induction of autoantibodies
Induction of interferon-neutralizing antibodies
In patients with advanced hepatitis/cirrhosis
    susceptibility to bacterial infections
    worsening of liver function

of autoimmune hepatitis in individuals who are genetically predisposed to develop autoimmune liver disease[33,34]. The presence of interferon-neutralizing antibodies is often of no clinical importance, but when present in large amounts this can counteract the effects of IFN-α. In the presence of advanced hepatitis, IFN-α may cause worsening of liver function. Because of this, and of the increased susceptibility to bacterial infection, IFN-α should be used only under close monitoring in patients with mild or moderate hepatic decompensation.

THYMOSIN-α_1 (T-α_1)

T-α_1 is a synthetic polypeptide of 28 amino acids originally isolated from thymosin fraction 5. It is an immunomodulator with multiple modes of action. It primarily increases the efficiency of T-cell maturation[35]. It also acts on T cells after maturation, inducing an increased production of cytokines, e.g. interferon-γ, interleukin-2[36]. Thirdly it up-regulates the expression of cytokine receptors[37]. In a study involving woodchucks infected with the woodchuck hepatitis virus, 12 woodchucks were randomized to receive T-α_1 twice weekly or no treatment for 6 months[38]. The viral titres remained high in the control animals while viral titres became undetectable in four of the six treated animals, and were reduced to 1% of entry values in the remaining two animals.

In a phase II trial on patients with chronic hepatitis B, seven patients received thymosin fraction 5 or T-α_1 while five patients received subcutaneous placebo injections twice weekly for 6 months[39]. Eighty-six per cent of the thymosin-treated patients cleared HBV-DNA from their sera compared to only 20% in the control group ($p < 0.04$). The same proportion of patients showed absence of replicative forms of HBV-DNA in the liver biopsies. Response to thymosin therapy was associated with improvement in peripheral lymphocyte, CD3 and CD4 counts, and in interferon-γ production. The serological improvements were sustained during follow-up.

Currently an American phase III clinical trial is being analysed after completion. The preliminary results have been published in an abstract[40]. Ninety-nine patients were recruited in this multicentre randomized controlled trial. Since the response to thymosin may be delayed up to 12 months after cessation of therapy, the authors decided to analyse the results at 12 months (i.e. 6 months after therapy), and at a later period. At 12 months, 14% of 49 thymosin-treated patients were negative for HBeAg and HBV-DNA, compared to 4% of 50 placebo patients ($p = 0.084$). At the latest follow-up visit, 25% of the treated patients had responded, compared to 12% of placebo patients ($p < 0.11$). These preliminary results suggest a trend in favour of T-α_1, but are far less promising than the phase II trial results.

Other phase III trials are being performed in Taiwan and Singapore, the former having completed recruitment with 158 subjects. Any definitive conclusions concerning the usefulness of T-α_1 must await the final outcome of these phase III trials.

The effect of combining T-α_1 with lymphoblastoid IFN was tested in 15 patients. Preliminary data showed loss of HBV-DNA in 60% of the patients and loss of HBsAg in 40%[41]. Again, firm conclusions will have to await further trials.

Concerning the safety of T-α_1, to date *no* adverse events have been reported in over 1000 subjects who had received the drug, including normal subjects and patients with hepatitis B and C, autoimmune hepatitis, acquired immunodeficiency syndrome and cancers.

THERAPEUTIC VACCINES

Patients who clear HBV develop a strong HLA class I-restricted response; whereas this response is weak in HBsAg carriers. Both IFN-α and the withdrawal of steroid probably act by inducing cytotoxic T lymphocytes (CTL).

A therapeutic vaccine, Theradigm-HBV, has been designed to induce a CLT response to HBV[42]. Theradigm-HBV consists of three components. The hepatitis B core antigen (HBcAg) peptide 18–27 is chosen as the CTL peptide epitope. Since peptides tend to be poor immunogens, two additional components are added to enhance immunogenicity: tetanus toxoid peptide 830–843 as the T helper peptide epitope and two palmitic acid molecules as the lipid component. HBcAg peptide 18–27 is selected because it has been shown to be recognized by CTL obtained from patients with acute HBV infection[43,44].

A dose escalation trial in 26 normal subjects showed that Theradigm-HBV was safe, and able to induce a primary HBV-specific CTL response with the first dose and a booster effect with the second dose given 28–35 days later.

A phase II study is under way to determine the efficacy of vaccinating HBsAg carriers with two doses of Theradigm-HBV.

FAMCICLOVIR

Famciclovir is the oral derivative of penciclovir. It is converted to penciclovir in the intestinal wall and in the liver after absorption[45]. Penciclovir is a guanine analogue that inhibits viral DNA chain elongation by competing for viral DNA polymerase in its active intracellular triphosphate form[46]. It has potent effect against the herpes simplex and zoster viruses[47].

Famciclovir suppresses the replication of the duck hepatitis B virus in the Pekin duck very effectively; and is also found to be effective against human HBV replication in human hepatoma cells transfected with the HBV genome[48]. In a double-blind placebo-controlled pilot study, 17 patients were randomized to receive famciclovir 250 mg t.d.s. or 500 mg t.d.s., or placebo[49]. Of the 11 evaluable patients who received famciclovir, six had > 90% reduction in HBV-DNA levels compared with none of the patients who received placebo. In four of the responders the fall in HBV-DNA was sustained throughout the 10-day treatment, and in two of these the fall persisted for a further 2 weeks. More prolonged courses of famciclovir are now being further assessed for its effect on HBV replication in phase III trials.

The use of famciclovir in the treatment of HBV recurrence after liver transplantation will be discussed later.

Famciclovir is found to be remarkably safe in multiple clinical trials for patients with herpes zoster and genital herpes[47]. The commonest adverse effects, of headache, nausea and diarrhoea, occurred with equal frequency in patients receiving famciclovir and in patients receiving placebo.

LAMIVUDINE

Lamivudine (the (–) enantiomer of 2′-deoxy-3′-thiacytidine) is a 2′3′-dideoxynucleoside similar in structure to 3′-azido-3′-deoxythymidine (AZT), 2′3-dideoxycytidine (ddC) and 2′3-dideoxyinosine (ddI), drugs used for the treatment of patients with human immunodeficiency virus (HIV) infection. Like these agents, lamivudine inhibits DNA synthesis by chain termination of the nascent proviral DNA. It also interferes with the reverse transcriptase activity of HIV and HBV. It was approved for use in HIV patients in late 1995 because of its synergistic effect with AZT in these patients[50].

Lamivudine inhibits the replication of HBV in human HBV-transfected cell lines[51], but withdrawal of lamivudine results in the reappearance of replicative HBV-DNA[52]. It is also very effective *in vivo* when given to infected ducks and chimpanzees[53].

Multiple phase II dose-ranging trials with[54] or without[55,56] placebo have been performed in both Caucasian and Oriental HBsAg carriers. Oral daily doses of 5–600 mg were given for 4–12 weeks. The conclusions from these trials are essentially identical. Within 1 week of therapy, HBV-DNA dropped to very low levels. For doses of 25 mg daily or below, the suppression of HBV-DNA was suboptimal; but 100% of patients receiving 100 mg daily or more of lamivudine had almost complete suppression of HBV-DNA (95–100% of pretreatment levels). This was associated with a decrease in HBeAg and HBsAg titres (Glaxo, unpublished data) and normalization of ALT levels[55]. These reductions occurred irrespective of the pretreatment HBV-DNA and ALT levels, in both Caucasians and Orientals[54,55]. In the majority of patients, HBV-DNA, HBeAg and HBsAg returned to pretreatment levels 4–8 weeks after treatment. However, in 19% of the patients on 12 weeks of lamivudine, HBV-DNA suppression was sustained[55]. HBeAg disappeared in 12% of patients.

Several large-scale multicentre controlled trials are now being performed in Southeast Asia, in Europe and in the United States, comparing lamivudine with or without IFN, and with placebo. In one trial the patients will be treated for at least 3 years. Since the phase II trials show that the majority of patients have a rebound of the HBV-DNA on cessation of therapy, lamivudine will probably have to be given on a long-term basis. Averett and Mason have emphasized that suppression of viral replication *per se* is not enough; there must be a corresponding decline in the number of productively infected hepatocytes[57]. The latter process, i.e. the reduction in the number of infected hepatocytes, will depend on the spontaneous death of infected hepatocytes and possibly on the inefficient passage of covalently closed circular DNA (ccc DNA) of HBV from other infected hepatocytes which proliferate to replace the dying cells[58]. This means that viral suppressors will probably have to be administered over many months, if not years. With lamivudine being taken orally once daily, patient compliance should be good. One conceivable endpoint for cessation of therapy would be the complete eradication of HBV, i.e. the disappearance of HBsAg and HBV-DNA in the serum (and the liver) as shown by PCR assays[57].

It is potentially dangerous to stop lamivudine prematurely. One case report describes the occurrence of a rise in ALT 4 weeks after discontinuing lamivudine[59]. This rose to 100 times the upper limit of normal 4 months later, associated with jaundice, a fall in clotting factors and hepatic collapse on liver biopsy. The authors postulate a reinfection of hepatocytes with a subsequent severe immune reaction. The patient was treated with a course of prednisone; he survived with HBV-DNA and HBeAg clearance. According to the authors such rise of ALT occurs in 16% of patients within 8–24 weeks after cessation of treatment. It appears from this report that, in future use, lamivudine may have to be maintained on a long-term basis until there is evidence of complete viral eradication, as indicated above.

Otherwise, lamivudine is a remarkably safe drug. It is unlike fialuridine (FIAU), which caused severe hepatic failure and lactic acidosis in seven out of 15 patients, five of whom died[60]. FIAU probably causes the above toxicity because it contains a free 3′-hydroxyl group which allows its incorporation into DNA, including mitochondrial DNA, at internucleotide linkages[61]. Lamivudine lacks this free 3′-hydroxyl group.

Compared to other non-FIAU nucleoside analogues, lamivudine also has fewer potential side-effects. Drugs such as AZT and ddC can cause myopathy and marrow hypoplasia[62,63]. It has been shown in rats that AZT, though not incorporated into mitochondrial DNA, inhibits mitochondrial DNA, RNA and polypeptide synthesis[62]. In contrast, when tested in cell cultures, lamivudine has much less effect upon mitochondrial DNA content and on the activity of DNA polymerase γ, the enzyme responsible for the replication of mitochondrial DNA[48] (Glaxo, unpublished data).

The adverse events encountered with lamivudine in clinical settings are summarized in Table 5. These are the events reported in a total of 19 520 patients, of whom 631 had HBV infection and 18 889 patients had HIV infection. A large proportion of the latter patients had been receiving lamivudine for over 2 years. (The data have been kindly supplied to the author, with permission to use it, by Glaxo Research and Development Ltd.)

Table 5 Adverse events of lamivudine observed in 19 520 patients (data kindly supplied by Glaxo Research and Development Ltd)

	HIV infection	*HBV infection*	*Percentage of total population*
No. of patients	**18 889**	**631**	
Adverse events			
haematological	103	1	0.53
neurological	54	0	0.28
pancreatitis	52	0	0.27
other hepatobiliary complications	23	5	0.14
gastrointestinal	39	0	0.20
endocrine	26	2	0.14
musculoskeletal	8	1	0.05
psychiatric	3	–	0.02

The haematological abnormalities were mild anaemia, neutropenia or thrombocytopenia. They were reported in only one patient with HBV infection, and that patient had liver transplantation. Neurological events mostly comprised muscle weakness. Some patients developed elevations of creatine kinase levels, but most of these were not associated with symptoms.

Pancreatitis has so far been reported only in patients with HIV infection. About one-third of the patients who developed pancreatitis had a history of pancreatitis prior to lamivudine treatment. It was often difficult to decide whether the pancreatitis was causally related to lamivudine, whether it was a complication of HIV infection or whether it was due to concomitant drug treatment, e.g. steroid or AZT.

Other hepatobiliary complications included elevation of transaminases (not related to withdrawal of lamivudine), bilirubin, lipase and amylase. These were mostly without clinical symptoms. Finally, the occasional patients had diarrhoea, nausea, hypoglycaemia and myalgia. In total, around 1.6% of the patients were reported to have complications, most of them mild. Lamivudine is a very safe drug.

VIRAL SUPPRESSORS IN LIVER TRANSPLANTATION

Hepatitis B immune globulin (HBIG) is the only agent proven to be of use for the prevention of HBV recurrence after liver transplantation for end-stage hepatitis B cirrhosis. In a study of 372 HBsAg-positive patients, by Samuel and his colleagues[64], the 3-year actuarial risk of recurrence of HBV infection was 83% in patients positive for HBV-DNA, 66% in patients negative for HBV-DNA but positive for HBeAg, and 58% in patients negative for both HBV-DNA and HBeAg. With long-term administration of HBIG, the 3-year risk of recurrence was significantly reduced ($p < 0.001$) but was still 36%. Furthermore, the dosing of HBIG is difficult, requiring constant monitoring of anti-HBs titres. Its cost also is considerable (estimated to be US$30 000 per year).

Recently, very encouraging results have been achieved with the three viral suppressors, ganciclovir, famciclovir and lamivudine.

The first two agents have been used in patients with recurrent HBV infection despite HBIG treatment. In one series, ganciclovir was given intravenously to eight of these patients (and to one patient with *de-novo* HBV infection) for 3–10 months[65]. In all the patients, serum HBV-DNA levels dropped, the mean drop being 90%. ALT levels also decreased. Hepatic expression of HBV antigens and HBV-DNA was reduced in three of six patients assessed. After discontinuation of ganciclovir, HBV-DNA recurred or increased in all the patients except in the patient with *de-novo* infection. Four patients underwent retreatment with success.

A similar study was performed using famciclovir. After finding that famciclovir was useful when preceded by a 2-week course of intravenous prostaglandin E[66], Krüger and his colleagues used famciclovir as the sole agent, given orally, in 38 patients with HBV reinfection following liver transplantation[67]. There was a median reduction in serum HBV-DNA of 91% in 83% of evaluable patients. Eight patients were on famciclovir for over 1 year without significant side-effects.

Lamivudine has been used as a prophylactic agent to *prevent* hepatitis B reinfection following liver transplantation. It is used as a single agent without HBIG and is given orally for at least 4 weeks prior to transplantation. In one of the first published abstracts, 12 patients were transplanted, with one early post-operative death[68]. Before transplantation, all the patients were positive of HBV-DNA using PCR assay. After transplantation, only one patient had recurrent HBV infection. The other 10 surviving patients all became negative for HBV-DNA in the serum and for HBsAg and HBcAg in the liver biopsies. Six of these patients also lost HBsAg in the serum. The drug was well tolerated except for one patient, who developed sensorimotor neuropathy and myopathy.

Viral suppressors thus appear to provide an effective alternative to HBIG in both the prevention and treatment of HBV reinfection, after liver transplantation for HBsAg-positive subjects.

CONCLUSIONS

For the treatment of chronic hepatitis B, IFN-α is only of limited use, especially in the Oriental population. The use of newer immunomodulators such as T-α_1 and therapeutic vaccines is now being assessed clinically. So far, the effectiveness of T-α_1 appears to be modest.

A number of suppressors of the replication of HBV have also been assessed. Of these lamivudine proves to be the most potent. However, viral suppressors probably have to be taken on a long-term basis for an effective decline in the number of productively infected hepatocytes.

Viral suppressors have also been found to be useful in the treatment and in the prevention of the recurrence of HBV after liver transplantation for end-stage hepatitis B liver diseases. When given prophylactically (i.e. before the transplantation), a substantial proportion of patients will lose HBsAg after the transplantation.

References

1. Sherlock S. Hepatitis B: the disease. Vaccine. 1990;8:S6–9.
2. Margolis HS, Alter MJ, Hadler SC. Hepatitis B: evolving epidemiology and implications for control. Semin Liver Dis. 1991;11:84–92.
3. Bloom BS, Hillman AL, Fendrick AM, Schwartz JS. A reappraisal of hepatitis B virus vaccination strategies using cost-effectiveness analysis. Ann Intern Med. 1993;118:298–306.
4. Krahn M, Detsky AS. Should Canada and the United States universally vaccinate infants against hepatitis B? A cost-effectiveness analysis. Med Decis Making. 1993;13:4–20.
5. Kane MA. Progress on the control of hepatitis B infection through immunization. Gut. 1993;34:S10–12.
6. Maynard JE, Kare MA, Alter MJ, Hadler SC. Control of hepatitis B by immunization: global perspective. In: Zukerman AJ, editor. Viral hepatitis and liver disease. New York: Alan R Liss, 1988:967–69.
7. Beasley RP, Hwang L-Y. Overview on the epidemiology of hepatocellular carcinoma. In: Hollinger FB, Lemon SM, Margolis H, editors. Viral hepatitis and liver disease. Baltimore: Williams & Wilkins, 1991:532–5.
8. Eddleston ALW. Overview of HBV pathogenesis. In: Hollinger FB, Lemon SM, Margolis HS, editors. Viral hepatitis and liver disease. Baltimore: Williams & Wilkins; 1991:234–7.
9. Wong DKH, Cheung AM, O'Rourke K, Naylor CD, Detsky AS, Heathcote J. Effect of alpha-interferon treatment in patients with hepatitis B e antigen-positive chronic hepatitis B. A meta-analysis. Ann Intern Med 1993;119:312–23.

10. Wong JB, Koff RS, Tine F, Pauker SG. Cost-effectiveness of interferon-α2b treatment for hepatitis B e antigen-positive chronic hepatitis B. Ann Intern Med. 1995;122:664–75.
11. Chen DS, Sung JL. Hepatitis B e antigen and its antibody in chronic type B hepatitis. J Gastroenterol Hepatol. 1987;2:255–70.
12. Su IJ, Lai MY, Hsu HC, Chen DS, Yang PM, Chuang SM. Diverse virological, histo-pathological and prognostic implications of seroconversion from hepatitis B e antigen to anti-HBe in chronic hepatitis virus infection. J Hepatol. 1986;3:182–9.
13. Chen DS. Natural history of chronic hepatitis B virus infection: new light on an old story. J Gastroenterol Hepatol. 1993;8:470–5.
14. Wu PC, Lai C-L, Lam KC, Ho J. Prednisolone in HBsAg-positive chronic active hepatitis: histologic evaluation in a controlled prospective study. Hepatology. 1982;2:777–83.
15. Tur-Kaspa R, Burk R, Shaul Y et al. Hepatitis B virus DNA contains a glucorticoid-responsive element. Proc Natl Acad Sci USA. 1987;84:6417–21.
16. Hanson RG, Peters MG, Hoofnagel JH. Effects of immunosuppressive therapy with prednisone on B and T lymphocyte function in patients with chronic type B hepatitis. Hepatology. 1986;6:173–9.
17. Perrillo RP, Schiff ER, David GL et al. A randomized, controlled trial of interferon alfa-2b alone and after prednisone withdrawal in the treatment of chronic hepatitis B. N Engl J Med. 1990;323:295–301.
18. Nair PV, Tong MJ, Stevenson D, Rozkamp D, Boone C. Effect of short-term, high-dose prednisone treatment with HBsAg-positive chronic active hepatitis. Liver. 1985;5:8–12.
19. Perrillo RP, Regenstein FG. Corticosteroid therapy for chronic active hepatitis B: is a little too much? Hepatology. 1986;6:1416–18.
20. Lau JYN, Lai C-L, Lin HJ et al. Fatal reactivation of chronic hepatitis B virus infection following withdrawal of chemotherapy in lymphoma patients. Q J Med. 1989;73:911–17.
21. Koga Y, Kumashiro R, Yasumoto K et al. Two fatal cases of hepatitis B virus carriers after corticosteroid therapy for bronchial asthma. Intern Med. 1992;31:208–13.
22. Beasley RP. Hepatitis B virus as the etiologic agent in hepatocellular carcinoma: epidemiologic considerations. Hepatology. 1982;2:S21–6.
23. Beasley RP, Hwang LY. Postnatal infectivity of hepatitis B surface antigen-carrier mothers. J Infect Dis. 1983;147:185–90.
24. Lok ASF, Lai C-L, Wu PC, Leung EKY. Long-term follow-up in a randomized controlled trial of recombinant alpha-interferon in Chinese patients with chronic hepatitis B infection. Lancet. 1988;2:298–302.
25. Lok ASF, Wu PC, Lai C-L. A controlled trial of interferon with or without prednisone priming for chronic hepatitis B. Gastroenterology. 1992;102:2091–7.
26. Lai C-L, Lok ASF, Lin HJ, Wu PC, Yeoh EK, Yeung CY. The effect of recombinant alpha 2 interferon in Chinese HBsAg carrier children. Lancet. 1987;2:877–80.
27. Lai C-L, Lin HJ, Lau JYN et al. Effect of recombinant alpha 2 interferon with or without prednisone in Chinese HBsAg carrier children. Q J Med. 1991;78:155 -63.
28. Korenman J, Baker B, Waggoner J, Everhart JE, Di Bisceglie AM, Hoofnalge JH. Long-term remission of chronic hepatitis B after alpha-interferon therapy. Ann Intern Med. 1991;114:629–34.
29. Carreno V, Castillo I, Molina J, Porres JC, Bartolome J. Long-term follow-up of hepatitis B chronic carriers who responded to interferon therapy. J Hepatol. 1992;15:102–6.
30. Lok ASF, Chung HT, Liu VWS, Ma OCK. Long-term follow-up of chronic hepatitis B patients treated with interferon alfa. Gastroenterology. 1993;105:1833–8.
31. Chung HT, Lok ASF, Lai C-L. Re-evaluation of α-interferon treatment of chronic hepatitis B using polymerase chain reaction. J Hepatol. 1993;17:208–14.
32. Burman P, Totterman TH, Oberg K, Anders-Karlsson F. Thyroid autoimmunity in patients on long term therapy with leukocyte-derived interferon. J Clin Endocrinol Metabol. 1986;63:1086–90.
33. Vento S, Di Perri G, Garofano T et al. Hazards of interferon therapy for HBV-seronegative chronic hepatitis. Lancet. 1989;334:926.
34. Lisker-Melman M, Di Bisceglie AM, Usala SJ, Weintraub B, Murray LM, Hoofnagle JH. Development of thyroid disease during therapy of chronic viral hepatitis with interferon alfa. Gastroenterology. 1992;102:2155–60.
35. Schulof R. Thymic peptide hormones: basic properties and clinical applications in cancer. CRC Crit Rev Oncol Haematol. 1985;3:309–76.

36. Serrate S, Schulof R, Leondaridis L. Modulation of human natural killer cell cytotoxic activity, lymphokine production, and interleukin 2 receptor expression by thymic hormones. J Immunol. 1990;139:2338–43.
37. Leichtling K, Serrate S, Sztein M. Thymosin alpha 1 modulates the expression of high affinity interleukin-2 receptors on normal human lymphocytes. Int J Immunopharmacol. 1990;12:19–29.
38. Korba BE, Tennant BC, Cote PJ, Mutchnick MG, Gerin IL. Treatment of chronic woodchuck hepatitis virus infection with thymosin alpha 1. Hepatology. 1990;12:880 (abstract).
39. Mutchnick MG, Appelman HD, Chung HT *et al*. Thymosin treatment of chronic hepatitis B: A placebo-controlled pilot trial. Hepatology. 1991;14:409–15.
40. Mutchnick MG, Lindsay KL, Schiff ER, Cummings GD, Appelman HD. Thymosin α_1 treatment of chronic hepatitis B: a multicenter, randomized placebo-controlled double blind study. Gastroenterology. 1995;108:A1127 (abstract).
41. Rasi G, Mutchnick MG, DiVirgilio D *et al*. Combination low dose lymphoblastoid interferon (L-IFNα) and thymosin α_1 (Tα_1) in the treatment of chronic hepatitis B. Hepatology. 1994;20:299A (abstract).
42. Vitiello A, Ishoka G, Grey HM *et al*. Development of a lipopeptide-based therapeutic vaccine to treat chronic HBV infection. 1. Induction of a primary cytotoxic T lymphocyte response in humans. J Clin Invest. 1995;95:341–9.
43. Bertoletti A, Ferrari C, Fiaccadori F *et al*. HLA class I-restricted human cytotoxic T cells recognize endogenously synthesized hepatitis B virus nucleocapsid antigen. Proc Natl Acad Sci USA. 1991;88:10445–9.
44. Guilhot S, Fowler P, Portillo G *et al*. Hepatitis B virus (HBV) specific cytolytic T cell response in humans. Production of target cells by stable expression of HBV-encoded proteins in immortalized human B cell lines. J Virol. 1992;66:2670–8.
45. Vere Hodge RA, Perkins RM. Mode of action of 9-(4-hydroxy-3-hydroxymethylbut-1-yl) guanine (BRL 39123) against herpes simplex virus in MRC-5 cells. Antimicrob Agents Chemother. 1989;33:223–9.
46. Vere Hodge RA, Cheng YC. The mode of action of penciclovir. Antiviral Chem Chemother. 1993;4(Suppl. 1):13–24.
47. Saltzman R, Jurewicz R, Boon R. Safety of famciclovir in patients with herpes zoster and genital herpes. Antimicrob Agents Chemother. 1994;38:2454–7.
48. Korba BE, Gerin JL. Use of a standardized cell culture assay to assess activities of nucleoside analogs against hepatitis B virus replication. Antiviral Res. 1992;19:55-70.
49. Main J, Brown JL, Karayiannis P *et al*. A double blind, placebo-controlled study to assess the effect of famciclovir on virus replication in patients with chronic hepatitis B infection. J Hepatol. 1994:21(Suppl. 1):S32 (abstract).
50. Eron JJ, Benoit SL, Jemsek J *et al*. Treatment of lamivudine, zidovudine, or both in HIV-positive patients with 200 to 500 CD4 + cells per cubic millimeter. N Engl J Med. 1995;333:1662–9.
51. Doong SL, Tsai CH, Shinazi RF, Liotta DC, Cheng YC. Inhibition of the replication of hepatitis B virus in vitro by 2'3'-dideoxy-3'-thiacytidine and related analogues. Proc Natl. Acad Sci USA. 191;88:8495–9.
52. Ashman C, Larkin D, Cammack N, Boehme RE, Cameron JM. Lamivudine inhibits hepatitis B virus (HBV) production in the HBV transfected cell line 2.2.15. Sixth International Symposium on Viral Hepatitis, Madrid, 1994 (abstract P-65).
53. Tyrell DLJ, Fischer K, Sayani K. Treatment of chimpanzees and ducks with lamivudine, 2'3'dideoxy3'thiacytidine results in a rapid suppression of hepadnaviral DNA in sera. Clin Invest Med. 1993;16(Suppl. 4):B77 (abstract).
54. Lai C-L, Ching CK, Tung A *et al*. Lamivudine is effective in suppressing HBV DNA in Chinese HBsAg carriers: a placebo-controlled trial. Hepatology. 1996 (in press).
55. Dienstag JL, Perillo RP, Schiff ER, Bartholomew M, Vicary C, Rubin M. A preliminary trial of lamivudine for chronic hepatitis B infection. N Engl J Med. 1995;333:1657–61.
56. Tyrell DLJ, Mitchell MC, De Man RA *et al*. Phase II trial of lamivudine for chronic hepatitis B. Hepatology. 1993;18:112A (abstract).
57. Averett DR, Mason WS. Evaluation of drugs for antiviral activity against hepatitis B virus. Viral Hep Rev. 1995;1:129–42.
58. Fourel I, Cullen JM Saputelli J *et al*. Evidence that hepatocyte turnover is required for rapid clearance of duck hepatitis B virus during antiviral therapy of chronically infected ducks. J Virol. 1994;68:8321–30.

59. Honkoop P, De Man RA, Heÿtink RA, Schalm SW. Hepatitis B reactivation after lamivudine. Lancet. 1995;346:1156–7.
60. McKenzie R, Fried MW, Sallie R *et al.* Hepatic failure and lactic acidosis due to fialuridine (FIAU), an investigational nucleoside analogue for chronic hepatitis B. N Engl J Med. 1995;333:1099–105.
61. Cui L, Yoon S, Schinazi RF, Sommadossi J-P. Cellular and molecular events leading to mitochondrial toxicity of 1(2-deoxy-2-fluoro-1-β-D-arabinofuranosyl)-5-iodouracil in human. J Clin Invest. 1995;95:555–63.
62. Lewis W, Gonzalez B, Chomyn A, Papoian T. Zidovudine induces molecular, biochemical, and ultrastructural changes in rat skeletal muscle mitochondria. J Clin Invest. 1992;89:1354–60.
63. Thompson MB, Dunnick JK, Sutphin ME, Giles HD, Irwin RD, Prejean JD. Hematologic toxicity of AZT and ddc administered as single agents and in combination to rats and mice. Fund Appl Toxicol. 1991;17:159–76.
64. Samuel D, Muller R, Alexander G *et al.* and the investigators of the European Concerted Action on Viral Hepatitis Study. Liver transplantation in European patients with the hepatitis B surface antigen. N Engl Med. 1993;329:1842–7.
65. Gish RG, Lau JYN, Brooks L *et al.* Ganciclovir treatment of hepatitis B virus infection in liver transplant patients. Hepatology. 1996;23:1–7.
66. Boker KHW, Ringe B, Krüger M, Pichlmayr R, Manns MP. Prostaglandin E plus famciclovir – a new concept for the treatment of severe hepatitis B after liver transplantation. Transplantation. 1995;57:1706–8.
67. Krüger M, Angus P, Neuhaus P, Manns MP and the Famciclovir Liver Transplant Group. An open study to assess the effect of famciclovir on hepatitis B replication in patients with orthotopic liver transplantation. J Hepatol. 1995;23(Suppl. 1):173 (abstract).
68. Grellier L, Brown D, McPhilips P, Burroughs A, Rolles K, Dusheiko G. Lamivudine prophylaxis: a new strategy for prevention of reinfection in liver transplantation for hepatitis B DNA positive cirrhosis. Hepatology. 1995;22:224A (abstract).

Section II
Toxic and Metabolic Liver Diseases

8
Pathogenesis and treatment of alcoholic liver disease

C. S. LIEBER

PATHOGENESIS

Respective role of malnutrition and direct hepatotoxicity of ethanol

Experimental studies

Originally, the concept prevailed that ethyl alcohol was not more toxic to the liver than sugar, based largely on experimental work in rats given ethanol in drinking water[1]. With this technique, however, alcohol, when given with an adequate diet, resulted in negligible ethanol levels in the blood[2,3]. By its incorporation in a totally liquid diet the amount of ethanol consumed was increased to 36% of total energy; isocaloric replacement of carbohydrate or fat by ethanol in these nutritionally adequate diets consistently produced a 5–10-fold increase in hepatic triglycerides[2,3], with associated ultrastructural changes in mitochondria and endoplasmic reticulum[4] and plasma membranes[5], whereas no such lesions developed in pair-fed control animals. The ultrastructural lesions of the mitochondria have functional counterparts in terms of striking impairment of respiration and energy production[6–8], fatty acid oxidation[9] and susceptibility to acetaldehyde toxicity[10]. Continuous intragastric infusion of alcohol-containing liquid diets to rats also resulted in some fibrosis, whereas animals given isocaloric amounts of the control diet remained normal[11]. However, regarding alcohol-induced liver fibrosis, the baboons were found to mimic the human lesion more closely than the rodent. Indeed, cirrhosis was observed in 14 of a total of 67 baboons fed ethanol with adequate diets usually for 5 years or more, with septal fibrosis developing in an additional 14 animals. No lesions appeared in the corresponding pair-fed controls[12–16].

Clinical research

The hepatotoxicity of alcohol has also been demonstrated in humans. Individuals with a morphologically normal liver developed a fatty liver when given ethanol, either in addition to a normal diet, or as an isocaloric substitution for carbohydrates in a variety of non-deficient diets[2,3], both by morphological examination[2,3] and by direct measurement of the lipid content of the liver biopsies[17–19]. Even with a high-protein, vitamin-supplemented diet there were significant increases in hepatic triglycerides[18]. Electron microscopic studies conducted in some of the above-cited investigations, as well as by Lane and Lieber[20], showed that alcohol also causes injury to the mitochondria and the endoplasmic reticulum.

Epidemiology

The aetiological role of alcohol was also demonstrated in epidemiological studies. As reviewed elsewhere[21], a variety of investigations have clearly linked the incidence of cirrhosis and associated mortality to the amount and duration of alcohol consumed. Of course, factors other than ethanol also play a role, such as genetic make-up, viruses, other toxins and dietary composition. In particular, the influence of other hepatotoxins[22] and malnutrition[23] in alcoholic liver disease has been recognized. However, in addition to these other factors, and even in their absence, ethanol and/or its metabolite acetaldehyde exert hepatotoxic effects, some of which have now been well defined.

Mechanism of alcohol-induced liver damage

ADH-mediated redox changes

Ethanol, unlike other drugs, is consumed in massive amounts that readily overwhelm the liver's capacity for detoxification[24]. The primary pathway for ethanol metabolism involves hepatic cytosolic *alcohol dehydrogenase* (ADH) isozymes (Fig. 1). Extrahepatic tissues also contain isozymes of ADH, but these have a much lower affinity for ethanol than the hepatic ones; as a consequence, at the levels of ethanol achieved in the blood, these extrahepatic enzymes are inactive; therefore, extrahepatic metabolism of ethanol is negligible, with the exception of the gastric one, as discussed elsewhere[25].

In ADH-mediated oxidation of ethanol, acetaldehyde is produced and hydrogen is transferred from ethanol to the cofactor nicotinamide adenine dinucleotide (NAD), which is converted to its reduced form (NADH)[26]. The acetaldehyde produced again loses hydrogen and is converted to acetate, most of which is released into the blood stream. The large amounts of reducing equivalents produced overwhelm the hepatocyte's ability to maintain redox homeostasis and a number of metabolic disorders ensue. These include alterations in the metabolism of lipids, carbohydrates, proteins, and purines[26–29] (Fig. 1).

Role of cytochrome P450 2E1

Ethanol is also oxidized in liver microsomes by an ethanol-inducible cytochrome P450[27–29] that contributes to ethanol metabolism and tolerance, and activates xenobiotics to toxic radicals, thereby explaining the increased vulnerability of the heavy drinker to industrial solvents, anaesthetic agents (e.g. enflurane), commonly prescribed drugs (e.g. isoniazid), over-the-counter analgesics (e.g. acetaminophen, also called paracetamol), chemical carcinogens, and

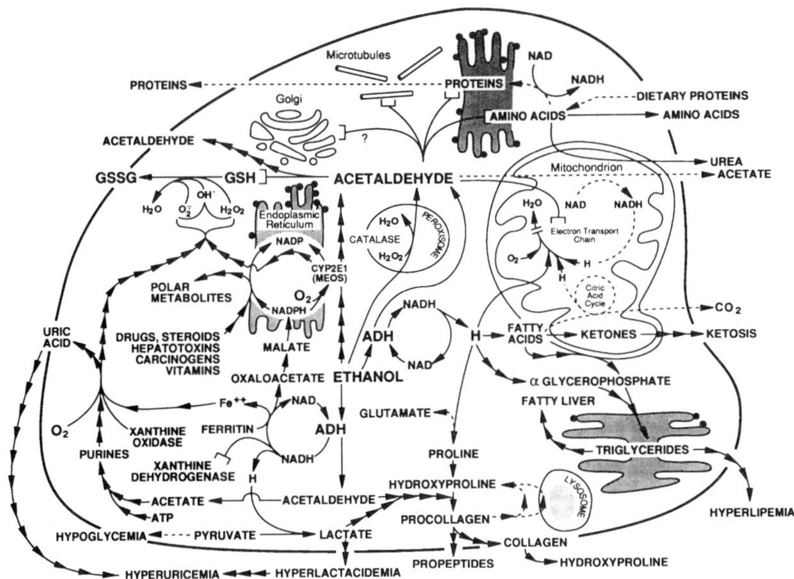

Fig. 1 Oxidation of ethanol in the hepatocyte. Many disturbances in intermediary metabolism and toxic effects can be linked to: (1) ADH-mediated generation of NADH; (2) the induction of the activity of microsomal enzymes, especially the MEOS containing P450 2E1 (CYP2E1) and (3) acetaldehyde, the product of ethanol oxidation. GSH, reduced glutathione GSSG, oxidized glutathione – – –, pathways that are depressed by ethanol; →→→ stimulation or activation; –[, interference or binding

even nutritional factors, such as vitamin A[30]. The specific form of cytochrome P450 involved (P450 2E1) has now been purified in rabbits[31], rats[32], and humans[33].

Role of acetaldehyde

Acetaldehyde, the active metabolite of ethanol, promotes lipid peroxidation and covalently binds to protein[22,26], resulting in alterations of microtubules, plasma membranes and mitochondria, and the formation of protein adducts, with enzyme inactivation, decreased DNA repair, and antibody production.

Immunohistochemical studies have documented the presence of *acetaldehyde–protein adducts* in the liver of alcoholics[34], particularly in the perivenular zones where the hepatocellular injury is most severe and the fibrosis begins. As the liver injury progresses, the adducts extend, particularly in areas with inflammation and active fibrogenesis[35]. Similar adducts were visualized in patients with non-alcoholic liver disease[35], who can develop increased levels of acetaldehyde from endogenous sources[36]. In both types of patients the serum antibodies against *in-vitro*-produced acetaldehyde-modified epitopes increase and correlate with the severity of the liver injury[37,38]. A liver protein that triggers this immune response has been identified as a protein–acetaldehyde adduct of approximately 200 kDa found in the liver cystolic fraction of alcoholics and non-alcoholics with liver disease[39], as well as in rats with experimentally induced cirrhosis[40,41]. Immune complexes of these adducts reacted with anti-collagen antibodies[40,41], indicating that the target protein is a form of collagen. This adduct was readily produced *in vitro* by incubation of liver cytosolic proteins with acetaldehyde at concentrations lower than those needed to produce other protein adducts[39,41]. Since the adduct was also found in the cytosol of rat hepatocytes isolated by collagenase digestion of cirrhotic livers[40], the acetaldehyde-induced modification must occur, at least in part, intracellularly, where procollagens could be one of the target proteins. In cirrhotic rats the major increase in the immunoreactive adduct was found in the microsomal fractions, and had a molecular weight lower than 180 kDa, consistent with procollagen[41].

During and after secretion, procollagen is converted into collagen by splitting off the non-helical propeptides at the carboxy and amino ends, both of which exert feedback inhibition of collagen synthesis[42–44]. It has been shown that the carboxyterminal propeptide is internalized and specifically inhibits procollagen gene transcription[43,45], a major mechanism for feedback regulation of collagen synthesis. The propeptide exerts a concentration-dependent inhibition of procollagen synthesis in cultured Ito cells, and markedly decreases the accumulation of collagen in the media. However, when the same amount of the acetaldehyde-modified propeptide was added to the culture media, the inhibition of procollagen synthesis in lipocytes was significantly less than that produced by the unmodified propeptide[46]. The lesser inhibition of procollagen synthesis in the cells was associated with a greater accumulation of collagen in the media, comparable to the one we previously reported to be produced in these cells upon incubation with acetaldehyde[47]. Since incubation with similar concentrations of acetaldehyde resulted in the formation of procollagen–acetaldehyde adducts, it is likely that the acetaldehyde-induced stimulation of collagen synthesis could be mediated, at least in part, by releasing collagen synthesis from its normal feedback regulation due to the decreased capacity of the acetaldehyde-modified propeptide to inhibit collagen synthesis. Indeed, the abundance of these adducts correlated with the activity of the disease[39], and may account for the immuno-histochemical association of acetaldehyde–protein adducts with areas of enhanced fibrogenesis in the liver of patients with alcoholic and, to a lesser extent, non-alcoholic liver diseases[35].

Oxidative stress

Binding of acetaldehyde with cysteine and/or *glutathione* (GSH), inhibition of GSH synthesis and loss from the liver, all contribute to a depression of liver glutathione[48] (Fig. 2). Ethanol-induced depletion of glutathione has been shown to be particularly striking in primates[48–50]. The ultimate precursor of cysteine, one of the amino acids of the tripeptide GSH, is methionine but, in patients with liver disease, the enzyme which activates methionine to *S*-adenosylmethionine is depressed (Fig. 2)[51], thereby contributing to the GSH depletion.

GSH offers one of the mechanisms for the scavenging of toxic free radicals. Although GSH depletion is not necessarily sufficient to cause lipid peroxidation, it is generally agreed that it may favour the peroxidation produced by other

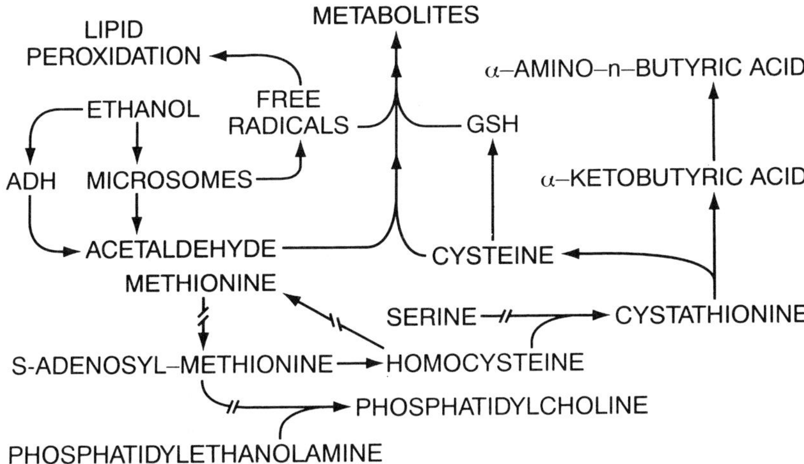

Fig. 2 Link between accelerated acetaldehyde production and increased free radical generation by the 'induced' microsomes, resulting in glutathione (GSH) depletion and enhanced lipid peroxidation, with metabolic blocks due to alcohol, folate deficiency and/or alcoholic liver disease. Possible beneficial effects of GSH, its precursors (including *S*-adenosylmethionine) and of phosphatidylcholine are illustrated (from ref. 49)

factors. As for tissue damage due to other aetiological agents, alcohol-induced liver damage causes a fibrotic response which, when excessive, may result in scarring, culminating in cirrhosis. The scarring process can be promoted by the inflammatory cell reaction which is associated with liver injury, especially alcoholic hepatitis; it may also be directly influenced by acetaldehyde itself. Indeed, acetaldehyde was found to increase collagen production in cultured myofibroblasts[52] and lipocytes[47], in association with an increase in mRNA for collagen[53]. Excess collagen production may also be favoured by the products of lipid peroxidation[54].

Impairments in antioxidant protective mechanisms have been reported in alcoholics, including alterations of GSH (see above), selenium[55,56] and vitamin E[56–58], especially in cirrhotics[59] (Fig. 3). Hepatic lipid peroxidation is significantly increased after chronic ethanol feeding in rats receiving a low vitamin E diet[60], indicating that dietary vitamin E is an important determinant of hepatic lipid peroxidation induced by chronic ethanol feeding. The lowest hepatic α-tocopherol was found in rats receiving a combination of low vitamin E and ethanol: both low dietary vitamin E and ethanol feeding significantly reduced hepatic α-tocopherol content; the latter, in part, because of increased conversion of α-tocopherol to α-tocopherylquinone[60]. These deficient defence systems, coupled with increased acetaldehyde and oxygen radical generation by the ethanol-induced microsomes (Figs 1 and 2), may contribute to liver damage via lipid peroxidation and also via enzyme inactivation.

Iron overload may play a contributory role, since chronic alcohol consumption results in increased iron uptake by hepatocytes[61] and since ferric citrate-induced lipid peroxidation is accentuated in microsomes from ethanol-fed

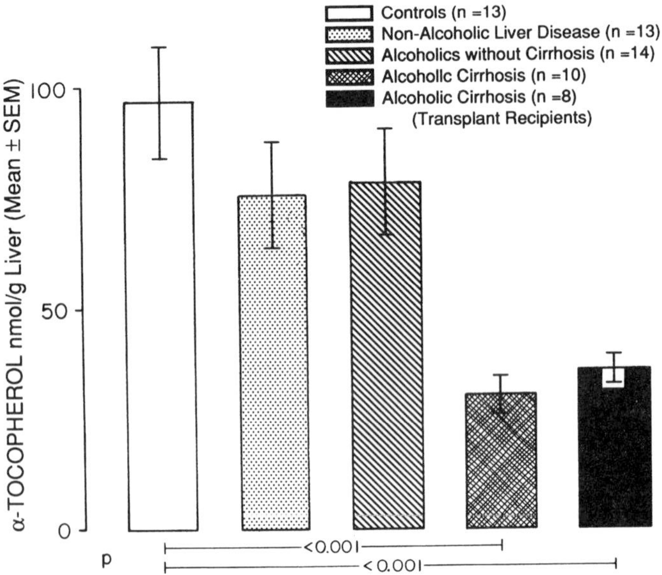

Fig. 3 Effects of various liver diseases on total hepatic tocopherol levels. Only the two cirrhotic groups had significantly lowered α-tocopherol levels (from ref. 60)

rats. Iron overload, as well as iron deficiency, in the alcoholic have been reviewed elsewhere, in conjunction with other mineral abnormalities[23].

Role of stellate cell activation

Stellate cells (also called lipocytes, Ito or fat-storing cells), are 'activated' after chronic alcohol consumption and appear to play a major role in fibrogenesis[62,63]. These cells in culture produce collagen. When acetaldehyde is added to these cells they respond with a further increase in collagen accumulation (see above).

Collagen accumulation results from an imbalance between *collagen degradation* and collagen production. Thus cirrhosis might, in part, represent a relative failure of collagen degradation to keep pace with synthesis. Interestingly, polyunsaturated phosphatidylcholine (PPC) may affect this balance. Indeed, addition of PPC to transformed lipocytes was found to prevent the acetaldehyde-mediated increase in collagen accumulation, possibly by stimulation of collagenase activity[64]. The active ingredient was identified as dilinoleoylphosphatidylcholine[15]. The role of collagenase was also shown indirectly in humans by the correlation of the development of alcoholic fibrosis with increased activity of the circulating tissue inhibitor of metalloproteinase (TIMP)[65]. Indeed, serum TIMP was significantly increased in alcoholic cirrhosis and may not only play a role in its pathogenesis through inhibition of collagenase activity, but can also serve as a marker of precirrhotic and cirrhotic states, since this test was more sensitive in detecting either perivenular fibrosis or septal fibrosis, and offered better discrimination from fatty liver than serum procollagen peptide (PIIIP). The stimulation of collagenase activity may explain, at least in part, why PPC attenuates the development of fibrosis (including cirrhosis) after chronic alcohol administration[14], an effect confirmed using more purified extracts, which again pointed to dilinoleoylphosphatidylcholine as the active ingredient[15]. In the latter studies the control livers remained normal, whereas 10 of 12 baboons fed alcohol without PPC developed septal fibrosis or cirrhosis, with transformation of $81\pm3\%$ of the hepatic lipocytes to collagen-producing transitional cells. By contrast, none of the eight animals fed alcohol with PPC developed septal fibrosis or cirrhosis, and only $48\pm9\%$ of their lipocytes were transformed. PPC resulted in a correction of the hepatic phospholipid depletion and restoration of the activity of phosphatidylcholine methyltransferase, which was found to decrease after alcohol (Fig. 3), both in non-human[66] and human[51] primates. In addition, the substrate for the enzyme is also decreased after chronic ethanol consumption because of a block in the activation of methionine to S-adenosylmethionine[51] (Fig. 2).

SYMPTOMATOLOGY AND TREATMENT

Fatty liver

Fat accumulation in the liver cells is the earliest and most common response to alcohol. In massive steatosis the hepatocytes are uniformly filled by large fat droplets, the cell nucleus may be eccentrically placed and when the cell membranes between adjacent hepatocytes rupture, fatty cysts are formed. Increased hepatic lipid content may be demonstrated by biochemical measurements before it becomes histologically apparent. Evidence of necrosis is usually sparse, but sometimes hepatocytes are surrounded by mononuclear cells, indicating a mild inflammatory response. When pronounced, these formations are called 'lipogranulomas'. Sometimes there is massive microvesicular steatosis which may resemble those seen in Reyes' syndrome and in acute fatty liver of pregnancy[67].

Ultrastructural changes reveal enlarged and distorted mitochondria with shortened cristae containing crystalline inclusions[68]. The endoplasmic reticulum shows vacuolar dilatation and proliferation. Alcohol has been shown to induce these alterations in rats, baboons and in both alcoholic and non-alcoholic human volunteers despite adequate nutrition[19,20].

The clinical spectrum of alcoholic fatty liver may extend from silent non-symptomatic hepatomegaly to severe hepatocellular failure with cholestasis and portal hypertension[67–70]. Most of the patients with pure fatty liver are virtually asymptomatic. Hepatomegaly is the commonest clinical sign. In more advanced cases hepatic tenderness, anorexia, nausea, emesis, jaundice, fluid accumulation and even spider angiomas are present. Severe forms of fatty liver may present a clinical picture mimicking extrahepatic obstructive jaundice, especially if associated with dark urine and acholic stools[69,70]. Typical abnormalities in laboratory tests are slightly or moderately elevated γ-glutamyltransferase (GGT) and serum transaminases (AST and ALT). In contrast to more advanced alcoholic liver injury, all the abnormalities in laboratory tests tend to return to normal rapidly within the first days of hospitalization. Thus, alcoholic steatosis is completely reversible in most instances. In some extremely severe cases, alcoholic fatty liver may have a fatal outcome[71], but as a rule even those patients needing hospitalization improve within a few days or weeks after cessation of alcohol consumption. In view of the role of dietary fat in the production of the alcoholic fatty liver[17,72], decreasing the fat content in the diet might be beneficial, but this has not been systematically assessed.

Perivenular fibrosis

Although it can occur anywhere in the hepatic acinus, the earliest deposition of fibrous tissue is generally seen around the central veins and venules, now called terminal hepatic venules. Such perivenular fibrosis (Fig. 4) has been described in alcoholic hepatitis and is often associated with a necrotizing process called sclerosing hyaline necrosis[73]. When intensive, it may obliterate the terminal hepatic veins and lead to postsinusoidal portal hypertension with ascites prior to the development of cirrhosis[74].

It is important to note that perivenular fibrosis can also be seen in the absence of widespread inflammation and necrosis, in association with what most pathologists would label as 'simple' fatty liver. Of 75 hospitalized alcoholic subjects in whom the diagnosis of simple fatty liver had been made on liver biopsy, 40% were found to have perivenular fibrosis on the basis of a review of the histology. There was no evidence of diffuse alcoholic hepatitis. Once perivenular fibrosis

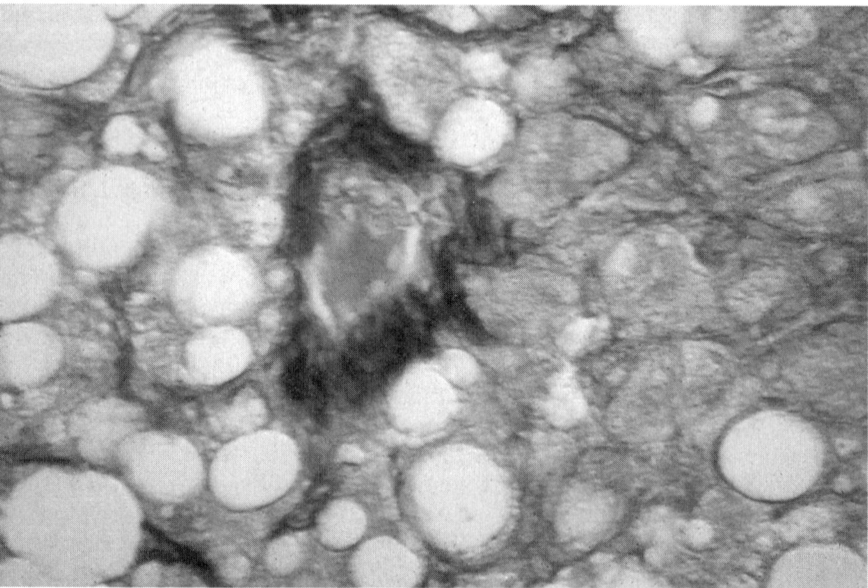

Fig. 4   Sirius red stain of a liver biopsy from a patient with alcoholic fatty liver without evidence of alcoholic hepatitis. Note the fibrous rim around the terminal hepatic venule (perivenular fibrosis). Some fibrous strands surround the adjacent hepatocytes (perisinusoidal and pericellular fibrosis) and sinusoid (×250) (from ref. 107)

has developed, it indicates that the patient has already entered the fibrotic process, and that upon continuation of drinking he or she will rapidly develop more severe stages, including cirrhosis[75]. Thus, this lesion can be considered a marker of vulnerability to the development of subsequent cirrhosis and therefore can be used as an indication for active intervention. Indeed, although fibrosis as a result of necrosis and inflammation is thought to be the underlying mechanism of alcoholic cirrhosis, cirrhosis commonly develops without an apparent intermediate stage of alcoholic hepatitis, both in alcoholics[75] and in baboons given alcohol[12,14,15]. It is obvious that among the alcohol users there is a subpopulation of very heavy drinkers who are particularly at risk of developing alcoholism and its complications. Because major complications (such as cirrhosis) do not develop in all heavy drinkers, there is a need for early detection of those susceptible individuals before their social or medical disintegration, to prevent, rather than simply treat, their major somatic complications. Screening for heavy drinkers is now facilitated by biological markers of excessive alcohol consumption[76,77]. Of the various markers studied, carbohydrate-deficient transferrin is particularly useful[78,79]. Among individuals at risk, namely these heavy drinkers, the physician can recognize lesions in the liver, such as perivenular fibrosis, which already at a very early precirrhotic stage allow prediction of which subjects are prone to undergo rapid progression to the cirrhotic stage upon continuation of drinking[75,80]. Perivenular fibrosis is commonly associated with perisinusoidal and pericellular fibrosis, and correlates with collagenization of the Disse space, but these other changes are more difficult to quantify on routine light microscopy. In addition, independently of necrosis and inflammation, alcohol (via acetaldehyde) directly affects lipocytes in the liver. Long-term alcohol consumption transforms stellate cells into collagen-producing myofibroblast-like cells[62,63,81], and acetaldehyde stimulates collage synthesis in these cells (see above), causing the deposition of collagen, the characteristic protein of the fibrous tissue.

Originally, treatment of liver disease complicating alcoholism appeared to be relatively simple, because it was attributed exclusively to associated malnutrition. Indeed, nutritional deficiences are common in the alcoholic and, when present, should be corrected. Over the past two decades the realization of the intrinsic toxicity of ethanol shifted the emphasis of treatment from the correction of nutritional deficiences to the control of alcohol consumption. More recently, however, the pendulum is swinging back to a more comprehensive approach. Indeed, at a biochemical cellular level, both 'toxic' and 'nutritional' effects are often intertwined. Therapeutically, some agents that can be viewed as 'supernutrients' were found to be effective in non-human primates, e.g. *S*-adenosylmethionine for the treatment of early aspects of alcohol-induced liver injury and polyunsaturated lecithin for the prevention of fibrosis. Both compounds are now being tested in humans. Indeed, agents that replenish glutathione, such as *S*-adenosylmethionine, were found to be effective in the initial stage of alcohol-induced liver injury[82].

Alcoholic hepatitis

This stage is characterized by the appearance of necrosis with an inflammatory reaction, including polymorphonuclear cells. From either clinical or pathological signs this inflammatory response of the liver to alcohol has been called 'florid cirrhosis', 'acute hepatic insufficiency', 'progressive alcoholic cirrhosis', or 'steatonecrosis Mallory body type'. The term 'alcoholic hepatitis' is nowadays widely accepted by most pathologists and clinicians. While the incidence of fatty liver in alcoholics is very common, alcoholic hepatitis develops in only a fraction of heavy drinkers, even after decades of abuse. The long-term incidence of cirrhosis in patients with alcoholic hepatitis is nine times higher than in those with fatty liver[83]. Thus, traditionally, alcoholic hepatitis has been viewed as the precursor lesion of alcoholic cirrhosis but, as mentioned above, alcoholic cirrhosis can also develop in the absence of alcoholic hepatitis.

Histological characteristics of alcoholic hepatitis are ballooning and great disarray of hepatocytes, predominantly in perivenular areas, parenchymal and portal infiltration with polymorphonuclear leucocytes, varying degrees of steatosis, necrosis, fibrosis, and cholestasis. Lymphocytes are seen in perivenular zones or within the parenchyma in direct contact with the plasma membranes of the hepatocytes. Mallory's alcoholic hyaline irregular cytoplasmic bodies can be considered as a diagnostic hallmark but are not always present. Ultrastructural changes in alcoholic hepatitis are similar to, but more severe than, the ones seen in fatty liver[68]. Collagenous material may be found in the space of Disse and associated with loss of microvilli that normally project from the hepatocyte[84].

On rare occasions the liver pathology resembles that of chronic active hepatitis[85,86]. Whether the latter lesion is related to alcohol, or merely represents the coincidental appearance of another disease process in an alcoholic, has not been settled, but recent evidence suggests involvement of hepatitis non-A–non-B, particularly C.

The spectrum of alcoholic hepatitis may thus range from mild anicteric hepatomegaly to fatal disease with jaundice, ascites, liver coma, gastrointestinal haemorrhage and with all the complications of severe hepatic insufficiency. In general there is a correlation between the severity of the histological features of alcoholic hepatitis (hepatocellular necrosis, leucocytic infiltration, frequency of alcoholic hyaline) and the degree of hepatomegaly, leucocytosis and elevations of serum transaminases and the intensity of symptoms. An AST/ALT ratio greater than 2.0 is considered indicative for alcoholic liver injury. However, this ratio may be less helpful in the presence of cirrhosis[87].

The depression of serum albumin and prolongation of the prothrombin time has been shown to correlate with the severity of the histological lesion[88].

Other common laboratory findings include serum bilirubin elevations[90]. It should, however, be remembered that serum bilirubin may also be increased in the absence of alcoholic hepatitis (for instance, because of haemolysis or alcoholic pancreatitis).

In patients with hepatic encephalopathy or a high value for Maddrey's discriminant function (based on the prothrombin and bilirubin level), prednisolone improves short-term survival[89]. Oxandrolone may benefit moderately malnourished patients[90]. Propylthiouracil has been suggested for the treatment of alcoholic hepatitis[91], and colchicine for alcoholic cirrhosis[92], but additional controlled trials are needed to establish their efficacy.

Cirrhosis

Microscopically, scar tissue distorts the normal architecture of the liver by forming bands of connective tissue joining portal and central zones. At first, nodules are regular in size and shape. In more advanced cirrhosis, nodules become larger and frequently irregular.

One of the most characteristic features of cirrhosis is the change in the hepatic blood circulation. Endophlebitis[93] and perivenular fibrosis[94] may impair outflow from the sinusoids, and the regenerative nodules may compress the hepatic veins, resulting in post-sinusoidal portal hypertension. The total blood flow is reduced by extrahepatic portasystemic shunts and the effective circulation is limited by neovascularization of connective tissue septa which form ana-stomoses between the afferent branches of the portal vein and hepatic artery and the efferent tributaries of the hepatic veins[95,96]. Collagen deposits in the space of Disse[84], and reduction in the number of patent fenestrations[97], may further increase the resistance to blood flow and isolate the hepatocyte from its blood supply. As a result of these changes, marked deterioration in residual hepatic function may occur, especially if either the cardiac output or the circulating blood volume changes.

In addition to fibrosis, various admixtures of fat, inflammatory reactions, and cholestasis may be seen. Histologically stainable iron deposits are common in cirrhotic livers, especially in alcoholic subjects[98,99]. However, total iron stores are very seldom increased and never exceed 179 mmol (10 g). The differentiation from primary haemochromatosis is possible by measuring the total hepatic iron content from liver biopsies.

Typically, serum electrophoresis reveals a decrease in serum albumin and pre-albumin and a broad elevation of the β- and γ-globulins. Frequently, Iga and also IgG and IgM are elevated. Serum transaminases and alkaline phosphatases are usually only mildly elevated.

Hepatocellular carcinoma (HCC) has become a relatively frequent finding in liver cirrhosis, presumably because of improved management and prolonged survival[100]. Pathogenetically it has been traditionally related to cirrhosis, but possible carcinogenic properties of alcohol must also be considered, since primary hepatocellular carcinoma can complicate non-cirrhotic alcoholic liver disease[101]. Furthermore, at least in some studies, there appears to be a significant interaction between alcohol and viral hepatitis (especially hepatitis C) in hepatocarcinogenesis[102,103].

Autopsy studies show that cirrhosis may remain unrecognized antemortem in 40% of cirrhotic patients, and in about 20% it is discovered fortuitously on routine examination, or during the evaluation of some other, unrelated, disease.

Low-grade and continuous fever is also common in decompensated cirrhosis. Jaundice and hepatomegaly are typical primary physical signs of cirrhosis. Secondary phenomena include portal hypertension with splenomegaly, oedema and ascites, encephalopathy, gastrointestinal haemorrhage from oesophageal or gastric varices and bleeding tendencies due to clotting factor abnormalities. Tertiary complications include spontaneous peritonitis caused by anaerobic bac-teria and possibly associated alcoholic hepatitis (see above). Most patients are detected when they seek treatment for these complications. Finally, liver transplantation, originally not an option for patients with alcoholic liver disease, is now being considered for alcoholics who have stopped drinking[104].

PROSPECTS

The clinical course and ultimate outcome of alcoholic liver disease is still dismal. Indeed, in a prospective survey of 280 subjects with alcoholic liver injury[105] it was found that, within 48 months of follow-up, more than half of those with cirrhosis, and two-thirds of those with cirrhosis plus alcoholic hepatitis, had died. This effect is compounded by age. In a study of patients with alcoholic cirrhosis, the mortality rate at 1 year was 50% among those who were over 60 years of age, as compared with 7% among the younger subjects[106]. This dismal outcome is more severe than that of many cancers, yet it is attracting much less concern, both among the public and the medical profession. This may be due, at least in part, to a pervasive and pernicious perception that not much can be done about this major public health issue. One purpose of this review is to reveal how concepts about alcoholic liver disease have evolved, and how elucidation of the biochemical effects of ethanol is resulting in improvement of both diagnosis and treatment.

Acknowledgements

This review is based on a lecture presented at the Falk Symposium 90, 29 February 1996, in Hong Kong. Original studies reviewed here were supported, in part, by the Department of Veterans Affairs and NIH grants AA05934, AA07275, and AA03508.

References

1. Best CH, Hartroft WS, Lucas CC, Ridout JH. Liver damage produced by feeding alcohol or sugar and its prevention by choline. Br Med J. 1949;2:1001–6.
2. Lieber CS, Jones DP, Mendelson J, DeCarli LM. Fatty liver, hyperlipemia and hyperuricemia produced by prolonged alcohol consumption, despite adequate dietary intake. Trans Assoc Am Phys. 1963;76:289–300.
3. Lieber CS, Jones DP, DeCarli LM. Effects of prolonged ethanol intake: production of fatty liver despite adequate diets. J Clin Invest. 1965;44:1009–21.
4. Iseri OA, Lieber CS, Gottlieb LS. The ultrastructure of fatty liver induced by prolonged ethanol ingestion. Am J Pathol. 1966;48:535–55.
5. Yamada S, Mak KM, Lieber CS. Chronic ethanol consumption alters rat liver plasma membranes and potentiates release of alkaline phosphatase. Gastroenterology. 1985;88:1799–806.
6. Cederbaum AI, Lieber CS, Rubin E. Effects of chronic ethanol treatment on mitochondrial functions. Arch Biochem Biophys. 1974;165:560–9.
7. Cederbaum AI, Lieber CS, Rubin E. Effect of chronic ethanol consumption and acetaldehyde on partial reactions of oxidative phosphorylation and CO_2 production from citric acid cycle intermediates. Arch Biochem. 1976;176:525–38.
8. Arai M, Leo MA, Nakano M, Gordon ER, Lieber CS. Biochemical and morphological alterations of baboon hepatic mitochondria after chronic ethanol consumption. Hepatology. 1984;4:165–74.
9. Cederbaum AI, Lieber CS, Beattie DS, Rubin E. Effect of chronic ethanol ingestion on fatty acid oxidation by hepatic mitochondria. J Biol Chem. 1975;250:5122–9.
10. Matsuzaki S, Lieber CS. Increased susceptibility of hepatic mitochondria to the toxicity of acetaldehyde after chronic ethanol consumption. Biochem Biophys Res Commun. 1977;75:1059–65.

11. Tsukamoto H, French SW, Benson N *et al.* Severe and progressive steatosis and focal necrosis in rat liver induced by continuous intragastric infusion of ethanol and low fat diet. Hepatology. 1985;5:224–32.
12. Lieber CS, DeCarli LM, Rubin E. Sequential production of fatty liver, hepatitis and cirrhosis in sub-human primates fed ethanol with adequate diets. Proc Natl Acad Sci USA. 1975;72:437–41.
13. Lieber CS, Leo MA, Mak KM, DeCarli LM, Sato S. Choline fails to prevent liver fibrosis in ethanol-fed baboons but causes toxicity. Hepatology. 1985;5:561–72.
14. Lieber CS, DeCarli LM, Mak KM, Kim C-I, Leo MA. Attenuation of alcohol-induced hepatic fibrosis by polyunsaturated lecithin. Hepatology. 1990;12:1390–8.
15. Lieber CS, Robins S, Li J *et al.* Phosphatidylcholine protects against fibrosis and cirrhosis in the baboon. Gastroenterology. 1994;106:152–9.
16. Popper H, Lieber CS. Histogenesis of alcoholic fibrosis and cirrhosis in the baboon. Am J Pathol. 1980;98:695–716.
17. Lieber CS, Spritz N. Effects of prolonged ethanol intake in man: role of dietary, adipose, and endogenously synthesized fatty acids in the pathogenesis of the alcoholic fatty liver. J Clin Invest. 1966;45:1400–11.
18. Lieber CS, Rubin E. Alcoholic fatty liver. Am J Med. 1968;44:200–6.
19. Rubin E, Lieber CS. Alcohol-induced hepatic injury in non-alcoholic volunteers. N Engl Med. 1968;278:869–76.
20. Lane BP, Lieber CS. Ultrastructural alterations in human hepatocytes following ingestion of ethanol with adequate diets. Am J Pathol. 1966;49:593–603.
21. Lieber CS, DeCarli LM. Hepatotoxicity of ethanol. J Hepatol. 1991;12:394–401.
22. Lieber CS. Mechanisms of ethanol–drug–nutrient interactions. J Toxicol Clin Toxicol. 1994;32:631–81.
23. Lieber CS. The influence of alcohol on nutritional status. Nutr Rev. 1988;46:241–5.
24. Lieber CS. Alcohol metabolism. In: P Hall, editor. Alcoholic liver disease: pathology and pathogenesis, 2nd edn. Australia: Edward Arnold, A division of Hodder & Stoughton Publishers; 1995:17–40.
25. Lieber CS, Gentry RT, Baraona E. First pass metabolism of ethanol. In: Saunders JB, Whitfield JB, editors. The biology of alcohol problems. Oxford: Elsevier (In press).
26. Lieber CS. Alcohol and the liver: 1994 update. Gastroenterology. 1994;106:1085–1105.
27. Lieber CS, DeCarli LM. Ethanol oxidation by hepatic microsomes: adaptive increase after ethanol feeding. Science. 1968;162:917–18.
28. Lieber CS, DeCarli LM. Hepatic microsomal ethanol oxidizing system. *In vitro* characteristics and adaptive properties *in vivo*. J Biol Chem. 1970;245:2505–12.
29. Ohnishi K, Lieber CS. Reconstitution of the microsomal ethanol-oxidizing system: qualitative and quantitative changes of cytochrome P-450 after chronic ethanol consumption. J Biol Chem. 1977;252:7124–31.
30. Leo MA, Lieber CS. Hypervitaminosis A: a liver lover's lament. Hepatology. 1988;8:412–17.
31. Koop DR, Morgan ET, Tarr GE, Coon MJ. Purification and characterization of a unique isozyme of cytochrome P-450 from liver microsomes of ethanol-treated rabbits. J Biol Chem. 1982;257:8472–80.
32. Ryan DE, Ramanthan L, Iida S *et al.* Characterization of a major form of rat hepatic microsomal cytochrome P450 induced by isoniazid. J Biol Chem. 1985;260:6385–93.
33. Lasker JM, Raucy J, Kubota S, Bloswick BP, Black M, Lieber CS. Purification and characterization of human liver cytochrome P-450-ALC. Biochem Biophys Res Commun. 1987;148:232–8.
34. Niemelä O, Juvonen T, Parkkila S. Immunohistochemical demonstration of acetaldehyde-modified epitopes in human liver after consumption. J Clin Invest. 1991;87:1367–74.
35. Holstege A, Bedossa P, Poynard T *et al.* Acetaldehyde-modified epitopes in liver biopsy specimens of alcoholic and non-alcoholic patients: localization and association with progression of liver fibrosis. Hepatology. 1994;19:367–74.
36. Uppal R, Rosman A, Hernández R, Baraona E, Lieber CS. Effects of liver disease on red blood cell acetaldehyde in alcoholics and non-alcoholics. Alcohol Alcoholism. 1991 (Suppl. 1):323–6.
37. Hoerner M, Behrens UJ, Worner TM *et al.* The role of alcoholism and liver disease in the appearance of serum antibodies against acetaldehyde adducts. Hepatology. 1988;8:569–74.

38. Koskinas J, Kenna JG, Bird GL, Alexander GJM, Williams R. Immunoglobulin A antibody to a 200-kilodalton cytosolic acetaldehyde adduct in alcoholic hepatitis. Gastroenterology. 1992;103:1860–7.
39. Svegliati-Baroni G, Baraona E, Lieber CS. Collagen acetaldehyde adducts in alcoholic and non-alcoholic liver diseases. Hepatology. 1994;20:111–18.
40. Behrens UJ, Ma XL, Bychenok S, Baraona E, Lieber CS. Acetaldehyde collagen adducts in CCl_4-induced liver injury in rats. Biochem Biophys Res Commun. 1990;173:111–19.
41. Baraona E, Liu W, Ma XL, Svegliati-Baroni G, Lieber CS. Acetaldehyde-collagen adducts in N-nitrosodimethylamine-induced liver cirrhosis in rats. Life Sci. 1993;52:1249–55.
42. Wiestner M, Krieg T, Hörlein D, Gianville RW, Fietzek P, Müller PK. Inhibiting effect of procollagen peptides on collagen biosynthesis in fibroblast cultures. J Biol Chem. 1979;254:7016–23.
43. Wu CH, Donovan CB, Wu GY. Evidence for pretranslational regulation of collagen synthesis by procollagen propeptides. J Biol Chem. 1986;261:10482–4.
44. Fouser L, Sage EH, Clark J, Bornstein P. Feedback regulation of collagen gene expression: a Trojan horse approach. Proc Natl Acad Sci USA. 1991;88:10158–62.
45. Wu CH, Walton CM, Wu GY. Propeptide-mediated regulation of procollagen synthesis in IMR-90 human lung fibroblast cell cultures. Evidence for transcriptional control. J Biol Chem. 1991;266:2983–7.
46. Ma X, Svegliati-Baroni G, Zhou J, Baraona E, Lieber CS. Acetaldehyde carboxypropeptide adducts attenuate feedback inhibition of collagen synthesis in Ito cells. Alcoholism Clin Exp Res. 1994;18:514.
47. Moshage H, Casini A, Lieber CS. Acetaldehyde selectively stimulates collagen production in cultured rat liver-storing cells but not in hepatocytes. Hepatology. 1990;12:511–18.
48. Shaw S, Jayatilleke E, Ross WA, Gordon ER, Lieber CS. Ethanol induced lipid peroxidation: potentiation by long-term alcohol feeding and attenuation by methionine. J Lab Clin Med. 1981;98:417–25.
49. Lieber CS. Pathogenesis and treatment of liver fibrosis: 1995 update. Dig Dis. (In press).
50. Lieber CS, Casini A, DeCarli LM et al. S-adenosyl-L-methionine attenuates alcohol-induced liver injury in the baboon. Hepatology. 1990;11:165–72.
51. Duce AM, Ortiz P, Cabrero C, Mato JM. S-adenosyl-L-methionine synthetase and phospholipid methyltransferase are inhibited in human cirrhosis. Hepatology. 1988;8:65–8.
52. Savolainen E-R, Leo MA, Timpl R, Lieber CS. Acetaldehyde and lactate stimulate collagen synthesis of cultured baboon liver myofibroblasts. Gastroenterology. 1984;87:777–87.
53. Casini A, Cunningham M, Rojkind M, Lieber CS. Acetaldehyde increases procollagen type I and fibronectin gene transcription in cultured rat fat-storing cells through a protein synthesis-dependent mechanism. Hepatology. 1991;13:758–65.
54. Chojkier M, Houglum K, Solis-Herruzo J, Brenner DA. Stimulation of collagen gene expression by ascorbic acid in cultured human fibroblast. A role for lipid peroxidation? J Biol Chem. 1989;264:16957–62.
55. Korpela H, Kumpulainen J, Luoma PV, Arranto AJ, Sotaniemi EA. Decreased serum selenium in alcoholics as related to liver structure and function. Am J Clin Nutr. 1985;42:147–51.
56. Tanner AR, Bantock I, Hinks L, Lloyd B, Turner NR, Wright R. Depressed selenium and vitamin E levels in an alcoholic population: possible relationship to hepatic injury through increased lipid peroxidation. Dig Dis Sci. 1986;31:1307–12.
57. Bjørneboe GEA, Bjørneboe A, Hagen BF, Morland J, Drevon CA. Reduced hepatic alpha-tocopherol content after long-term administration of ethanol to rats. Biochem Biophys Acta. 1987;918:236–41.
58. Bjørneboe GEA, Johnsen J, Bjørneboe A et al. Some aspects of antioxidant status in blood from alcoholics. Alcoholism Clin Exp Res. 1988;12:806–10.
59. Leo MA, Rosman A, Lieber CS. Differential depletion of carotenoids and tocopherol in liver disease. Hepatology. 1993;17:977–86.
60. Kawase T, Kato S, Lieber CS. Lipid peroxidation and antioxidant defense systems in rat liver after chronic ethanol feeding. Hepatology. 1989;10:815–21.
61. Zhang H, Loney LA, Potter BJ. Effect of chronic alcohol feeding on hepatic iron status and ferritin uptake by rat hepatocytes. Alcoholism Clin Exp Res. 1993;17:394–400.
62. Mak KM, Leo MA, Lieber CS. Alcoholic liver injury in baboons: transformation of lipocytes to transitional cells. Gastroenterology. 1984;87:188–200.

63. Mak KI, Lieber CS. Lipocytes and transitional cells in alcoholic liver disease: a morphometric study. Hepatology. 1988;8:1027–33.
64. Li JJ, Kim CI, Leo MA, Mak KM, Rojkind M, Lieber CS. Polyunsaturated lecithin prevents acetaldehyde-mediated hepatic collagen accumulation by stimulating collagenase activity in cultured lipocytes. Hepatology. 1992;15:373–81.
65. Li JJ, Rosman AS, Leo MA, Nagai Y, Lieber CS. Tissue inhibitor of metalloproteinase is increased in the serum of precirrhotic and cirrhotic alcoholic patients and can serve as a marker of fibrosis. Hepatology. 1994;19:1418–23.
66. Lieber CS, Robins SJ, Leo MA. Hepatic phosphatidylethanolamine methyltransferase activity is decreased by ethanol and increased by phosphatidylcholine. Alcoholism Clin Exp Res. 1994;18:592–5.
67. Uchida T, Kao H, Quispe-Sjogren M, Peters RL. Alcoholic foamy degeneration a pattern of acute alcoholic injury of the liver. Gastroenterology. 1983;84:683–92.
68. Svoboda DJ, Manning RT. Chronic alcoholism with fatty metamorphosis of the liver. Am J Pathol. 1964;44:645–62.
69. Ballard H, Bernstein M, Farrar JT. Fatty liver presenting as obstructive jaundice. Am J Med. 1961;30:196–201.
70. Phillips GB, Davidson CS. Liver disease of the chronic alcoholic simulating extrahepatic biliary obstruction. Gastroenterology. 1957;33:236–44.
71. Randall B. Fatty liver and sudden death. Hum Pathol. 1980;11:147–53.
72. Lieber CS, Spritz N, DeCarli LM. Role of dietary, adipose and endogenously synthesized fatty acids in the pathogenesis of the alcoholic fatty liver. J Clin Invest. 1966;45:51–62.
73. Edmondson HA, Peters RL, Reynolds TB, Kuzma OT. Sclerosing hyaline necrosis of the liver. A recognizable clinical syndrome. Ann Intern Med. 1963;59:646–73.
74. Reynolds TB, Hidemura R, Michel H et al. Portal hypertension without cirrhosis in alcoholic liver disease. Ann Intern Med. 1969;70:497–506.
75. Worner TM, Lieber CS. Perivenular fibrosis as precursor lesion of cirrhosis. J Am Med Assoc. 1985;254:627–30.
76. Rosman AS, Lieber CS. Biochemical markers of alcohol consumption. Alcohol Health Res World 1990; 210–18.
77. Litten R, Allen J. Measuring alcohol consumption; psychosocial and biochemical methods. Totowa, NJ: Humana; 1992.
78. Stibler H, Borg S, Joustra M. Micro anion exchange chromatography of carbohydrate-deficient transferrin in serum in relation to alcohol consumption (Swedish Patent 8400587-5). Alcohol Clin Exp Res. 1986;10:535–44.
79. Behrens UJ, Worner TM, Braly LF, Schaffner F, Lieber CS. Carbohydrate-deficient transferrin (CDT), a marker for chronic alcohol consumption in different ethnic populations. Alcohol Clin Exp Res. 1988;12:427–32.
80. Nakano M, Worner T, Lieber CS. Perivenular fibrosis in alcoholic liver injury: ultrastructure of histologic progression. Gastroenterology. 1982;83:777–85.
81. Friedman SL. The cellular basis of hepatic fibrosis: mechanisms and treatment strategies. N Engl J Med. 1993;328:1828–35.
82. Lieber CS, Williams R, editors. Recent advances in the treatment of liver disease. Drugs, Vol. 40, Suppl. 3. Auckland, New Zealand: Addis International, 1990:1–138.
83. Sörensen TIA, Orholm M, Bentsen KD, Hoyby G, Eghoje K, Christoffersen P. Prospective evaluation of alcohol abuse and alcoholic liver injury in man as predictors of development of cirrhosis. Lancet. 1984;2:241–4.
84. Klion FM, Schaffner F. Ultrastructural studies in alcoholic liver disease. Digestion. 1968;1:2–14.
85. Goldberg SI, Mendenhall CL, Connell AM, Chedid A. Non-alcoholic chronic hepatitis in the alcoholic. Gastroenterology. 1977;72:598–604.
86. Hodges JR, Millward-Sadler GH, Wright R. Chronic active hepatitis: the spectrum disease. Lancet. 1982;1:550–2.
87. Williams AL, Hoofnagle JH. Ratio of serum aspartate to alanine aminotransferase in chronic hepatitis. Relationship to cirrhosis. Gastroenterology. 1988;95:734–9.
88. Helman RA, Temko MH, Nye SW, Fallon HJ. Alcoholic hepatitis: natural history and evaluation of prednisolone therapy. Ann Intern Med. 1971;74:311–21.
89. Ramond MJ, Poynard T, Rueff B et al. A randomized trial of prednisolone in patients with severe alcoholic hepatitis. N Engl J Med. 1992;326:507–12.

90. Mendenhall CL, Anderson S, Garcia-Pont *et al.* Short-term and long-term survival in patients with alcoholic hepatitis treated with oxandrolone and prednisolone. N Engl J Med. 1984;311:1464–70.

91. Orrego H, Blake JE, Blendis LM, Compton KV, Israel Y. Long-term treatment of alcoholic liver disease with propylthiouracil. N Engl J Med. 1987;317:1421–7.

92. Kershenobich D, Vargas F, Garcia-Tsao G, Tomayo RP, Gent M, Rojkind M. Colchicine in the treatment of cirrhosis of the liver. N Engl J Med. 1988;318:1709–13.

93. Goodman ZD, Ishak KG. Occlusive venous lesions in alcoholic liver disease. A study of 200 cases. Gastroenterology. 1982;83:786–96.

94. Van Waes L, Lieber CS. Early perivenular sclerosis in alcoholic fatty liver: an index of progressive liver injury. Gastroenterology. 1977;73:646–50.

95. Bradley SE, Ingelfinger FJ, Bradley GP. Hepatic circulation in cirrhosis of the liver. Circulation. 1952;5:419–29.

96. Popper H. The pathogenesis of alcoholic cirrhosis. In: Fisher MM, Rankin JG, editors. Alcohol and the liver. New York: Plenum Press; 1977:289–305.

97. Mak KM, Lieber CS. Alterations in endothelial fenestrations in liver sinusoids of baboons fed alcohol: a scanning electron microscopic study. Hepatology. 1984;4:386–91.

98. Bell ET. Relation of portal cirrhosis to haemochromatosis and to diabetes mellitus. Diabetes. 1955;4:435–46.

99. Powell LW. The role of alcoholism in hepatic iron storage disease. Ann NY Acad Sci. 1975;253:124–34.

100. Lee FI. Cirrhosis and hepatoma in alcoholics. Gut. 1966;7:77–85.

101. Lieber CS, Seitz HK, Garro AJ, Worner TM. Alcohol related diseases and carcinogenesis. Cancer Res. 1979;39:2863–86.

102. Ohnishi K, Iida S, Iwama S *et al.* The effect of chronic habitual alcohol intake on the development of liver cirrhosis and hepatocellular carcinoma. Cancer. 1982;49:672–7.

103. Bréchot C, Nalpas B, Couroucé AM *et al.* Evidence that hepatitis B virus has a role in liver-cell carcinoma in alcoholic liver disease. N Engl J Med. 1982;306:1384–7.

104. Kumar S, Stauber RE, Gavaler JS *et al.* Orthotopic liver transplantation for alcoholic liver disease. Hepatology. 1990;14:159–64.

105. Chedid A, Mendenhall CL, Garside P, French SW, Chen T, Rabin L and the VA Cooperative Group. Prognostic factors in alcoholic liver disease. Am J Gastroenterol. 1991;82:210–16.

106. Potter JF, James OFW. Clinical features and prognosis of alcoholic liver disease in respect of advancing age. Gerontology. 1987;33:380–7.

107. Lieber CS. Alcoholism: a disease encompassing all of medicine. Resident Staff Phys. 1995;41:15–28.

9
Drug-associated hepatitis

J. NEUBERGER

INTRODUCTION

Adverse drug reactions involving the liver are uncommon. The great majority of adverse drug reactions are relatively benign and, provided the patient or physician is aware of the possible drug involvement in the patient's illness, early and prompt withdrawal of the drug usually leads to rapid resolution. However, in some cases, such as drug-associated benign or malignant liver tumours (for example associated with the use of oral contraceptive), the adverse drug reaction may present several years after drug ingestion. In other examples, as with the vanishing bile duct syndrome associated with the use of some penicillins, liver damage may progress for several months despite withdrawal of the drug.

SPECTRUM OF DRUGS CAUSING HEPATOTOXICITY

While it is generally accepted that all pharmaceutical agents may be associated with adverse reactions affecting the liver and other organs, it is often forgotten, both by the profession and the general public, that other, non-pharmacological agents may also be associated with liver damage. It is generally assumed that naturally occurring compounds, such as vitamins or herbal remedies, are not likely to be hepatotoxic; the physician often fails to enquire fully about all treatments. Thus, in any patient presenting with liver damage of unknown cause, the physician should enquire not only about conventional medicines but also herbal remedies, vitamin supplementation and possible exposure to environmental toxins (Table 1). It must also be remembered that the so-called 'recreational drugs', such as cocaine or ecstasy, may also be associated with drug toxicity, and the patient is less likely to offer a history of drug ingestion.

EPIDEMIOLOGY OF DRUG REACTIONS

Prior to the introduction of any new pharmacological agent to the market place, many normal subjects and patients have been tested, and those agents associated

Table 1   Spectrum of agents causing hepatitis

Medicinal agents
Herbal remedies, e.g. mistletoe, *Senecio*
Herbal teas, e.g. Chinese herbal teas
Mushrooms, e.g. *Amanita phalloides*
Plants, e.g. sassafras
'Recreational' drugs, e.g. cocaine, ecstasy
Environmental toxins, e.g. pesticides
Vitamins, e.g. vitamin A

with significant liver damage are well identified and, depending on the cost/benefit ratio, may be withdrawn from sale. The limitations of clinical studies in identifying significant adverse drug reactions have been summarized by Bruppacher[1], who has defined the five 'toos' of clinical trials:

1. *Too few patients*: clinical studies have been too small to detect rare events. For example, to detect an adverse reaction affecting 1 in 1000 with a power of 0.95, it is necessary to screen just under 3000 patients; if the adverse event has an incidence of 1 in 10 000, it will be necessary to observe 30 000 treated patients.
2. *Too median aged*: the young and old end of the spectrum of the normal population are usually not well represented in the clinical studies; indeed, most studies will specifically exclude such people. With some drugs, toxicity may be greatest in these people.
3. *Too simple*: trials are focused on assessing the efficacy or otherwise of the drug, and thus give too little attention to other variables which may be related to toxicity.
4. *Too narrow*: complicated therapeutic situations tend to be excluded from the trial and, therefore, a toxic effect may be missed.
5. *Too brief*: clinical trials are usually driven in part by commercial considerations and may be too short to detect those toxicities associated with accumulative or late adverse reactions.

Finally, it must be remembered that the presence of the disease being treated may mask drug toxicity. This is well illustrated by the recent trial with fialuridine (FIAU) for the treatment of chronic viral hepatitis B[2]. This nucleoside analogue was subsequently withdrawn because of serious hepatotoxicity, which was recognized comparatively late because many of the patients were already suffering from significant liver disease and the toxicity of the drug was initially attributed to the underlying progressive, severe liver disease.

The reporting of adverse drug reactions is often sporadic and many countries, including the United Kingdom, rely primarily on voluntary adverse drug reaction reporting. This system, whilst it is undoubtedly highly effective, suffers from a number of significant disadvantages:

1. Reporting of a suspected adverse drug reaction does not prove causality and, therefore, careful scrutiny of the records is required to estimate causality.

2. The system is dependent on the alertness and public-spirit of the doctor, who has no personal benefit from reporting the adverse drug reaction and, therefore, many suspected reactions are not reported.
3. Many known adverse drug reactions are not reported and it may, therefore, be difficult to establish the true prevalence.
4. Because an adverse drug reaction may be rare, the clinicians may be slow to detect a new reaction.

There have been a number of studies looking at reported adverse drug reactions. For example, the Danish Committee on Adverse Drug Reactions[3] published the reported reactions received by them between 1978 and 1987. Hepatic injuries accounted for just under 6% of all adverse drug reactions reported, but for 14.7% of all fatal drug reactions. Of the total adverse drug reactions affecting the liver, 14% were classified as acute hepatotoxic, 16% as acute cholestatic, and 27% as abnormalities of liver function. Halothane in particular accounted for the majority of the reactions, and indeed fatalities. A similar report by Bem *et al.*, on 1600 cases reported to the Committee on Safety of Medicines in the UK[4], indicated that about 1600 cases of adverse drug reactions were reported each year, of which hepatic reactions accounted for 3.5%. Of these hepatic reactions, 7% were fatal. As with the Danish ADR report, the majority of drug reactions were jaundice and hepatitis; the commonest drugs implicated were halothane, antibiotics and oral contraceptives. The commoner drugs reported to cause hepatitis are listed in Table 2.

There have been other approaches to identify adverse drug reactions. Some studies have looked at admissions to hospital and have tried retrospectively to identify those instances which may be due to drugs. An alternative approach is to use computerized databases. However, retrospective analyses often contain incomplete data, and looking at rare events is often difficult. While such an approach may be helpful in assessing the incidence of a known adverse drug reaction, it may be less successful in identifying a previously unrecognized one. Therefore, it is likely that the degree and extent of adverse drug reaction reporting will remain far from ideal.

DIAGNOSIS OF DRUG REACTIONS

There are three basic guidelines for drug reactions which must be borne in mind in their diagnosis:

1. Virtually all forms of liver damage may be induced by drugs and other medications; therefore, unless the diagnosis is clear, a drug cause for the liver damage should always be considered.
2. One drug may be associated with more than one pattern of liver damage.
3. The diagnosis of drug-induced liver damage is, in general, one of exclusion.

A recent meeting[5] has drawn attention to clinical, serological and histological diagnostic criteria to identify drug-associated acute hepatitis (Table 3). As the diagnosis of an adverse drug reaction is one of exclusion of other causes, involvement of the as-yet-unidentifiable hepatitis viruses can, as yet, be excluded.

Table 2   Some drugs which may cause acute hepatitis

Anaesthetic agents
  enflurane
  halothane
  methoxyflurane
	Cardiovascular drugs
	  amiodarone
	  methyldopa
	  diltiazem
	  nifedepine
	  perhexiline
	  minocycline
	  ACE inhibitors

Analgesics
  Acetaminophen (paracetamol)
  NSAIDs
  diclofenac	

Anticonvulsants
  phenytoin
  valproate
	Endocrine agents
	  glipizide
	  acetohexamide
	  propylthiouracil
	  tamoxifen

Antimicrobials
  penicillins
  sulphonamides
  ketoconazole
  rifampicin/isoniazid
  metronidazole
  amphotericin
  nitrofurantoin
  cephalosporins
	Neurological drugs
	  amineptine
	  cocaine
	  tricyclic antidepressants

Antineoplastic drugs
  etoposide
  fluorouracil
  methotrexate
  vincristine
  doxorubicin
  nitrosourea
	Others
	  disulfiram
	  cyclosporin A
	  vitamin A
	  cimetidine
	  etretinate
	  coumarin anticoagulants

Some authors have advocated a challenge test whereby the drug is administered again under controlled conditions to a patient. This is rarely justified, may be fatal and may indeed prove misleading. Perhaps the best example of a fatal, although often inadvertent challenge is with the anaesthetic agent halothane, where a significant number of patients who have developed jaundice following one halothane exposure are given, for a variety of different reasons, a repeat halothane anaesthetic and in such cases there may be a fatal outcome[6]. Furthermore, the challenge may be misleading and may give false-negative and false-positive results[7].

Table 3   Criteria for diagnosing acute drug-associated hepatitis (from ref. 5)

Feature		Initial treatment	Subsequent treatment
Suggestive	from starting	5 to 90 days	1 to 15 days
Compatible	from starting from stopping	<5 or >90 days <15 days	>15 days <15 days
Incompatible	from starting from stopping	Drug taken after onset of reaction >15 days*	

* Except for slowly metabolized drugs.

PATTERNS OF DRUG-INDUCED HEPATITIS

The clinical presentation of drug-induced hepatitis resembles other forms of hepatitis, and there are no reliable features to indicate a drug aetiology. There may be a short prodromal illness which is rapidly followed by the onset of pale stools, dark urine and jaundice. Anorexia and right upper quadrant pain may be a prominent feature, and indeed has misled some clinicians to make an inappropriate diagnosis of gallstone disease. Laparotomy in such a situation may have disastrous effects on the clinical course of disease. The spectrum of hepatitis, however, ranges from a minor and asymptomatic derangement of liver function tests to fulminant hepatic failure.

The histological features of drug-associated hepatitis are also non-specific. The types of liver cell injury are shown in Table 4. Panacinar spotty degeneration and necrosis resembles typical viral hepatitis involving all acinar zones, with degeneration and spotty necrosis of the hepatocytes. In this case cholestasis is usually minimal. Liver cell injury may be manifest by ballooning of the liver cell with features of apoptosis. Small areas of necrosis are distributed randomly throughout the lobule. The Kupffer cells are hypertrophied. The inflammatory response is variable, ranging from totally absent to a significant infiltration by eosinophils and neutrophils.

More severe damage is associated with submissive necrosis, and is characterized by central necrosis, again with ballooning of hepatocytes with degeneration and apoptosis. Inflammation is again variable, but cholestasis is usually mild. Fat accumulation may be present. Massive necrosis, in the case of drug-associated liver cell damage, resembles that caused by fulminant viral hepatitis, with liver damage occurring throughout the lobule. Eosinophilic infiltrate is characteristic but not diagnostic of drug hepatitis. It is unusual for histological features to be diagnostic of a drug aetiology of acute hepatitis. Indeed, in many clinical situations, liver biopsy is rarely required: however, it may be useful in excluding other causes of acute hepatitis.

PATTERNS OF DRUG REACTIONS

Conventionally, acute hepatitic reactions are divided into type A and type B (Table 5). Type A reactions are the predictable reactions which are dose-dependent and host-independent. The classic example of this type of drug reaction is paracetamol toxicity (see below). The greater the quantity of drug

Table 4 Liver histological features suggestive of a drug aetiology

Zonal necrosis
Prominent eosinophilic infiltrate
Microvesicular steatosis
Periportal cholestasis
Granulomas
Destructive bile duct lesions

Table 5 Classification of acute drug-associated hepatitis

Characteristic	Predictable	Idiosyncratic	
		Immune	Metabolic
Dose-dependent	Yes	No	No
Gender	M=F	F>M	M=F
Latent period	4–20 weeks	2–10 weeks	4–20 weeks
Response to challenge	Slow	Rapid	Slow
Animal models	Yes	No	Variable
Incidence	Varies	<0.001%	0.1–1%

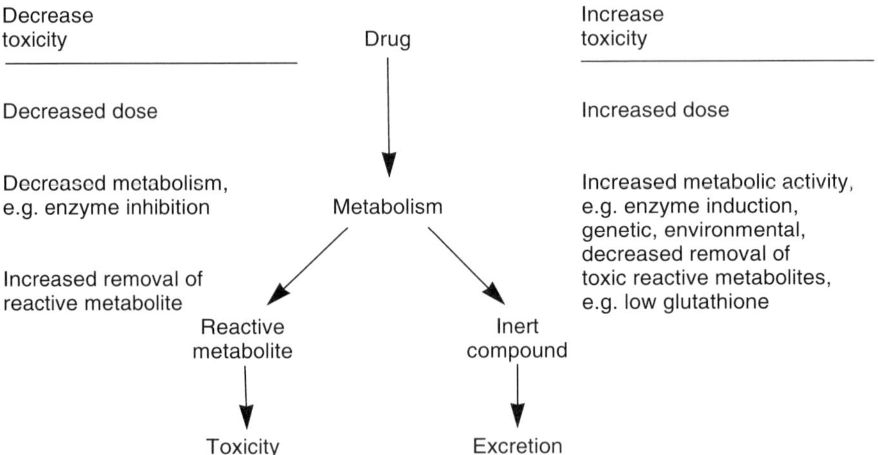

Fig. 1 Factors which may affect predictable drug toxicity

ingested, the greater the probability of liver damage occurring although, as will be illustrated below, there are many factors which may modify host susceptibility to predictable drug reactions (Fig. 1).

The idiosyncratic drug reactions are host-dependent and dose-independent. Broadly, these may be divided into two groups: those which are dependent on abnormal metabolism and those in which immune mechanisms have been implicated. The metabolic idiosyncratic drug reactions usually involve either metabolism of a drug (or metabolite) through a usually minor pathway, or else failure of detoxification of a drug. Immune reactions are characterized by other features of hypersensitivity (Table 6). This type of reaction is typified by halothane hepatitis (see below).

PARACETAMOL TOXICITY – AN EXAMPLE OF A PREDICTABLE HEPATOTOXIN

Paracetamol (acetaminophen) is an antipyretic analgesic which is usually, in therapeutic doses, well tolerated and with few side-effects. Liver damage from

Table 6   Characteristics of immune-mediated drug hepatitis

Fever
Rash
Arthralgia
Lymphadenopathy
Peripheral/tissue eosinophilia
Autoantibodies (organ non-specific)
Tissue granuloma
Blood dyscrasias

paracetamol overdose has now become one of the commonest causes of drug-induced liver injury, and of fulminant hepatic failure[8]. The mortality rate associated with paracetamol overdose is dependent both on the dose taken and the effectiveness of intervention.

The metabolism of paracetamol metabolism is now well defined (Fig. 1). In the healthy adult more than 90% of the oral dose is eliminated by conjugation within the hepatocyte to the glucuronic or sulphate metabolite. Some metabolism also occurs in the kidneys, lung and intestine. Less than 5% of the administered dose is metabolized by cytochrome P450 2E2 to produce an electrophilic metabolite, N-acetyl-P-benzoquinone imine (NAPQI). NAPQI is rapidly conjugated to glutathione and so eliminated. Ingestion of larger amounts of paracetamol leads to saturation of the sulphate and glucuronidation pathways, so that a greater proportion of the drug is metabolized through the P450 system. This results in depletion of glutathione, and unconjugated NAPQI reacts with a variety of cellular macromolecules, resulting in calcium mobilization and an increase in intracellular calcium, and so cell death.

Understanding of the mechanism of paracetamol metabolism and detoxification has allowed for design of strategies for therapeutic intervention. Since depletion of glutathione to remove excess NAPQI is a crucial step in the pattern of toxicity, it would seem desirable to provide the cell with increased glutathione. Intravenously administered glutathione is non-permeable to the cell and, therefore, treatment with N-acetylcysteine intravenously, or oral methionine, is shown to be both theoretically and practically effective. All Accident and Emergency Departments need to be aware of the benefits of early intervention with major improvements in survival. Guidelines for the threshold for treatment of paracetamol overdose are now widely available, but patients are still developing liver failure because of misuse of the available guidelines. The interpretation is dependent on knowing accurately when the patient took the overdose, and cannot be used when the overdose was taken over a period of hours. Susceptibility to paracetamol is affected by many other factors, as discussed below. Because of the excellent safety profile of N-acetylcysteine, it is usually far safer to give the agent than not, if there is any significant risk of liver failure developing. Oral methionine is also very effective in preventing liver cell necrosis.

The dose of paracetamol reported to cause liver damage is very variable. Of course, the patient may not be aware how much paracetamol has been ingested; some of the paracetamol may not be absorbed because of vomiting, which may be iatrogenically induced.

The therapeutic dose is approximately 10–15 mg/kg, whereas the threshold for liver damage[9] is about 250 mg/kg. However, liver damage has been reported in patients taking as little as 12 g of paracetamol. It must also be emphasized that paracetamol is contained in drug combinations.

RISK FACTORS FOR PARACETAMOL HEPATOTOXICITY

As would be anticipated from knowledge of the pathways of paracetamol toxicity, patients who have enzyme induction are likely to be at greater risk of toxicity. Alcohol is perhaps the best-known of these enzyme inducers which induces, particularly, cytochrome P450 2E1. Bray and colleagues at King's College Hospital[10] have retrospectively examined patients with significant paracetamol toxicity, and studied the alcohol consumption. In men who drank more than 168 g of alcohol per week, and women who drank more than 112 g per week, mortality was greater than in those who drank less. Nonetheless, in a subsequent study, the same group at King's College Hospital showed that mortality rates in alcohol abusers and non-abusers are similar[11]. They also confirmed that there was a lack of correlation between the dose of paracetamol ingested and the outcome, suggesting that, once a certain level of liver damage had been achieved, additional drug had little further adverse effect. Others have shown other enzyme inducers, such as phenobarbitone and phenytoin, may also be associated with an increased risk of hepatotoxicity[12,13].

The involvement of anticonvulsants in enhancing hepatoxicity may be related to the fact that other cytochromes, including 1A2 and 3A4, may be involved in the generation of NAPQI, and that these cytochrome isozymes are enhanced by anticonvulsants. More recently there has been an increased association of hepatotoxicity with isoniazid[14,15], and in patients with AIDS, which is thought to be potentiated by treatment with zidovudine[16].

It has been suggested that cimetidine, a weak enzyme inhibitor, may be involved in hepatoprotection. Although data in animals were encouraging, this has not been fully substantiated in humans. This presumably relates to the relatively weak enzyme inhibition of cimetidine, and in the clinical situation the agent would have to be given before the patient ingested paracetamol. This observation remains of theoretical rather than practical value.

INCREASED SUSCEPTIBILITY TO PARACETAMOL TOXICITY

Severe hepatic injury and liver cell failure have been reported in patients taking therapeutic levels of paracetamol. While it is not possible in some cases to exclude either intentional or inadvertent overdose, it is probable that chronic ill-health is associated with a reduction in the levels of glutathione and, thus, increasing susceptibility[17,18]. Hence, patients who are malnourished, for whatever reason, are more likely to present with toxicity at lower doses[19].

OTHER FACTORS WHICH DETERMINE DRUG SUSCEPTIBILITY

As might be expected, there will be many factors that determine susceptibility of an individual to drug hepatotoxicity. Rates of absorption and deposition of the drug may vary considerably within individuals. There are many isozymes of the cytochrome P450s and, therefore, differences in different enzyme activities are associated with increased or decreased susceptibility to drug toxicity (Table 7)[20]. Furthermore, induction or inhibition of different cytochromes by external agents, including co-administered drugs, may also alter the susceptibility to drug reactions. Other P450 enzymes are also involved, and these include the N-acetyltransferase enzymes; flavin mono-oxygenases[21–23] and glucuronyl-transferases and epoxide hydrolases[24] where genetic variations are associated with toxicity.

In immune reactions, host HLA type and other immune responsive genes may also be important. Thus, HLA A11 and Aw24-Bw5-DR2 have been associated with halothane-associated liver damage; DR6 and DR2 in nitrofurantoin hepatitis, DR6 in chlorpromazine hepatitis and A11 in diclofenac hepatitis[25]. However, HLA associations must be interpreted with care, since many reports have been based on serological techniques for tissue typing, which may give up to 25% false results, the diagnosis of the drug reaction may be uncertain and the patient population may be genetically mixed.

Other factors which may influence susceptibility to drug reactions are shown in Table 8. There is uncertainty as to the importance of age on drug toxicity: very young rats are unable to metabolize paracetamol well, and so are protected from the effects of overdose. Other animal studies have suggested that some enzyme activities may be reduced in the elderly, but whether this has any significant clinical effect is uncertain. While several reports have suggested that drug reactions requiring hospital admissions are more frequent in the elderly, it remains to be shown that this is due to increased susceptibility rather than other factors; for example, it is this group of people who tend to take more medication and cannot tolerate illness so well.

Sex probably has a relatively small role in determining susceptibility to drug toxicity, although females are more susceptible to immune-mediated drug

Table 7 Genetic variations in drug-metabolizing enzymes which may be associated with hepatotoxic reactions

Enzyme	*Drugs associated with toxicity*
Cytochrome CYP1A2	Acetaminophen, Tacrine
Cytochrome CYP2C9	Tienilic acid, phenytoin
Cytochrome CYP2D6	Perhexiline
Cytochrome CYP2E1	Ethanol, enflurane
Cytochrome CYP3A4	Amiodarone, cyclosporin, cocaine
N-acetyltransferase	Isoniazid
Sulphoxidation	Chlorpromazine
Glucuronyltransferase	Diclofenac
Epoxide hydrolase	Phenytoin

Table 8 Some host factors which affect susceptibility to drug toxicity

Age
Gender
Nutritional status
Co-administered drugs
Coexisting disease
Pregnancy
Immune factors such as HLA
Genetic variability in drug-metabolizing enzymes
Environmental factors
Past history/family history of adverse drug reaction

toxicity. Nutritional status does have an effect in some patients, since glutathione stores are reduced and cytochrome P450 2E1 activity is induced.

Finally, the presence of liver and extrahepatic disease may affect drug susceptibility. Azathioprine-induced liver damage, for example, is more common in patients with renal impairment, and liver disease may increase the risk of toxicity from antimetabolites, possibly because of reduced biliary excretion.

IMMUNE-MEDIATED DRUG REACTIONS

Almost all drugs and agents require metabolism before manifestation of hepatotoxicity. The association of drug reactions with markers of hypersensitivity has raised the possibility of immune mechanisms being involved in the liver damage. The best example of this is halothane hepatitis. Severe liver damage following halothane exposure is an idiosyncratic and dose-independent drug reaction, occurring particularly in patients who are middle-aged, fat and female[26,27]. It is not clear whether these patient characteristics represent those undergoing anaesthesia, or implies a certain risk factor. Farrell and Prendergast Murray[28] have suggested that there is a genetic contribution in that the majority of patients, and a proportion of their first-degree relatives, have lymphocytes which show enhanced sensitivity from electrophilic metabolites of phenytoin. The nature of the genetic abnormality is not clear, and the study requires confirmation. Furthermore, it has not been shown that those patients with such increased susceptibility are at greater risk of halothane toxicity.

Direct evidence of an immune response to halothane-altered metabolites came from studies by Vergani and colleagues[29]. Rabbits were exposed to halothane, and after 24 hours were sacrificed, their livers removed and hepatocytes isolated for *in-vitro* studies. Using serum from patients with presumed halothane hepatitis, immunofluorescence and indirect cytotoxicity studies showed that the patients' serum contained an antibody which reacted with halothane-altered liver cell determinants. Further studies have shown that those exposed to halothane but without developing liver damage have no comparable antibody. Subsequent studies by Kenna and colleagues[30,31] have further characterized these antigens using immunoblotting techniques, and have now identified over eight antigens with molecular masses between 54 and 100 kDa. Some of these antigens have been defined more closely, and they include a cytochrome P450 antigen, a protein disulphide isomerase, and a microsomal carboxylesterase. The significance of these reactions is unclear. It still remains to be shown whether the presence of these immune responses occurs as part of the hepatotoxic response, or merely as a consequence of the liver damage.

Other studies taking liver from patients exposed to halothane, but who have not developed liver damage, show that these antigens are present in the liver, and suggest that the susceptibility to halothane hepatitis is a consequence of immune recognition rather than antigen presentation or production[32]. Whether the mechanism of liver cell necrosis is antibody-dependent, directly cytotoxic or complement-mediated has not been shown. It is possible to give a diagrammatic representation of this form of liver damage (Fig. 2).

As yet there are no therapeutic implications as a consequence of these observations. A number of anecdotal studies have described treatment of patients with established halothane hepatitis using immunosuppression, but none has yet been effective. Transplantation remains the only therapeutic option in those with advanced liver failure.

OTHER EXAMPLES OF POSSIBLE IMMUNE-MEDIATED HEPATOTOXICITY

There are a few other examples of drug toxicity in which immune mechanisms have been implicated in the pathogenesis of the liver damage. Drug reactions associated with antibodies to cellular organelles include minocycline, papaverine, fenobrate, clometacin and oxyphenisatin. The associated autoantibodies are antinuclear, antimitochondrial and antiactin (smooth muscle). Homberg and colleagues[33] have identified another autoantibody, termed antiliver/kidney

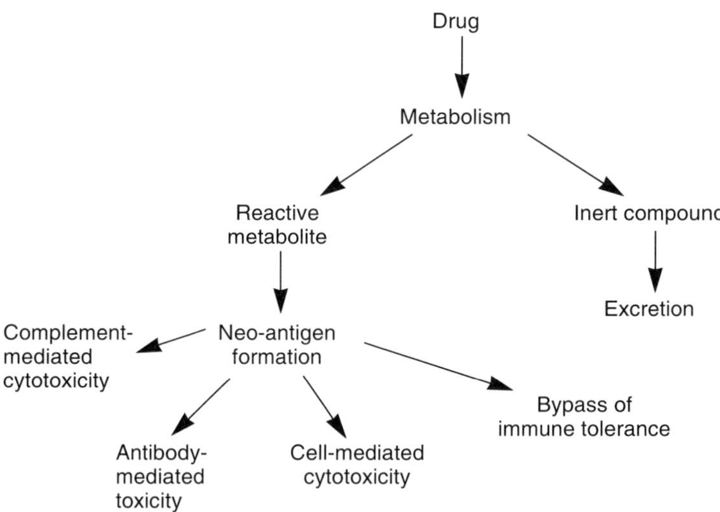

Fig. 2 Possible mechanism of immune-mediated drug hepatotoxicity

microsomal antibody. This antibody was found in association with hepatitis associated with the uricosuric diuretic, tienilic acid. The antibody was termed LKM-2, to distinguish it from the LKM-1 associated with the predominantly childhood variant of autoimmune hepatitis, and LKM-3 associated with hepatitis D viral infection. This antibody has subsequently been identified as reacting with cytochrome P450 2C9, the major drug-metabolizing enzyme for the drug.

Other drugs which are associated with an immune basis include dihydralazine, phenytoin and carbamazepine.

It has been suggested that the *in-vitro* lymphocyte transformation test may be of value in the diagnosis of immune-mediated drug injury; however, this approach is not without problems[35]. It was suggested by Berg and Becker[35] that any information from such tests should be interpreted with caution and the results considered of clinical relevance if they are consistent with the clinical observations, done within 4 weeks of the reaction, and done using a wide range of drug concentration and, when tested 3–6 months later, prove negative.

CLINICAL PROBLEMS

As indicated above, in the majority of cases a high index of suspicion will usually lead to the correct diagnosis and management of drug reactions. A full history and examination is required to assess the severity of liver damage and exclude other causes for the hepatitis. The need for a liver biopsy is limited; however, the major dilemma facing the clinician is antituberculous therapy. The introduction of isoniazid resulted in a dramatic fall in the mortality from tuberculosis, but shortly after the widespread introduction of the drug cases of hepatitis began to appear. Studies have shown that between 10% and 35% of patients receiving isoniazid develop transient and asymptomatic elevation of serum transaminases. In the majority of instances these abnormal liver tests occur within 2 months after institution of therapy, and resolve without discontinuation of the drug. However, about 1 in 100 will develop severe hepatitis and, if the agent is not stopped, severe liver cell damage will occur, with the development of fulminant hepatic failure, and with a mortality approaching 10%. There remains controversy as to whether weekly blood tests will help in early reduction of mortality.

The frequency of isoniazid hepatitis is dependent on several factors which include older (>50 years) age, those with a history of chronic alcohol ingestion, and those taking other drugs such as rifampicin. In contrast, factors associated with a higher mortality include older age, black women, surgery and other drugs. The combination of isoniazid and rifampicin appears to be especially hepatotoxic: whether this is due to the fact that both agents are hepatotoxic and have a synergistic effect, or whether rifampicin exerts its effect as an enzyme inducer, is still uncertain. Pyrazinamide co-administration also appears to have a deleterious effect on the outcome of liver failure associated with isoniazid[34]. There remains controversy whether slow or fast acetylators are more susceptible.

Isoniazid hepatotoxicity fulfils the criteria for an idiosyncratic reaction, although there are no features to implicate immune mechanisms. A toxic metabolite may be involved. Isoniazid is metabolized by *N*-acetyltransferase to acetyl isoniazid; about half of which is hydrolysed to acetyl hydrazine. This is then metabolized to several compounds including diacetyl hydrazine (by *N*-acetyltransferase) and to toxic *N*-hydroxy derivative metabolites by the cytochrome P450 system (especially 2E1). Variations in acetylator phenotype appear to have little effect on hepatotoxicity.

The clinician looking after a patient with abnormal liver tests while taking antituberculous therapy is faced with a difficult dilemma – should medication be continued, with the possibility of fatal liver damage, or should the drugs be stopped, with the risk of reactivation of the tuberculosis? There is little help in the literature to guide the clinician. Most would advocate close monitoring of the liver function tests and, if they become more abnormal, then all treatment should be stopped; when the liver tests have normalized then treatment without isoniazid should be reinstituted.

SUMMARY

Acute hepatitis from adverse drug reactions remains a diagnosis of exclusion. Serious complications from drug reactions are relatively rare, but may ultimately prove to be fatal unless the causal agent is rapidly identified and, where appropriate, withdrawn. Close monitoring is important.

References

1. Bruppacher R. Epidemiological identification and evaluation of hepatic adverse drug reactions. Semin Liver Dis. 1995;15:301–8.
2. McKenzie R, Fried M, Sallie R *et al*. Hepatic failure and lactic acidosis due to fialuridine (FIAU), an investigational nucleoside analogue for chronic hepatitis B. N Engl J Med.1995;333:1099–1105.
3. Friis H, Andreason PB. Drug induced hepatic injury: analysis of 1100 cases reported to the Danish Committee on Adverse Drug Reactions between 1971 and 1978. J Intern Med. 1992;232:133–8.
4. Bem JL, Mann R, Rawlins M. Review of yellow cards. Br Med J. 1988;296:1319.
5. Benichou C. Criteria for drug induced liver disorders. Report of an International Consensus Conference. J Hepatol. 1990;11:272–6.
6. Neuberger J, Williams R. Halothane anaesthesia and liver damage. Br Med J. 1984;289:1136–9.
7. Farrell GC. Drug induced liver disease. Edinburgh: Churchill Livingstone; 1994.
8. Vickers C, Neuberger J, Buckels J, McMaster P, Elias E. Transplantation of the liver in adults and children with fulminant hepatic failure. J Hepatol. 1988;7:143–50.
9. Tolman KG. Hepatotoxicity of antirheumatic drugs. J Rheumatol. 1990;17:6–20.
10. Bray GP, Mowat C, Muir D *et al*. The effect of chronic alcohol intake on prognosis and outcome in paracetamol overdosage. Hum Exp Toxicol. 1991;10:435–50.
11. Makin A, Wendon J, Williams R. A seven year experience of severe acetaminophen induced hepatotoxicity (1987–1993). Gastroenterology. 1995;109:1907–16.
12. Bray GP, Harrison P, O'Grady J, Williams R. Long-term anticonvulsant therapy worsens outcome in paracetamol-induced fulminant hepatic failure. Hum Exp Toxicol. 1992;11:265–70.
13. Pirotte JH. Apparent potentiation by phenobarbital of hepatotoxicity from small doses of acetaminophen. Ann Intern Med. 1984;101:403–7.
14. Murphy R, Swartz R, Watkins PB. Severe acetaminophen toxicity in a patient receiving isoniazid. Ann Intern Med. 1990;113:799–802.
15. Crippen JS. Acetaminophen hepatotoxicity: potentiation by isoniazid. Am J Gastroenterol. 1993;88:590–3.
16. Shriner K, Goetz MB. Severe hepatotoxicity in a patient receiving both acetaminophen and zidovudine. Am J Med. 1992;93:94–6.

17. Bonkovsky H, Kane S, Jones D *et al.* Acute hepatic and renal toxicity from low doses of acetaminophen in the absence of alcohol abuse or malnutrition. Hepatology. 1994;19:1141–4.
18. Seeff L, Cuccherini B, Zimmerman H *et al.* Acetaminophen hepatotoxicity in alcoholics: a therapeutic misadventure. Ann Intern Med. 1986;104:399–404.
19. Patel M, Tang B, Kalow W. Variability of acetaminophen metabolisms in Caucasians and Orientals. Pharmacogenetics. 1992;2:28–33.
20. Fontana R, Watkins P. Genetic predisposition to drug-induced liver disease. Gastro Clin N Am. 1995;24:811–38.
21. Weber WW, Hein DW. *N*-acetylation pharmacogenetics. Pharmacol Rev. 1985;37:25–79.
22. Grant DM. Molecular genetics of the *N*-acetyltransferases. Pharmacogenetics. 1993;3:45–50.
23. Ziegler DM. Recent studies on the structure and function of multisubstrate flavin-containing monooxygenases. Annu Rev Pharmacol Toxicol. 1993;33:179–99.
24. Omiecinski C, Aicher L, Swenson L. Developmental expression of human microsomal epoxide hydrolase. J Pharmacol Exp Ther. 1994;289:417–23.
25. Berson A, Larrey D, Lepage V *et al.* Possible role of HLA in hepatotoxicity. J Hepatol. 1994;20:336–42.
26. Ray DC, Drummond G. Halothane hepatitis. Br J Anaesth. 1991;67:84–9.
27. Kenna J, Neuberger J, Williams R. Specific antibodies to halothane induced liver antigens in halothane-associated hepatitis. Br J Anaesth. 1987;59:1286–90.
28. Farrell G, Prendergast Murray M. Halothane hepatitis. Detection of a constitutional susceptibility factor. N Engl J Med. 1985;313:1310–14.
29. Vergani D, Mieli-Vergani G, Alberti A *et al.* Antibodies to the surface of halothane-altered rabbit hepatocytes in patients with severe halothane-associated hepatitis. N Engl J Med. 1980;303:66–71.
30. Kenna J, Martin J, Satoh H, Pohl L. Factors affecting the expression of trifluoracetylated liver microsomal neoantigens in rats treated with halothane. Drug Metab Disp. 1990;18:788–93.
31. Van Pelt F, Kenna J. Formation of trifluoracetylated protein antigens in cultured rat hepatocytes exposed to halothane *in vitro*. Biochem Pharmacol. 1994;48:461–71.
32. Kenna J, Neuberger J, Williams R. Evidence for expression in human liver of halothane-induced neoantigen recognized by antibodies in sera from patients with halothane hepatitis. Hepatology. 1988;8:1635–41.
33. Homberg J, Abuaf N, Hemly-Khalid S *et al.* Drug-induced hepatitis associated with anti-cytoplasmic organelle autoantibodies. Hepatology. 1985;5:722–7.
34. Durand F, Bernuau J, Pessayre D *et al.* Deleterious influence of pyrazinamide on the outcome of patients with fulminant or subfulminant liver failure during antituberculous treatment including isoniazid. Hepatology. 1995;21:929–32.
35. Berg P, Becker EW. The lymphocyte transformation test – a debated method for the evaluation of drug allergic hepatic injury. J Hepatol. 1995;22:115–18.

10
Haemochromatosis

J. W. HALLIDAY

BACKGROUND

Haemochromatosis (HC), sometimes called hereditary or genetic haemo-chromatosis, refers to a genetic disorder in which a progressive increase in body iron stores eventually leads to the deposition of excessive amounts of iron in the *parenchymal* cells of the liver, pancreas, heart and other organs. The excess iron deposition eventually results in cellular damage and functional insufficiency of the involved organs. An inappropriate increase in intestinal iron absorption is detectable early in the disease. A similar degree of iron overload may arise as a consequence of ineffective erythropoiesis (as in thalassaemia), when increased iron absorption is also present.

The amount of iron in the body is controlled largely at the point of entry, i.e. the intestinal mucosa. The lack of a major excretory pathway for iron in humans means than any increase in iron intake, either by a prolonged increase in iron absorption or as a consequence of the administration of parenteral iron, will produce an increase in iron stores in the body unless there is a concomitant pathological increase in iron losses, e.g. by blood loss.

HC is inherited as an autosomal recessive trait and the susceptibility locus is tightly linked to the HLA locus on chromosome 6[1-3]. The gene frequency is approximately 1 in 10 to 1 in 20, with a homozygote frequency in Caucasian populations (particularly of Celtic ancestry) of 1 in 300[4]. In Australia, where a high meat intake is relatively common, the majority of relatives predicted by HLA typing to be homozygous for the gene will eventually exhibit full bio-chemical and clinical expression of the disease[5]. Heterozygotes do not develop a progressive increase in iron stores to the extent seen in homozygotes, but may show some biochemical abnormality such as an increase in transferrin saturation.

Until recently a diagnosis of HC was made only in patients who presented with clinical signs and symptoms of the disease, such as the classic triad of skin pigmentation, hepatomegaly and diabetes described by Sheldon in 1935[6]. Loss of libido and testicular atrophy were common, and cardiac manifestations occurred in 5–15% of symptomatic patients[7]. The diagnosis is now frequently made in asymptomatic subjects (especially in family studies) where an elevated serum iron, serum transferrin saturation and serum ferritin concentration have been detected[8,9]. A liver biopsy with chemical determination of the hepatic iron concentration permits the hepatic iron index to be calculated (hepatic iron concentration in μmol/g dry weight $\div$ age in years). An index greater than 1.9 is usually present in adult homozygous subjects and less than 1.5 in heterozygotes[10,11]. The relative risk of hepatocellular cancer (HCC) in patients with iron overload who are already cirrhotic is 200-fold[12]. Weekly venesection in precirrhotic patients removes the excess iron and prevents the subsequent development of cirrhosis and of HCC. Early detection is thus very important and all first-degree relatives should be offered screening by transferrin saturation and serum ferritin. HLA typing of the family can be used for the detection of those relatives of a proband who are at risk of developing iron overload. Recently a more detailed haplotype analysis has been shown to be useful (see later).

DIAGNOSIS

While the classical clinical features of the disease are diagnostic in advanced iron overload, in the early stages laboratory investigations are often the first indicators of excess iron stores. These include an elevated serum iron level >30 μmol/L (>170 μg/100 ml) associated with an elevated transferrin saturation (>50%) and an elevated serum ferritin concentration[9,13,14]. The serum ferritin may also be elevated by hepatocellular necrosis, especially in alcoholic liver disease, or by other inflammatory processes, and several families in which the serum ferritin concentration has been normal despite unequivocal increases in body iron stores have been reported[15–18].

Liver biopsy allows definition of the extent of tissue damage and both histochemical and biochemical assessments of tissue iron, but other methods have been investigated[19–24]. Serum ferritin concentration, hepatic iron concentration and retrospective calculation of iron removed when iron stores are depleted are all useful in calculating the degree of excess iron stores[19,20]. Hepatic iron concentrations may exceed 400 μmol/g in advanced symptomatic disease.

HLA typing is of no use as a screening test in the general population. It is extremely useful, however, in families, and particularly in siblings of a proband, to predict the risk of developing iron overload[25,26].

PATHOLOGY

The major pathological findings in *advanced* HC relate to the massive amounts of iron found in the parenchymal cells of most organs, particularly liver, pancreas, heart and endocrine glands. The liver is enlarged and nodular and, along with the pancreas, presents a striking reddish-brown colour. On histological examination, iron is found in large amounts in the parenchymal cells. Only in the late stages of the disease is iron also seen in Kupffer cells, macrophages and biliary epithelial cells – a useful factor in the differential diagnosis. Extensive iron deposition is associated with dense fibrosis in the liver and pancreas; in the liver the fibrosis leads eventually to a mixed macro-micronodular cirrhosis[27].

THE BIOCHEMICAL DEFECT

The underlying biochemical defect in HC is unknown, but iron absorption is always inappropriately high in relation to the body iron stores. Theoretically, this could result from a defect in the intestinal mucosal cells of the upper small intestine, in the liver, the reticuloendothelial system or a more generalized defect. A defect in the known iron proteins transferrin or ferritin, or their receptors, in a hitherto unknown transport protein, or an abnormality in the regulation of a transport protein, could also occur.

The intestinal mucosal cell

It is a well-known fact that iron absorption is increased soon after stimulation of the bone marrow to increase erythropoiesis, as occurs after haemorrhage and hypoxia and also in iron deficiency, but the mechanism remains unclear. Several observations have suggested that the intestinal mucosal cell itself functions abnormally in HC, and that the cell is behaving as if the body is iron-deficient[28,29].

Two new membrane iron-binding proteins have been described, one by Teichmann and Stremmel[30] and one by Conrad and colleagues[31]. The former is a 160 kDa iron-binding protein (a trimer of 54 kDa monomers) which was localized to brush-border plasma membranes, was present in human intestinal mucosa and was found in liver and heart but not in the oesophagus. An antibody against this protein inhibited Fe^{3+} uptake by more than 50%. Studies also indicated that the protein was up-regulated in HC and remained so after phlebotomy therapy[32]. The iron-binding protein described by Conrad *et al.*[31] is a 56 kDa molecule seen in the apical cytoplasm of rat duodenal mucosa. These two iron-binding proteins remain as potentially important sources of the defect, but their biological significance remains to be confirmed.

At least two *in-vivo* studies have provided data which indicate that the defective control of iron absorption in this disease is mediated at the level of intestinal cell transfer to the plasma (i.e. serosal transfer as opposed to mucosal uptake). These data are supported by a recent study by McLaren *et al.*[33], in which mucosal iron kinetics were analysed using a compartmental model of intestinal iron absorption and systemic ferrokinetics. In subjects with HC the transfer of mucosal iron to the plasma was inappropriately high, although still inversely related to body iron stores as in normal subjects. This increase in mucosal iron transfer rate appeared to be the major determinant of increased iron absorption.

There have been major recent advances in the elucidation of the coordinate regulation by iron of both ferritin synthesis and transferrin receptor (TfR) expression[34–37]. These proteins have now been shown to be coordinately regulated by means of at least two binding proteins (IRP) which bind to the iron regulatory elements in the mRNA of both TfR and ferritin. This coordinate regulation appears to be intact in HC, and the gene for the protein lies on chromosome 9, not 6 as for the HC gene. However, in subjects with HC, intestinal mucosal H and L ferritin, as well as immunohistochemically detectable ferritin, fail to rise in parallel with the serum ferritin levels[38,39]. It has also been shown that the steady-state mRNA for both H and L ferritin is inappropriately low, while the mRNA for TfR is inappropriately increased[40], and there is sustained activity of an iron-regulatory factor[41]. These observations merely suggest: (a) that the coordinate regulation of the genes for TfR and for ferritin in the gut is still intact, (b) that the levels of iron in the gut cells are inappropriately low for reasons not clear, and (c) that the demonstrated abnormality in intestinal ferritin in HC is secondary to a primary abnormality elsewhere in the mucosal cell, to a more remote defect (for example in the liver or the monocyte/macrophage system), or to a more generalized cellular or membrane defect.

The genes for transferrin and its receptor are located on chromosome 3, and numerous studies have concluded that both transferrin and its receptor function normally in HC[40,42]. Recent work supports the hypothesis that the TfR on the gut cells is concerned more with the transport of iron *from* the plasma to the mucosal cell, presumably for use within the cell, especially during cell growth[43,44].

It has been suggested that HC relates to a failure to 'switch' from neonatal to adult control of iron absorption[45,46]. The hypothesis is attractive but so far unsubstantiated. Recent mapping and linkage studies[47] of an H-ferritin pseudo-gene on chromosome 6 place it centromeric to the HC locus, which makes this unlikely to be a candidate gene for the disease.

The liver

In HC, in contrast to secondary iron overload, the abnormal iron accumulation occurs in the hepatocytes, and it is only late in the disease that Kupffer cells, macrophages and biliary epithelial cells of the liver contain stainable iron. In addition, a high percentage saturation of circulating transferrin with iron is observed before the accumulation of large amounts of iron in the liver. The deposition of iron in hepatocytes and parenchymal cells of other organs could occur by other means. There are at least three mechanisms of iron delivery to hepatocytes in normal animals[48]. In conditions of iron overload, iron is also delivered to hepatocytes by non-transferrin-bound iron. The nature of this iron is ill-defined, but it probably includes a low-molecular-weight form, and could also include ferritin iron[49]. The production of a circulating regulator of iron absorp-tion has never been excluded, and both human and rat transplantation have been studied in iron overload in an attempt to further investigate this possibility[50–52]. Human liver transplants include some 22 subjects with HC successfully trans-planted for end-stage liver disease, and a further four instances in which a liver from an HC subject was inadvertently transplanted into a non-HC recipient. These cases have recently been reviewed[52]. The available results from these studies would be consistent either with a role for the intestinal mucosal cell in regulating iron uptake and body absorption according to its iron content, or with a role for a humoral factor in regulating iron transfer across the intestinal cell.

Non-transferrin-bound iron and hepatocyte membrane transport

Hepatic transferrin receptors are reportedly reduced in HC[53]. Recent attention has focused on the low-molecular-weight iron complexes referred to collectively as 'non-transferrin-bound' iron (NTBI). Although the NTBI accounts normally for less than 1% of the total serum iron, it may account for up to 35% of serum iron in subjects with HC[49]. Hepatic clearance of this form of iron is remarkably efficient[54], and is not reduced by hepatic iron loading[55]. Thus, NTBI may be quantitatively much more important than transferrin-bound iron in hepatic iron accumulation in HC. Using the isolated perfused liver model, Wright and colleagues[56] provided evidence that the hepatic uptake of NTBI is mediated by a membrane carrier, and occurs by an electron transfer mechanism in which there is a net movement of positive charge into the cell. These authors concluded that, since there is evidence that copper, zinc and manganese share a common carrier with iron, hepatic uptake and accumulation of these metal ions may be driven by similar transmembrane gradients[54,55]. However, uptake of NTBI did not appear to depend on the presence of transmembrane gradients for sodium, chloride or bicarbonate.

Against this background the recent demonstration of a membrane transport protein for copper that is defective in a disorder resulting from copper deficiency, Menke's disease, is of particular interest[57].

The reticuloendothelial system

The observation that Kupffer cells and intestinal macrophages contain little iron in subjects with HC has led to the suggestion that reticuloendothelial cells have a primary defect in iron metabolism, leading to reduced iron storage and the delivery of increased amounts of iron via the plasma to hepatocytes and other parenchymal cells. Kinetic studies involving reticuloendothelial function in HC lend support to this concept. A defect in storing iron, which is common to the two cell types, is certainly compatible with a number of observations in HC, including the paucity of iron present in these cells, the increased iron absorption, and the early rise in transferrin saturation.

A widespread parenchymal cell defect?

As discussed above, there is increasing evidence that HC results from a generalized membrane transport or other defect in multiple organs, as occurs in cystic fibrosis and other disorders. It is possible that a membrane iron-transport protein or proteins could reside on parenchymal cells of a number of organs and, if defective, lead to iron accumulation in those tissues. Alternatively, if confined to the intestine and monocyte/macrophage system (e.g. Kupffer cells of the liver), such a protein could be responsible for the rapid removal of iron from these cells, so that the cells respond to an apparent iron-deficient state, leading to a relative deficiency in ferritin and the concomitant increase in TfR concentration and sustained, inappropriately increased iron absorption.

GENETICS OF HAEMOCHROMATOSIS

The gene responsible for HC has not yet been identified, but it is known to be located on the short arm of chromosome 6 (6p) in close proximity to HLA-A, and HLA linkage has been used successfully to track the gene in affected pedigrees*.

The pattern of inheritance of HC within a particular family can be traced by HLA typing of first-degree relatives of the proband. Affected siblings of the proband usually have two HLA haplotypes identical to those of the proband, whereas unaffected siblings have one or neither haplotype identical to the proband[1–3,5,25].

The majority of homozygous relatives will eventually exhibit full clinical and biochemical expression of the disease, although this depends on oral iron intake and physiological (and pathological) blood loss. In a recent Australian study[5] 47 of 50 homozygous relatives (as determined by HLA studies) expressed the disease, either at first assessment or during a follow-up period of up to 8 years. In contrast, heterozygotes may demonstrate minor biochemical abnormalities of iron status, but do not develop a progressive increase in body iron stores of the order seen in homozygotes. In rare putative heterozygotes who appear to develop progressive iron overload, the possibility of either a chromosomal recombination, or a homozygous–heterozygous mating, resulting in misclassification of homozygotes as heterozygotes, must be considered[1–3,5,58].

The precise location of the HC gene on chromosome 6 has been difficult to ascertain, but the identification of short tandem repeat sequences (microsatellites) has now furnished a number of highly polymorphic markers. In 13 large pedigrees studied in an Australian population, there was a clear association between HC and specific alleles at HLA-A and D6S105, i.e. HLA-A3 and D6S105 allele 8. In an analysis of 82 unrelated HC patients and 82 unrelated healthy controls D6S105-8 was present in 93% of patients and 21% of controls ($\chi^2 = 86.46$; $p < 0.0001$). The approximate relative risk for this allele was 48.4. HLA-A3 was present in 62% of patients and 26% of controls ($\chi^2 = 22.8$, $p < 0.0001$). Approximate relative risk for A3 was 4.8. These results indicate that D6S105 is the closest marker to the HC gene so far reported[58]. A more recent haplotype analysis of chromosomes from 26 HC pedigrees containing multiply affected subjects was carried out in Australia[59]. A predominant ancestral haplotype allele 5-1-3-2-8 (marker order D6S248-D6S265-HLA-A-HLA-F-D6S105) was exclusively associated with HC (relative risk 903 for this haplotype), and was present in 33% of the 64 affected chromosomes. This provides strong evidence for a common mutation associated with HC in Australian patients and the probable introduction of HC into the population on an ancestral haplotype. An analysis of hepatic iron stores as assessed by chemical determination of the liver iron concentration and determination of the hepatic iron index in siblings was carried out in 22 sib pairs with HC[60]. A wide range of hepatic iron concentration (32–833 μmol/g dry weight) was found, and the hepatic iron index ranged from 1.65 to 14.4. These differences could not be

---

Note added in proof: A recent paper has described a novel gene (which has been called NLA-H) which is mutated in patients with haemochromatosis. 83% of 178 patients were homozygous for the mutation (Feder JN *et al*. Nature Genetics. 1996;13:399–413).

accounted for by differing exposure to the environmental factors that influence iron stores. However, a highly significant correlation for hepatic iron concentration ($r = 0.81$) and also for hepatic iron index ($r = 0.7$) was found between sibs of the same sex. These data provide strong evidence that genetic factors are the principal determinants of the amount of iron that accumulates in genetic HC. Recent evidence also suggests that HC patients with two copies of the ancestral haplotype show significantly more severe expression of the disorder[61]. Despite all the evidence cited above, the elucidation of the basic metabolic defect still awaits the cloning and sequencing of the HLA-A linked gene on the short arm of chromosome 6.

TREATMENT AND PROGNOSIS

There is now strong circumstantial evidence that venesection therapy prolongs life and at least partly reverses established tissue damage. This treatment should be undertaken as rapidly as possible, to minimize the risk of complications. In iron overload secondary to chronic anaemia, or in patients with severe heart failure who do not tolerate repeated venesection, iron-chelating agents should be used. The most cost-effective method of follow-up during therapy is to determine haemoglobin frequently with intermittent ferritin and transferrin saturation determinations.

In 1935[6], when treatment was limited to supportive measures for the complications of the disease such as diabetes, liver disease and heart failure, the mean survival after diagnosis was 4.4 years[7]. Primary liver cell cancer developed in 14% of patients at that time. By 1969, phlebotomy had improved the 5-year survival rate to 89%[62], and more recent studies show similar figures[63]. Strong evidence exists that the disease may be prevented by removal of excessive iron before tissue damage has occurred, providing reaccumulation of iron is prevented[1,64]; thus HCC does not appear to develop if the disease is treated before cirrhosis is present. The complications and natural course of the disease should be entirely preventable in patients and relatives with early iron overload.

References

1. Bassett ML, Halliday JW, Powell LW. HLA typing in idiopathic haemochromatosis: distinction between homozygotes and heterozygotes with biochemical expression. Hepatology. 1981;1:120–6.
2. Simon M, Alexandre JL, Bourel M, Le Marec B, Scordia C. Heredity of idiopathic haemochromatosis: a study of 106 families. Clin Genet. 1977;11:327–41.
3. Simon M, Bourel M, Genetet B, Fauchet R. Idiopathic haemochromatosis: demonstration of recessive transmission and early detection of family HLA typing. N Engl J Med. 1977;297:1017–21.
4. Leggett BA, Halliday JW, Brown NN, Bryant S, Powell LW. Prevalence of haemochromatosis amongst asymptomatic Australians. Br J Haematol. 1990;74:525–30.
5. Powell LW, Summers KM, Board PG, Axelsen E, Webb S, Halliday JW. Expression of haemochromatosis in homozygous subjects: implication for early diagnosis and prevention. Gastroenterology. 1990;98:1625–32.
6. Sheldon JH. Haemochromatosis. London: Oxford University Press; 1935.
7. Finch SC, Finch CA. Idiopathic haemochromatosis, an iron storage disease. A. Iron metabolism in haemochromatosis. Medicine. 1955;34:381.

8. Halliday JW, Russo A, Cowlishaw J, Powell LW. Serum ferritin in the diagnosis of early haemochromatosis: a study of 43 families. Lancet. 1977;2:621–3.

9. Bassett ML, Halliday JW, Bryan S, Dent O, Powell LW. Screening for haemochromatosis. Ann NY Acad Sci (New York). 1988;526:274–89.

10. Bassett ML, Halliday JW, Powell LW. Value of hepatic iron measurement in early haemochromatosis and determination of the critical iron level associated with fibrosis. Hepatology. 1986;6:24–9.

11. Summers KM, Halliday JW, Powell LW. Identification of homozygous haemochromatosis subjects by measurement of hepatic iron index. Hepatology. 1990;12:20–5.

12. Bradbear RA, Bain C, Siskind V *et al.* Cohort study of internal malignancy in genetic haemochromatosis and other chronic non-alcoholic liver diseases. J Natl Cancer Inst. 1985;75:81–4.

13. Halliday JW, Powell LW. Ferritin and cellular iron metabolism. Ann NY Acad Sci (New York). 1988;526:101–12.

14. Powell LW, Bassett ML, Axelsen E, Ferluga J, Halliday JW. Is all genetic (hereditary) haemochromatosis HLA-related? Ann NY Acad Sci (New York). 1988;526:23–33.

15. Edwards CQ, Carroll M, Bray P, Cartwright GE. Hereditary haemochromatosis. N Engl J Med. 1977;297:7–13.

16. Powell LW, Halliday JW. Serum ferritin in haemochromatosis. N Engl J Med. 1976;294:1185.

17. Wands JR, Rowe JA, Mezey SE *et al.* Normal serum ferritin concentrations in pre-cirrhotic haemochromatosis. N Engl J Med. 1976;294:302.

18. Feller ER, Pont A, Wands JR *et al.* Familial haemochromatosis. N Engl J Med. 1977;296:1422–6.

19. Grace ND, Powell LW. Iron storage disorders of the liver. Gastroenterology. 1974;64:1257–83.

20. Powell LW, Halliday JW, Cowlishaw JL. The relationship between serum ferritin and total body iron stores in idiopathic haemochromatosis. Gut. 1978;19:538–42.

21. Chapman RWG, Williams G, Bydder G, Dick R, Sherlock S, Kreel L. Computed tomography for determining liver iron content in primary haemochromatosis. Br Med J. 1980;1:440–2.

22. Gollan J. Diagnosis of haemochromatosis. Gastroenterology. 1983;84:418–31.

23. Howard JM, Ghent CN, Carey LS, Flanagan PR, Valberg LS. Diagnostic efficacy of hepatic computed tomography in the detection of body iron overload. Gastroenterology. 1983;84:209–15.

24. Brittenham GM, Farrell DE, Harris JW *et al.* Magnetic-susceptibility measurement of human iron stores. N Engl J Med. 1982;307:1671–5.

25. Bassett ML, Halliday JW, Powell LW. Early detection of idiopathic haemochromatosis: relative value of serum ferritin and HLA typing. Lancet. 1979;2:4–7.

26. Crawford DHG, Leggett BA, Powell LW, Halliday JW. Factors influencing disease expression in haemochromatosis. Annu Rev Nutr. 1995;16:139–60.

27. Searle J, Kerr JFR, Halliday JW, Powell LW. Iron storage disease. In: MacSween RNM, Anthony PP, Scheuer PJ, Portmann BC, Burt AD, editors. Pathology of the liver, 3rd edn. London: Churchill Livingstone; 1944:219–41.

28. Klausner RD. From receptors to genes – insights from molecular iron metabolism. Clin Res. 1988;36:494–500.

29. Bothwell TH. Iron deficiency. Med J Aust. 1972;2:433–8.

30. Teichmann R, Stremmel W. Iron uptake by human upper small intestine microvillus membrane vesicles. Indication for a facilitated transport mechanism mediated by a membrane iron-binding protein. J Clin Invest. 1990;86:2145.

31. Conrad ME, Umbreit JN, Moore EG, Peterson RDA, Jones MBA. A newly identified iron binding protein in duodenal mucosa of rats. J Biol Chem. 1990;265:5273–9.

32. Stremmel W, Arvailer D, Voerbuchep M, Teichmann R, Diede HE, Strohmeyer G. The membrane iron binding protein is enriched in the liver of patients with primary haemochromatosis. Hepatology. 1991;14:142A.

33. McLaren GD, Nathanson MH, Jacobs A, Trevett D, Thomson W. Regulation of intestinal iron absorption and mucosal iron kinetics in hereditary haemochromatosis. J Lab Clin Med. 1991;117:390–401.

34. Kuhn LC. mRNA–protein interactions regulate critical pathways in cellular iron metabolism. Br J Haematol. 1991;79:1–5.

35. Hentze MW, Caughman SW, Casey JW *et al*. A model for the structure and functions of iron-responsive elements. Gene. 1988;72:201–8.

36. Hentze MW, Seuanez HN, O'Brien SJ, Harford JB, Klausner RD. Chromosomal localization of nucleic acid-binding proteins by affinity mapping: assignment of the IRE-binding protein gene to human chromosome 9. Nucleic Acids Res. 1989;17:6103–8.

37. Hentze MW, Rouault TA, Harford JB, Klausner RD. Oxidation–reduction and the molecular mechanism of a regulatory RNA–protein interaction. Science. 1989;244:357–9.

38. Whittaker P, Skikne BS, Covell AM, Flowers C, Cooke A, Lynch SL. Duodenal iron proteins in idiopathic haemochromatosis. J Clin Invest. 1989;83:261–7.

39. Fracanzani AL, Fargion S, Romeno R, Piperno A, Arosio P, Fiorelli G. Immunohistochemical evidence for a lack of ferritin in duodenal absorptive epithelial cells in idiopathic haemochromatosis. Gastroenterology. 1989;6:1071–8.

40. Pietrangelo A, Rocchi E, Rigo G *et al*. Regulation of transferrin, transferrin receptor and ferritin gene expression in the duodenum of normal anaemic and siderotic subjects. Gastroenterology. 1992;102:802–9.

41. Pietrangelo A, Casalgrandi G, Quaglino D *et al*. Duodenal ferritin synthesis in genetic haemochromatosis. Gastroenterology. 1995;108:208–17.

42. Banerjee D, Falagan OR, Cluett J, Valberg LS. Transferrin receptors in the human gastrointestinal tract. Gastroenterology. 1986;91:861–9.

43. Anderson GJ, Powell LW, Halliday JW. Transferrin receptor distribution and regulation in the rat small intestine. Effect of iron stores and erythropoiesis. Gastroenterology. 1990;98:576–85.

44. Anderson GJ, Walsh MD, Powell LW, Halliday JW. Intestinal transferrin receptors and iron absorption in the neonatal rat. Br J Haematol. 1991;77:229–36.

45. Srai SKS, Epstein O, Denham ES, McIntyre N. The ontogeny of iron absorption and its possible relationship to pathogenesis of haemochromatosis. Hepatology. 1984;4:1033.

46. Srai SKS, Denham E, Epstein O. Development changes in the villous uptake of iron and enterocyte iron binding proteins in the guinea pig duodenum. Gut. 1987;28:A1333.

47. Summers KM, Tam KS, Bartley PB *et al*. Fine mapping of a chromosome 6 ferritin heavy chain gene: Relevance to haemochromatosis. Hum Genet. 1991;88:175–8.

48. Cook JD, Barry WE, Hershko C. Iron kinetics with emphasis on iron overload. Am J Pathol. 1973;72:337–43.

49. Batey RG, Pettit JE, Nicholas AW, Sherlock S, Hoffbrand A. Hepatic iron clearance from serum in treated haemochromatosis. Gastroenterology. 1978;75:856–9.

50. Adams PC, Reece AS, Powell LW, Halliday JW. Hepatic iron in the control of iron absorption in a rat liver transplantation model. Transplantation. 1989;48:19–21.

51. Adams PC, Zhong R, Haist J, Flanagan PR, Grant DR. Mucosal iron in the control of iron absorption in a rat transplantation model. Gastroenterology. 1991;100:370–4.

52. Powell LW. Does transplantation of the liver cure genetic haemochromatosis? J Hepatol. 1992;16:259–61.

53. Sciot R, Paterson AC, Van Den Oord JJ, Desmet VJ. Lack of hepatic transferrin receptor expression in haemochromatosis. Hepatology. 1987;7:831–7.

54. Brissot P, Wright TL, Ma W-L, Weisiger RA. Efficient clearance of non-transferrin bound iron by rat liver. J Clin Invest. 1985;76:1463–70.

55. Wright T, Brissot P, Ma W-L, Weisiger RA. Characterization of non-transferrin-bound iron clearance by rat liver. J Biol Chem. 1986;261:10909–14.

56. Wright T, Fitz JG, Weisiger RA. Non-transferrin-bound iron uptake by rat liver. J Biol Chem. 1988;263:1842–7.

57. Mercer JFB, Livingston J, Hall B *et al*. Isolation of a partial candidate gene for Menkes disease by positional cloning. Nat Genet. 1993;3:20–5.

58. Jazwinska EC, Lee SC, Webb SI, Halliday JW, Powell LW. Localization of the haemochromatosis gene close to D6S105. Am J Hum Genet. 1993;53:347–52.

59. Jazwinska EC, Pyper WR, Burt MJ *et al*. Haplotype analysis in Australian haemochromatosis patients: evidence for a predominant ancestral haplotype exclusively associated with haemochromatosis. Am J Hum Genet. 1995;56:428–33.

60. Crawford DHG, Halliday JW, Summers KM, Bourke MJ, Powell LW. Concordance of iron storage in siblings with genetic haemochromatosis: evidence for a predominantly genetic effect on iron storage. Hepatology. 1993;17:833–7.

61. Crawford DHG, Powell LW, Leggett BA *et al.* Evidence that the ancestral haplotype in Australian haemochromatosis patients may be associated with a common mutation in the gene. Am J Hum Genet. 1995;57:362–7.
62. Williams R, Smith PM, Spicer EJ, Barry M, Sherlock S. Venesection therapy in idiopathic haemochromatosis. Q J Med. 1969;38:1–16.
63. Niederau C, Fischer R, Sonnenberg A, Stremmel W, Trampish HJ, Strohmeyer G. Survival and causes of death in cirrhotic and in noncirrhotic patients with primary haemochromatosis. N Engl J Med. 1985;313:1256–62.
64. Bassett ML, Halliday JW, Ferris RA, Powell LW. Haemochromatosis: predictive accuracy of biochemical screening tests. Gastroenterology. 1984;87:628–33.

11
Wilson disease after cloning of the gene

J. L. GOLLAN

INTRODUCTION

It is more than 80 years since the London neurologist Samuel Alexander Kinnier Wilson defined the familial syndrome of progressive lenticular degeneration associated with cirrhosis of the liver. Considerable advances have been achieved in elucidating the clinical, biochemical, genetic and histological features, as well as in the management of patients with this disease[1]. With the recent cloning of the Wilson disease gene, our understanding of the disease has surged forward, although clarification of the pathogenetic defect and the application of genetic screening are among the problems yet to be resolved.

GENETICS

The gene for Wilson disease is distributed worldwide, and has been demonstrated in virtually all races. Current estimates indicate that the prevalence of the disease is approximately 1 in 30 000 livebirths, with an incidence ranging from 15 to 30 per million. The gene frequency varies between 0.3% and 0.7%, corresponding to a heterozygote carrier rate of slightly greater than 1 in 100.

Genetic studies of a large Israeli–Arab kindred identified a linkage between the Wilson disease locus and the red cell enzyme esterase D, thereby establishing that the gene mutation responsible for Wilson disease was located on chromosome 13[2]. Using multipoint linkage techniques the abnormal gene for Wilson disease was subsequently localized more specifically to 13q14-q21. In 1993 a candidate gene for Wilson disease (WND) was reported independently by several different groups of investigators, using slightly different positional cloning strategies[3–5]. The WND gene (designated ATP7B) consists of a transcript of approximately 7.5 kilobases, which is expressed primarily in liver, kidney and placenta; it also has been detected in heart, brain, lung, muscle and pancreas, albeit at much lower levels. The full-length cDNA sequence of the WND gene[3,5] predicts a 1411 amino acid protein, which is a member of the cation-transporting P-type ATPase subfamily, highly homologous to the Menkes disease gene product and the copper-transporting ATPase (cop A) found in copper-resistant strains of *Enterococcus hirae*. From sequence analysis of the cDNA, the WND protein is predicted to possess a metal-binding domain (containing five specific binding sites), an ATP-binding domain, a cation channel and phosphorylation region, and a transduction domain responsible for the conversion of the energy of ATP hydrolysis to cation transport.

To date, more than 40 unique mutations in the Wilson disease gene have been identified, the majority of which are single-base transversions or deletions. The wide spectrum of clinical manifestations in Wilson disease raises the question as to whether variability exists at the molecular level. The fact that Wilson disease is linked to chromosome 13 markers in all populations studied suggests that there is a single genetic locus for the disease, and it has been postulated that different mutations at that locus may explain the clinical variability. Indeed, physiological studies employing an animal model of Wilson disease reveal that a single gene mutation may inhibit copper transport at multiple locations within the cell. Hence, the variety of mutations identified in the Wilson disease gene potentially may affect copper transport to varying degrees, and at different cellular sites[6]. However, detailed genetic and epidemiological studies suggest that the variability in clinical expression observed in Wilson disease patients may not be solely a consequence of allelic heterogeneity, since marked differences in presentation, age of onset and disease course have been observed in family members who have inherited two identical mutant alleles.

DNA-BASED DIAGNOSIS

Developments involving the molecular genetics of Wilson disease have provided a means for carrier detection and early diagnosis[7,8]. In fact, several studies using haplotype analysis of relatives with closely linked markers have permitted precise carrier detection with less than 1–2% error. There is also a report of prenatal exclusion of Wilson disease by analysis of DNA polymorphism in a chorionic-villous biopsy performed at 9 weeks' gestation[9]. Unfortunately, the use of genetic techniques in the diagnosis of Wilson disease currently has significant limitations. DNA marker studies can be performed only within families, and under circumstances in which the diagnosis has already been established definitively in at least one family member by standard biochemical methods. The index patient's DNA is then used as a reference to recognize the disease-carrying chromosomes in other members of the family. However, spontaneous chromosomal rearrangements may cause such markers to be uninformative, thereby limiting the diagnostic reliability.

These findings indicate considerable potential difficulties for DNA-based genetic screening, since most patients will possess alleles with two different mutations of the Wilson disease gene[6]. Moreover, evaluation for Wilson disease by DNA marker analysis currently is not widely available, and frequently requires weeks before a result is available. Given the rapidity and accuracy of biochemical analyses in establishing the diagnosis of Wilson disease, as well as the aforementioned limitations of genetic testing, standard biochemical methods should continue to be utilized in the evaluation of the vast majority of suspected cases[6]. The most likely application of DNA linkage analysis will be in the uncommon situation in which biochemical methods do not provide a definitive answer, particularly under circumstances where patients have received prior chelation therapy. In addition, genetic screening of young presymptomatic family members of patients afflicted with the disorder would facilitate early diagnosis and permit initiation of therapy in the presymptomatic state[8].

PATHOGENESIS

It is postulated that the harmful effects of excess copper are mediated by the generation of free radicals, which deplete cellular stores of glutathione and oxidize lipids, enzymes and cytoskeletal proteins. Indeed, it has been shown that a number of intracellular systems are disrupted by elevated copper concentrations, including organellar membranes, DNA, microtubules, and various enzymes and proteins, although the principal cellular target of copper toxicity is unknown. In the earliest stages of hepatocellular injury, ultrastructural abnormalities involving the endoplasmic reticulum, mitochondria, peroxisomes and nuclei all have been identified[10]. These changes, in conjunction with diminished mitochondrial enzyme activities, may be important steps in the pathophysiological events leading to lipid peroxidation and triglyceride accumulation in the hepatocyte[10].

Wilson disease patients exhibit impaired biliary excretion of copper, which is believed to be the fundamental cause of the copper overload. The prompt reversal of abnormal copper metabolism in Wilson disease patients following orthotopic liver transplantation confirms that the primary defect resides in the liver. It has been proposed that the Wilson disease gene product is responsible for copper excretion from the liver cell, either across the canalicular (apical) membrane of the hepatocyte or more likely into a subcellular compartment that ultimately communicates with the bile canaliculus[5]. The latter is consistent with a Golgi-related or lysosomal defect underlying the diminished biliary excretion and systemic accumulation of copper observed in patients with Wilson disease[11]. In addition, in an animal model of Wilson disease, the Long–Evans Cinnamon rat, excessive hepatic copper accumulation occurs in the setting of diminished biliary excretion. These rodents exhibit impaired entry of copper into the lysosomes, with normal delivery of lysosomal copper to the bile[12]. The Long–Evans Cinnamon (LEC) rat is a mutant strain of the Long–Evans rat, which spontaneously develops fulminant hepatitis at 3–4 months of age, resulting in a 40% mortality rate. Surviving animals manifest chronic hepatic disease, low serum caeruloplasmin levels, and increased copper concentrations in the liver. Thus, the LEC rat shares many important clinical, biochemical and histological features with Wilson disease, and the recent availability of this animal model will probably provide new insight into the pathogenesis of the human disorder.

CLINICAL FEATURES

The biochemical defect which leads to the accumulation of copper in Wilson disease is present at birth; however, clinical symptoms are rarely observed before the age of 5 years. The initial signs of Wilson disease generally are detected in older children, adolescents and young adults. Patients typically present with hepatic and/or neurological dysfunction. In a large series of patients[13], the initial clinical manifestations were hepatic in 42%, neurological in 34%, psychiatric in 10%, haematological in 12% and renal in 1%. Less commonly, patients present with skeletal, cardiac, ophthalmological, endocrinological or dermatological symptoms (Table 1). Approximately 25% of the patients have involvement of two or more organ systems at initial evaluation, although with the advent of aggressive screening there has been a significant increase in the number of asymptomatic patients diagnosed.

Table 1 Clinical manifestations of Wilson disease

Hepatic	Cirrhosis, chronic active hepatitis, fulminant hepatic failure
Neurological	Bradykinesia, rigidity, tremor, ataxia, dyskinesia, dysarthria, seizures
Psychiatric	Behavioural disturbances, cognitive impairment, affective disorder, psychosis
Ophthalmological	Kayser–Fleischer rings, sunflower cataracts
Haematological	Haemolysis, coagulopathy
Renal	Renal tubular defects, diminished glomerular filtration, nephrolithiasis
Cardiovascular	Cardiomyopathy, arrhythmias, conduction disturbances, autonomic dysfunction
Musculoskeletal	Osteomalacia, osteoporosis, degenerative joint disease
Gastrointestinal	Cholelithiasis, pancreatitis, spontaneous bacterial peritonitis
Endocrinological	Amenorrhoea, spontaneous abortion, delayed puberty, gynaecomastia
Dermatological	Azure lunulae, hyperpigmentation, acanthosis nigricans

Adapted from Zucker SD., Gollan JL. Wilson's disease: pathophysiology and therapy. In: Prieto J, Rodés J, Shafritz DA, editors. Hepatobiliary diseases. Berlin: Springer-Verlag; 1992:809 (with permission).

HEPATIC MANIFESTATIONS

Hepatic involvement in Wilson disease tends to manifest at a younger age (mean of 8–12 years) than does neurological dysfunction, and is non-specific, mimicking the features of a variety of acute and chronic liver diseases. Three major clinical patterns of liver disease are observed: cirrhosis, chronic active hepatitis and fulminant hepatic failure. In the early asymptomatic phase of Wilson disease, or in the presence of inactive cirrhosis, liver tests may be normal or only minimally elevated. In the majority of cases, hepatic injury develops insidiously and, if untreated, pursues a chronic and relentless course to cirrhosis.

An estimated 5–30% of patients with Wilson disease exhibit clinical, biochemical and histological features similar to those observed in chronic active hepatitis[14,15]. The diagnosis may be overlooked in these patients, since a significant percentage, almost 50% in one series[14], have no evidence of neurological dysfunction or Kayser–Fleischer rings on ophthalmological examination. Serum caeruloplasmin levels may also be normal in the setting of severe hepatic inflammation. It has been estimated that Wilson disease represents the underlying aetiology in 5% of patients with idiopathic chronic active hepatitis who are under 35 years of age[15]. A distinctive feature of Wilsonian chronic active hepatitis is the relatively modest elevations of serum aminotransferase levels in the presence of severe hepatocellular necrosis and inflammation [15].

Wilson disease occasionally manifests as fulminant hepatic failure. These patients may be indistinguishable from individuals with viral-induced hepatic necrosis, and many of the biochemical tests used to establish the diagnosis of Wilson disease are abnormal in patients with other forms of fulminant hepatic failure[16]. The clinical features most suggestive of fulminant Wilsonian hepatitis include the presence of intravascular haemolysis, splenomegaly and Kayser–Fleischer rings. Biochemical markers indicative of Wilson disease include relatively mild elevations in serum transaminases despite massive hepatic necrosis, hyperbilirubinaemia with normal or low alkaline phosphatase levels, and a markedly elevated serum copper concentration[16]. The serum level of aspartate aminotransferase (AST) is typically higher than that of alanine aminotransferase (ALT), as a result of the associated haemolysis. Although uncommonly observed in Wilsonian fulminant hepatic failure, Kayser–Fleischer rings are not pathognomonic, since they are occasionally seen in patients with other cholestatic hepatic diseases. The presence of severe coagulopathy and hypercupriuria are not useful in distinguishing Wilsonian from non-Wilsonian hepatic failure[16]. Liver biopsy with measurement of quantitative copper may be helpful, although deranged clotting function may preclude this procedure or necessitate the transjugular approach. If a biopsy specimen is obtained, histological evidence of cirrhosis (predominantly micronodular) in a young patient with fulminant hepatitis is suggestive of Wilson disease, as is an elevated hepatic copper content.

Wilson disease patients with acute hepatic failure tend to be young and to have a fulminant clinical course, with survival generally no longer than days to weeks unless hepatic transplantation is performed[16,17]. Medical treatment is frequently unsuccessful, particularly when the disorder is associated with haemolysis and renal insufficiency. It should be noted, however, that there are reports of recovery from Wilsonian chronic active hepatitis with acute hepatic failure on medical therapy alone. Even when transplantation is unavailable, it remains imperative to make the diagnosis of Wilson disease for the purpose of aggressive medical therapy and family screening.

HEPATIC PATHOLOGY

Abnormal liver histology is evident in biopsy specimens from asymptomatic Wilson disease patients within the first decade of life. The earliest changes detectable on light microscopy include glycogen deposition in the nuclei of periportal hepatocytes, and moderate fatty infiltration. The lipid droplets, which are composed of triglycerides, progressively increase in number and size, in some cases resembling the steatosis induced by ethanol. Ultrastructural abnormalities in the liver cells may coexist with, or even precede, the changes observed by light microscopy. Hepatocyte mitochondria typically exhibit heterogeneity in size and shape, with increased matrix density, separation of the normally apposed inner and outer mitochondrial membranes, widened intercristal spaces, and an array of vacuolated and crystalline inclusions within the matrix. Although similar isolated abnormalities may be observed in other pathological conditions, the simultaneous occurrence of several of these anomalies in the same mitochondrion appears to be specific for patients with early Wilson disease. The mitochondrial changes generally become less pronounced or disappear after several years of therapy with D-penicillamine, indirectly supporting the notion that these abnormalities are a consequence of copper toxicity. Over time the ultrastructural abnormalities found in early Wilson disease usually regress as the liver disease progresses to hepatic fibrosis and, ultimately, cirrhosis.

The histochemical staining of liver biopsy specimens for copper is of little diagnostic value in patients with Wilson disease. This is because, during the initial stages of copper accumulation, the metal is distributed diffusely in the cytoplasm and is frequently undetectable by rhodamine or rubeanic acid staining. Orcein, which is believed to stain polymerized metallothionein sequestered in lysosomes, exhibits a characteristic granular pattern in only half of patients with early Wilson disease. As the disease becomes more advanced, copper is sequestered within hepatocyte lysosomes and is detectable by routine histochemical techniques, even though tissue concentrations are actually lower than in earlier stages of the disorder. In contradistinction to Wilson disease, other conditions in which hepatic copper is elevated (e.g. primary biliary cirrhosis, sclerosing cholangitis, biliary atresia, intrahepatic cholestasis of childhood, Indian childhood cirrhosis, idiopathic copper toxicosis, and the normal neonate) are nearly always associated with stainable copper. Due to the insensitivity of copper staining techniques, time-dependent changes in the distribution of copper within the liver cell, heterogeneity of hepatic copper deposition, and the lack of specificity of hepatocyte copper granules, histochemical staining for copper is unreliable in establishing the diagnosis of Wilson disease.

The rate of progression of the liver histology from fatty infiltration to cirrhosis is variable, although it tends to occur by one of two general processes, either with or without hepatic inflammation. Some Wilson disease patients develop a histological picture that is indistinguishable from chronic active hepatitis[14,15]. Pathological features include mononuclear cell infiltrates, which consist mainly of lymphocytes and plasma cells, piecemeal necrosis extending beyond the limiting plate, parenchymal collapse, bridging hepatic necrosis and fibrosis. If untreated, this may evolve into macronodular cirrhosis or progress rapidly to fulminant hepatitis. The development of cirrhosis may also occur in the absence of significant parenchymal inflammatory infiltrate or necrosis. It is notable that the vast majority of Wilson disease patients have evidence of fibrosis on liver biopsy, despite widely varying levels and patterns of hepatic inflammation and injury.

Hepatocellular carcinoma is uncommonly associated with Wilson disease, in contrast to haemochromatosis. It has been proposed that the diminished cancer risk is due to the relative dearth of an inflammatory component in the pathogenesis of Wilsonian cirrhosis. Indeed, animal studies suggest that copper may exert a protective effect against the development of malignancy. On the other hand, LEC rats exhibit a high incidence of hepatocellular carcinoma in the setting of marked hepatic copper accumulation[18], and this neoplastic potential is effectively abrogated by the administration of D-penicillamine. These observations have led to speculation that the low incidence of hepatocellular carcinoma in Wilson disease patients is attributable to chelation therapy, as long-term survival is uncommon in untreated patients.

DIAGNOSIS OF WILSON DISEASE

The simplest screening procedure includes a slit-lamp examination of the eyes, and measurement of serum caeruloplasmin and transaminase (ALT, AST) levels. If Kayser–Fleischer rings are present on ophthalmological examination and caeruloplasmin levels are below 20 mg/dl in a patient with neurological signs or symptoms, the diagnosis of Wilson disease is established. If a patient is asymptomatic, exhibits isolated liver disease, or lacks corneal rings, the co-existence of a hepatic copper concentration above 250 μg/g dry weight and a low serum caeruloplasmin level is also sufficient to make the diagnosis.

Serum caeruloplasmin

The normal serum concentration of caeruloplasmin is 20–40 mg/dl. Levels are low in the human newborn, although they gradually rise during the first 2 years of life, coincident with the postnatal decline in hepatic copper concentration. Although a decreased caeruloplasmin level *per se* is not diagnostic of Wilson disease, approximately 90% of all patients (85% of individuals presenting with hepatic manifestations of the disease) have levels of this glycoprotein that are below the normal range. Hypocaeruloplasminaemia may occasionally occur in other hepatic conditions, such as fulminant non-Wilsonian hepatitis, due to diminished hepatic synthetic function. Patients with nephrotic syndrome, protein-losing enteropathy, malabsorption, or severe malnutrition may also manifest low serum caeruloplasmin levels, although there is usually no diag-nostic difficulty in these cases.

Confusion may arise with regard to the 10% of heterozygous carriers of the gene for Wilson disease who manifest diminished serum levels of caerulo-plasmin, yet never develop clinical symptoms or signs of the disease. These individuals, who represent approximately 1 in 2000 persons in the general popu-lation, may present a difficult diagnostic dilemma if they fortuitously develop chronic active hepatitis or cirrhosis (of another aetiology), thereby mimicking the clinical, biochemical and histological features of Wilson disease.

Normal caeruloplasmin concentrations are found in up to 15% of patients with Wilson disease and active liver involvement[14]. This presumably is due to increased hepatic synthesis and release of the glycoprotein in response to hepatic inflammation, as caeruloplasmin is an 'acute phase reactant'. The caerulo-plasmin concentration declines to the low levels typically associated with Wilson disease as the inflammatory activity in the liver abates; a further reduction in the caeruloplasmin level generally follows the initiation of chelation therapy. Plasma concentrations are also influenced by a variety of humoral and hormonal agents, and elevated oestrogen levels, secondary to pregnancy or exogenous administration, may occasionally elevate previously low caerulo-plasmin levels into the normal range.

Urinary copper excretion

The urinary excretion of copper is greater than 100 μg/24 h (normal: <40 μg/24 h) in most patients with symptomatic Wilson disease, reflecting increased serum levels of the readily filterable fraction of non-caeruloplasmin copper. In patients with fulminant hepatic necrosis due to Wilson disease, urinary excretion of the metal may exceed 1000 μg/24 h, as hepatic copper stores are released into the systemic circulation. Unfortunately, the measurement of urinary copper is often misleading due to inaccuracies in collection and laboratory analysis, and care must be taken to use copper-free containers for storage of the urine samples. It should also be noted that asymptomatic Wilson disease patients do not necessarily exhibit elevated urinary copper concentrations. Moreover, urinary copper levels may be elevated in a variety of other hepatic disorders including cirrhosis, chronic active hepatitis and cholestatic disorders, such as primary biliary cirrhosis. The use of D-penicillamine to increase urinary copper excretion appears to be of little diagnostic value, since it does not reliably distinguish Wilson disease from other liver disorders. Thus, the quantification of urinary copper is of little value as a screening test for Wilson disease; although it may be useful as a means of confirming the diagnosis, and in evaluating compliance and the response to chelation therapy.

Hepatic copper concentration

If Kayser–Fleischer rings or neurological abnormalities are absent, a liver biopsy for quantitative copper determination is essential to establish the diagnosis of Wilson disease. Care must be taken to ensure that the biopsy needle and specimen container are free from copper contamination. It is recommended that a disposable needle made entirely of steel, or a Klatskin or Menghini needle washed in 0.1 mol/L EDTA and rinsed with demineralized water, be used. In addition, the syringe should contain 5% dextrose rather than saline solution, and an adequate-sized sample (2 cm core) should be sent for quantitative copper analysis. The normal hepatic copper concentration varies from 15 to 55 μg/g (0.24–0.87 μmol/g) dry liver. Virtually all untreated patients with Wilson disease have elevated hepatic copper levels, ranging from 250 to as high as 3000 μg/g dry liver. Values below 250 μg/g are usually attributable to the irregular distribution of copper in the liver, particularly in the presence of cirrhosis, when small fragmented biopsy samples are obtained.

The finding of a normal hepatic copper concentration effectively excludes the diagnosis of untreated Wilson disease. However, an elevated liver copper level alone is insufficient to establish the diagnosis of Wilson disease, since concentrations above 250 μg/g may be found in other chronic hepatic disorders (mostly cholestatic), including primary biliary cirrhosis, primary sclerosing cholangitis, extrahepatic biliary obstruction or atresia, intrahepatic cholestasis of childhood, chronic active hepatitis, Indian childhood cirrhosis, idiopathic copper toxicosis, and in vineyard sprayers inhaling copper salts. These patients are readily distinguished from those with Wilson disease on the basis of history, physical findings and biochemical testing. Moreover, in the great majority of individuals with prolonged cholestasis, serum caeruloplasmin concentrations are either normal or increased.

Incorporation of orally administered radiocopper into caeruloplasmin

Rarely, when a diagnostic dilemma remains or liver biopsy is contraindicated (e.g. severe coagulopathy), the radiocopper loading test may be useful[19]. Serum radioactivity is measured at 1, 2, 4 and 48 h after oral administration of the radionuclide (2 mg cupric acetate containing 0.3–0.5 mCi of ^{64}Cu, mixed in 100–150 ml fruit juice or ginger ale). In healthy subjects, and in patients with hepatic disorders that mimic Wilson disease, the plasma concentrations of radio-copper rise rapidly, are maximal within 1–2 h, and then fall and rise again over the ensuing 48 h, as the non-caeruloplasmin-bound radiocopper is incorporated into newly synthesized caeruloplasmin in the liver and then released into the circulation. Wilson disease patients, on the other hand, incorporate little or no radiocopper into nascent caeruloplasmin, even in the presence of normal caeruloplasmin concentrations. Heterozygotes have a pattern of incorporation that is intermediate between that of Wilson disease patients and healthy individuals.

Abdominal imaging

Despite advances in computerized tomography (CT) and magnetic resonance imaging (MRI), these radiological modalities are of little value in the diagnosis or evaluation of hepatic involvement in Wilson disease. While evidence of chronic liver disease (e.g. splenomegaly, heterogeneous liver parenchyma, varices) may be identified in patients with advanced disease, these findings are neither specific nor sensitive for Wilson disease.

DIAGNOSTIC SCREENING

The diagnostic approach to Wilson disease must be tailored according to the clinical presentation. It must be emphasized that, in the absence of definitive DNA haplotype analysis, the diagnosis of Wilson disease should not be based on the results of an individual laboratory test, and can be established only in the setting of confirmatory clinical and biochemical data. Patients with neurological or psychiatric manifestations should undergo slit-lamp examination of the eyes and determination of serum caeruloplasmin. The documentation of Kayser–Fleischer rings and a low serum caeruloplasmin concentration is sufficient to establish the diagnosis, which can be confirmed by the presence of an increased 24-h urinary copper excretion. A liver biopsy with quantification of hepatic copper is essential if either: (a) Kayser–Fleischer rings are absent (in order to exclude the possibility that the patient is heterozygous for the gene), or (b) caeruloplasmin levels are normal (as occurs in up to 15% of cases).

In patients who present primarily with hepatic dysfunction the diagnosis may be difficult, since caeruloplasmin levels may be falsely elevated and ophthalmo-logical findings absent. It is imperative that biochemical screening for Wilson disease be performed in all patients under 40 years of age who have clinical or histological findings compatible with chronic active hepatitis, and in whom autoimmune and viral hepatitis have been excluded. In patients with a high index of suspicion a serum caeruloplasmin concentration should be obtained, urinary copper excretion measured, and a liver biopsy performed (providing no contraindication exists). In the rare circumstance in which the diagnosis remains in doubt, a radiolabelled copper study may be confirmatory or, if feasible, haplotype analysis performed.

It is imperative that all first-degree relatives be screened, particularly siblings. Wilson disease may be clinically silent even in the presence of significant organ damage; hence, a delay in the diagnosis or in the initiation of therapy may lead to irreversible hepatic and/or neurological injury. Biochemical screening of children should not be performed prior to 3 or 4 years of age. The evaluation should consist of a careful history and physical examination, serological tests of liver function, a slit-lamp examination of the eyes, and a serum caeruloplasmin level, with liver biopsy and quantitative hepatic copper determination and/or DNA linkage analysis being reserved for diagnostic dilemmas. Once the diagnosis of presymptomatic Wilson disease is established, lifelong chelation therapy should be commenced immediately.

TREATMENT

Diet

The ubiquitous presence of copper in most foodstuffs makes stringent dietary copper restriction impractical. It is still suggested that patients avoid eating foods with a high copper content, such as liver, chocolate, nuts, mushrooms, legumes, and shellfish. Some authors also recommend the use of deionized or distilled water if the copper content of the patient's home drinking water exceeds 0.2 ppm, particularly during initial therapy. The use of domestic water softeners should be avoided, since these may substantially increase copper concentrations.

Pharmacological therapy

Penicillamine

Over the past three decades it has been well documented that oral D-penicillamine results in complete reversal or alleviation of hepatic, neurological and psychiatric abnormalities in most patients with Wilson disease, and this drug remains the 'gold standard' therapy for this disorder. The key to a successful outcome is early diagnosis and treatment, and clinical disease can be prevented indefinitely in asymptomatic patients, provided that they adhere to continuous maintenance therapy. Some individuals demonstrate a dramatic response within weeks of initiating D-penicillamine, while others may exhibit no clinical improvement, or even temporary neurological deterioration, for several months.

The precise mechanisms of action of D-penicillamine remain controversial. Although the logic for the use of this drug in the treatment of Wilson disease is based on its *in-vitro* copper-chelating properties, there is conflicting evidence regarding the ability of penicillamine to 'decopper' the liver and other organs. It has also been proposed that D-penicillamine detoxifies the liver by sequestering intracellular copper in an innocuous state, either through the direct formation of copper complexes or by the induction of metallothionein synthesis. The fulminant decompensation observed in previously compliant patients who discontinue D-penicillamine therapy for a relatively brief period of time offers support for this hypothesis. Other postulated mechanisms of action of D-penicillamine include inhibition of collagen crosslinking, enhancement of intracellular levels of reduced glutathione, and suppression of inflammation via effects on leukotriene and prostaglandin metabolism.

The standard dose of D-penicillamine is 1–2 g daily given orally in four divided doses 30 min before meals, although as much as 4 g/day can be administered to critically ill patients for brief periods of time. It is best taken on an empty stomach since food reduces its absorption. Most of the excess liver copper appears to be mobilized within the initial year of therapy, with urinary copper excretion approaching 2–5 mg/day during this period. After several years of treatment, urinary copper levels decline to approximately 0.5–1.0 mg daily, as hepatic copper concentrations approach normal levels. When symptoms have largely abated and a stable clinical course has been achieved, the maintenance dose of D-penicillamine may be reduced to 1 g daily. Liver function test abnormalities may persist for a year or more after the initiation of appropriate treatment. As they subside a corresponding resolution of hepatic histological and ultrastructural abnormalities is observed, although the regression of hepatic fibrosis and portal hypertension is less impressive.

A syndrome of acute deterioration has been described following the initiation of D-penicillamine therapy in as many as 20% of Wilson disease patients presenting with neurological symptoms. If observed, worsening of neurological dysfunction tends to occur within the first 4 weeks of therapy, and generally only in those patients who present with nervous system involvement, although the rare occurrence in asymptomatic patients has been reported. The cause of this exacerbation of neurological manifestations remains conjectural. However, the exacerbation of neurological sequelae associated with the initiation of treatment does not appear to be unique to penicillamine, as it has also been noted with all other forms of chelation therapy, including trientine. The dose of D-penicillamine should be reduced to 250 mg/day in any patient who exhibits an exacerbation of neurological symptoms following initiation of therapy. The dose should then be increased by 250 mg/day every 4–7 days until a urinary copper concentration of at least 2 mg/day is attained. Indeed, it may be prudent to introduce D-penicillamine in a low initial dose in *all* asymptomatic Wilson disease patients, or in those individuals presenting with mild symptomatology. Despite early clinical deterioration, continued treatment is mandatory in order to achieve subsequent improvement.

A variety of adverse effects of D-penicillamine have been recognized[1,13], although serious complications necessitating discontinuation of the drug are infrequent. Thus, D-penicillamine has been demonstrated to be effective and safe for use in the treatment of Wilson disease, and remains the first-line drug in this disorder.

Trientine

Trientine (triethylene tetramine dihydrochloride) was introduced in 1969 as an alternative chelating agent for cases in which serious toxic reactions to

D-penicillamine occur. It has been well established that 1–2 g administered orally in three divided doses induces negative copper balance and effects clinical improvement in patients with Wilson disease. As with penicillamine, trientine should be administered prior to meals, since food interferes with absorption. The exact mechanism of action of this drug remains unknown, although it has been shown to enhance urinary copper excretion and to decrease intestinal copper absorption. Unlike D-penicillamine, trientine causes the serum copper concentration to rise during cupriuresis, suggesting that the two agents may mobilize copper from different systemic pools. Most of the toxic side-effects necessitating conversion from D-penicillamine to trientine typically subside while on trientine. The exception is elastosis perforans serpiginosa, which may progress in some patients. Sideroblastic anaemia is the major side-effect attributed to this medication. Although trientine appears to cause minimal toxicity, it has less cupriuretic effect than D-penicillamine and, hence, is currently not recommended as primary therapy.

Zinc

The principal mode of action of zinc is postulated to be via the induction of intestinal metallothionein synthesis, which results in the sequestration of copper in intestinal epithelial cells, thereby preventing absorption into the portal circulation and enhancing faecal copper excretion. Zinc may also directly exhibit a protective effect on hepatocytes by inducing the synthesis of metallothionein in these cells. A minimum of 75 mg of zinc sulphate or zinc acetate per day, administered in two divided doses between meals, appears to maintain neutral or negative copper balance, although most studies have administered 50 mg thrice daily. Common side-effects of oral zinc include headaches and gastrointestinal upset, the incidence of which may be reduced by the use of zinc acetate, rather than zinc sulphate. Although long-term follow-up is limited, major complications have not been reported with the use of zinc for the treatment of Wilson disease.

Due to the slower onset of action as compared with other chelating agents, zinc is not recommended for the initial treatment of symptomatic Wilson disease. In fact, most of the published experience with zinc therapy has been in patients who previously had been decoppered with D-penicillamine. It has been suggested that zinc may be useful for presymptomatic or pregnant patients, as well as for maintenance therapy in individuals who have previously been decoppered with chelating drugs. However, there are data indicating that hepatic copper may continue to accrue in some Wilson disease patients treated with zinc alone[1]. Additionally, long-term follow-up studies are needed to determine whether the decoppered state is sustained with zinc therapy, and to monitor for untoward side-effects. Based on the information currently available, oral zinc should be used as a third-line therapy in the rare patients who develop intolerance to both D-penicillamine and trientine. There appears to be no synergistic effect of zinc in combination with a chelating agent; hence the concomitant administration of penicillamine or trientine and zinc is not currently recommended.

Thiomolybdates

Thiomolybdates appear to lower systemic copper levels by complexing lumenal copper, and thereby inhibiting intestinal absorption. In addition, the portion of the drug that is systemically absorbed may bind excessive serum copper and render it less available for cellular uptake, ultimately resulting in the removal of copper from intracellular stores. Moreover, in contrast to penicillamine and trientine, thiomolybdates exhibit a higher affinity for copper than metallothionein *in vitro*, suggesting that this drug may be able to more effectively remove copper from the cell. Limited studies of ammonium tetrathiomolybdate (60–100 mg daily in two divided doses) in Wilson disease patients in whom D-penicillamine and/or trientine was poorly tolerated or ineffective have demonstrated the drug to be highly successful in lowering hepatic copper concentrations[1]. Additional trials in a small number of patients have supported the efficacy and safety of ammonium tetrathiomolybdate in the initial treatment of Wilson disease, and have further suggested that this medication is less prone to precipitate the neurological decompensation observed with other chelating agents. Although these results appear promising, thiomolybdates have caused bone marrow suppression. Thus, further investigation is required before the routine use of this drug can be recommended.

Long-term management

Patients with Wilson disease require careful supervision during the first few months of therapy to ensure adequate copper excretion, and to monitor for the potential development of early adverse reactions to D-penicillamine. It is suggested that a physical examination be performed and a 24-h urinary copper excretion, complete blood count, urinalysis, and renal and liver function tests be checked on a weekly basis for the first 4–6 weeks following the initiation of chelation therapy. Bimonthly evaluations are then recommended through the first year, followed by at least yearly examinations thereafter. Lifelong chelation therapy, *without interruption*, is essential in all Wilson disease patients. Cessation of therapy may result in rapid and irreversible hepatic and neurological deterioration. In a study of 11 patients who discontinued treatment, eight patients died of fulminant hepatitis after an average period of only 2.6 years without treatment. Thus, it is imperative that an alternative agent be administered to any patient who is unable to continue D-penicillamine due to adverse effects[20].

Liver transplantation

Despite advances in medical therapy, significant mortality rates are still observed in specific subsets of patients with Wilson disease. These individuals, in whom orthotopic liver transplantation has proven most successful, generally present with acute fulminant hepatic failure associated with haemolysis and hypercupraemia (either as the initial presentation or following poor compliance with medical therapy), or with advanced cirrhosis and hepatic insufficiency, unresponsive to an adequate trial of chelation therapy and supportive measures. In the absence of severe hepatic disease, liver transplantation generally is not recommended for the management of refractory extrahepatic manifestations, such as neurological deterioration. In a series of 55 patients with Wilson disease who underwent hepatic transplantation, a 79% 1-year survival, and overall survival rate of 72% at 3 months to 20 years was reported[21]. Transplant recipients uniformly manifest complete reversal of the underlying defects in copper metabolism, and demonstrate significant improvement in most symptoms and signs of the disease.

References

1. Zucker SD, Gollan JL. Wilson's disease and hepatic copper toxicosis. In: Zakim D, Boyer TD, editors. Hepatology: a textbook of liver disease, 3rd edn. Philadelphia: Saunders; 1996:1105.
2. Frydman M, Bonne-Tamir B, Farrer LA *et al.* Assignment of the gene for Wilson's disease to chromosome 13: linkage to the esterase D locus. Proc Natl Acad Sci USA. 1985;82:1819.
3. Bull PC, Thomas GR, Rommens JM *et al.* The Wilson's disease gene is a putative copper transporting P-type ATPase similar to the Menkes gene. Nature Genet. 1993;5:327.
4. Petrukhin K, Fischer SG, Pirastu M *et al.* Mapping, cloning and genetic characterization of the region containing the Wilson disease gene. Nature Genet. 1993;5:338.
5. Tanzi RE, Petrukhin K, Chernov I *et al.* The Wilson disease gene is a copper transporting ATPase with homology to the Menkes disease gene. Nature Genet. 1993;5:344.
6. Schilsky ML. Identification of the Wilson's disease gene: clues for disease pathogenesis and the potential for molecular diagnosis. Hepatology. 1994;20:529.
7. Sternlieb I. The outlook for the diagnosis of Wilson's disease. J Hepatol. 1993;17:263.
8. Maier-Dobersberger T, Mannhalter C, Rack S *et al.* Diagnosis of Wilson's disease in an asymptomatic sibling by DNA linkage analysis. Gastroenterology. 1995;109:2015.
9. Cossu P, Pirastu M, Nucaro A *et al.* Prenatal diagnosis of Wilson's disease by analysis of DNA polymorphism. N Engl J Med. 1993;327:57.
10. Sternlieb I. Perspectives on Wilson's disease. Hepatology. 1990;12:1234.
11. Schilsky ML. Wilson disease: Genetic basis of copper toxicity and natural history. Sem Liver Dis. 1996;16:83.
12. Schilsky ML, Stockert RJ, Sternlieb I. Pleiotropic effect of the LEC mutation: a rodent model of Wilson's disease. Am J Physiol. 1994;266:G907.
13. Sternlieb I, Scheinberg IH. Wilson's disease. In: Wright R, Millward-Sadler GH, Alberti KGMM *et al.* editors. Liver and biliary disease. London: Saunders; 1985:949.
14. Scott J, Gollan JL, Samourian S *et al.* Wilson's disease, presenting as chronic active hepatitis. Gastroenterology. 1978;74:645.
15. Schilsky ML, Scheinberg IH, Sternlieb I. Prognosis of Wilsonian chronic active hepatitis. Gastroenterology. 1991;100:762.
16. McCullough AJ, Fleming R, Thistle JL *et al.* Diagnosis of Wilson's disease presenting as fulminant hepatic failure. Gastroenterology. 1983;84:161.
17. Mowat AP. Liver disorders in children: the indications for liver replacement in parenchymal and metabolic diseases. Transplant Proc. 1987;19:3236.
18. Sokol RJ. At long last: an animal model of Wilson's disease. Hepatology. 1994;20:533.
19. Sternlieb I, Scheinberg IH. The role of radiocopper in the diagnosis of Wilson's disease. Gastroenterology. 1979;77:138.
20. Scheinberg IH, Jaffe ME, Sternlieb I. The use of trientine in preventing the effects of interrupting penicillamine therapy in Wilson's disease. N Engl J Med. 1987;317:209.
21. Schilsky ML, Scheinberg IH, Sternlieb I. Liver transplantation for Wilson's disease: indications and outcome. Hepatology. 1994;19:583.

Section III
Cholestatic liver diseases

12
Mechanisms of cholestasis

J. L. BOYER

Knowledge of the basic cellular and molecular mechanisms of bile secretion is increasing rapidly and is beginning to facilitate an understanding of the pathophysiology of cholestasis. The present status of this knowledge has recently been reviewed[1,2].

Bile is formed by osmotic filtration in response to osmotic gradients created by the active excretion of organic and inorganic solutes from the hepatocyte into the bile canaliculus. These solutes include bile acids which determine the amount of bile acid-dependent bile flow, and HCO_3^-, and glutathione which account for the majority of bile acid-independent canalicular flow. Membrane transport systems at the basolateral membrane function to facilitate selective hepatic uptake of biliary constituents. These include the sodium taurocholate co-transporter (*ntcp*); the organic anion transport proteins (*oatp-1* and *2*; and the cholate/dicarboxylic acid exchangers)[3]. Transport proteins at the canalicular domain function to transport these and other solutes against concentration gradients into bile, and include the bile acid transporter (cBAT); a HCO_3^-/Cl^- exchanger; and glutathione and glutathione conjugate transporters) thereby creating the osmotic gradients that provide the driving force for bile salt-dependent and -independent bile production. Some of these transporters have been cloned (*ntcp, oatp-1* and *2*, and the canalicular GSH[4] and GSH conjugate transporters), the latter known as the canalicular multi-organic anion transporter or cMOAT, which may be identical to the cloned multi-drug-resistant protein, MRP[5-7].

During cholestatic liver injury, either from bile duct obstruction or intrahepatic cholestasis produced by oestrogens, endotoxin, or drug cholestasis, many of these transport systems on both basolateral and canalicular domains are impaired[2]. *Ntcp* is down-regulated by all of these processes[2]. Bile duct obstruction produces both transcriptional and post-transcriptional changes in *ntcp*, resulting in minimal expression of the transporter at the basolateral domain, and diminished uptake of bile acids[8]. The ATP-dependent canalicular bile acid transporter (cBAT) is inhibited by oestrogen and cyclosporin[9]. Transcytotic vesicles, which move across the cell on microtubules and deliver transport proteins to the apical canalicular domain, accumulate within the pericanalicular space[10]. Cytoskeletal elements are impaired, leading to a loss of cell polarity, a reduction in canalicular microvilli and a disordered microfilament array in the pericanalicular ectoplasm. Tight junction proteins are disordered (ZO–1 and occludin) and the paracellular pathway becomes 'leaky', resulting in dissipation of osmotic gradients in bile[11,12]. Signal transduction pathways, which normally help regulate and coordinate intracellular communications, are disrupted, including agonist-induced calcium signals and gap junction proteins (connexin 32 and 26), resulting in diminished canalicular contractility[13].

Clinical disorders of cholestasis often result from primary injury to the intrahepatic bile duct epithelium, known collectively as the vanishing bile duct diseases[14]. The physiology and pathophysiology of the transport systems on the bile duct epithelium are just beginning to be understood at the cellular and molecular level, a field that represents the 'new frontier' of biliary physiology and disease[15].

Together these cellular and molecular changes result in the syndrome of cholestasis.

Tauroursodeoxycholic acid (TUDCA) improves cholestatic liver injury in patients with cholestatic liver injury. While this bile acid may ameliorate cholestasis through several mechanisms, current evidence suggests that the primary beneficial effects of TUDCA result from the ability of this bile acid to stimulate canalicular bile secretion, possibly by augmenting exocytosis at the excretory domain by mobilizing intracellular and extracellular sources of calcium and stimulating protein kinase-C[16,17].

References

1. Boyer JL. The role of vesicle transport and exocytosis in bile formation and cholestasis: influence of cell volume, pHi, hormones and bile acids. In: Gentilini P, Arias IM, McIntyre N, Rodes J, eds. Cholestasis. Amsterdam: Elsevier; 1994:69–78.
2. Boyer JL. Molecular pathogenesis of cholestasis. In: Schmid R *et al.*, editors. Acute and chronic liver diseases: molecular biology and clinics. Dordrecht: Kluwer; 1996:87–95.
3. Meier PJ. Hepatocellular transport systems: from carrier identification in membrane vesicles to cloned proteins. J Hepatol. 1996;24:29–35.
4. Yi JR, Lu S, Fernandez-Checa J, Kaplowitz N. Expression cloning of a rat hepatic reduced glutathione transporter with canalicular characteristics. J Clin Invest. 1994;93:1841–5.
5. Keppler D, Mayer R, Kartenbeck J, Buchler M, Jedlitschky G, Leier I. Expression and localization of the MRP gene-encoded conjugate export pump in liver. In: Wehner F, Petzinger E, editors. Cell biology and molecular basis of liver transport. Dortmund:Projekt Verlag; 1995:161–7.
6. Muller M, de Vries EGE, Jansen PLM. Role of multidrug resistance protein (MRP) in glutathione S-conjugate transport in mammalian cells. J Hepatol. 1996;24:100–8.
7. Paulusma CC, Bosma PJ, Zaman GJR *et al.* Congenital jaundice in rats with a mutation in a multidrug resistance-associated protein gene. Science. 1996;271:1126–8.
8. Gartung C, Ananthanarayanan M, Rahman MA *et al.* Down-regulation of expression and function of the rat liver Na+/bile acid cotransporter in extrahepatic cholestasis. Gastroenterology. 1996;110:199–209.
9. Bohme M, Muller M, Leier I, Jedlitschky G, Keppler D. Cholestasis caused by inhibition of the adenosine triphosphate-dependent bile salt transport in rat liver. Gastroenterology. 1994;107:255–65.
10. Stieger B, Landmann L. Effects of cholestasis on membrane flow and surface polarity in hepatocytes. J Hepatol. 1996;24:128–34.
11. Fallon MB, Mennone A, Anderson JM. Altered expression and localization of the tight junction protein ZO-1 after common bile duct ligation. Am J Physiol. 1993;264:C1439–47.
12. Fallon MB, Nathanson MH, Mennone A, Saez JC, Burgstahler AD, Anderson JM. Altered expression and function of hepatocyte gap junctions after common bile duct ligation in the rat. Am J Physiol. 1995;37:C1186–94.

13. Nathanson MH, Burgstahler AD, Mennone A, Fallon MB, Gonzalez CB, Saez JC. Ca^{2+} waves are organized among hepatocytes in the intact organ. Am J Physiol. 1995;269:G167–71.
14. Desmet VJ. Vanishing bile duct disorder. In: Boyer JL, Ockner RK, editors. Progress in liver diseases. Philadelphia: Saunders; 1992:89–122.
15. Boyer JL. Bile duct epithelium: frontiers in transport physiology. Am J Physiol. 1996;270:G1–G5.
16. Beuers U, Nathanson MH, Isales CM, Boyer JL. Tauroursodeoxycholic acid stimulates hepato-cellular exocytosis and mobilizes extracellular Ca mechanisms defective in cholestasis. J Clin Invest. 1993;92:2984–93.
17. Beuers U, Throckmorton DC, Anderson MS *et al.* Tauroursodeoxycholic acid activates protein kinase C in isolated rat hepatocytes. Gastroenterology. 1996;110:1553–63.

13
Neonatal cholestasis: diagnostic and therapeutic approach

M. BURDELSKI

INTRODUCTION

The neonatal cholestasis syndrome represents an important clinical problem. It occurs in from 1:5000 to 1:10 000 livebirths[1]. The severity differs greatly from benign, self-limited physiological cholestasis to disorders with a progressive nature and an almost malignant course, such as in extrahepatic biliary atresia[2]. Between these extremes a variety of different pathophysiological entities may be found (Fig. 1). There are infectious, metabolic, idiopathic, genetic, structural and endocrine disorders resulting in cholestasis. The overlapping circles in Fig. 1 indicate that symptoms, clinical chemical findings and even ultrasound imaging results are very similar, despite different pathophysiological backgrounds. These clinical and clinical chemical differences between these disorders are the less striking, the smaller and younger these patients are. The

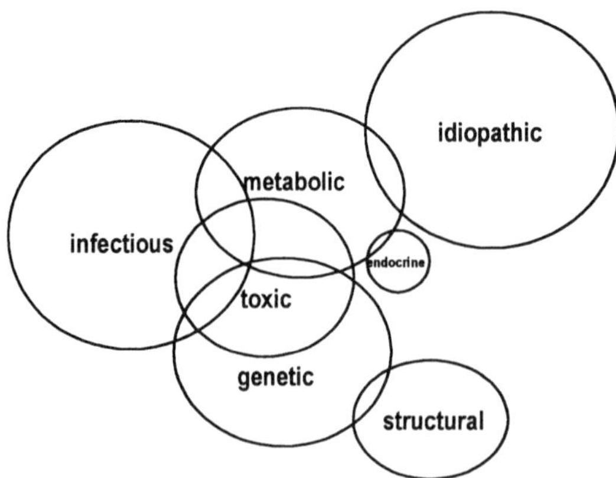

Fig. 1 The overlap of different causes of neonatal cholestasis

diagnostic challenge to any paediatrician is thus remarkable, especially if one takes into account that diagnosis has to be settled as soon as possible, and that imaging procedures such as ERCP, PTC and even CT (which are of great importance in adult cholestatic disorders) are difficult to perform in infants.

This review aims to elucidate a rational approach to differential diagnosis in cholestasis of infancy and to its therapy.

SPECIFIC DISORDERS

Infections

Increasing numbers of premature babies from very early gestational weeks receiving total parenteral nutrition (TPN) under intercurrent septicaemia and haemolysis present with cholestasis. These patients are seen more often than babies with perinatal infections, for instance due to cytomegalovirus, herpes simplex virus, toxoplasma or rubella virus. The pathophysiological background of cholestasis under TPN and infection remains to be elucidated. A hypothetical pathophysiological approach has been proposed, in which immaturity, decreased endocrine output in the gut and hypoxia lead to intestinal injury, hypomotility, small bowel overgrowth, and increased mucosal permeability, especially for toxins and endotoxins. These activate Kupffer cells, which respond with increased production of tumour necrosis factor (TNF), which is responsible for the resulting hepatic injury[3]. According to other authors the qualitative and quantitative imbalance of TPN solutions or consecutive changes in cell may be essential for the development of TPN-associated cholestasis[4].

Metabolic disorders

Hepatic-based metabolic disorders leading to cholestasis represent a second important aetiology: α_1-antitrypsin deficiency is the most frequent cause of cholestasis in this group, accounting for about 20% of cholestatic infants at King's College Hospital[5]. Patients with this disorder tend to present with intestinal haemorrhage due to vitamin K malabsorption[6]. All other metabolic disorders are comparatively rare and should be considered only if infection-like episodes, without proof of any infectious agent, are observed.

Genetic disorders

In this group the Alagille syndrome is one of the most important representatives. The characteristic clinical features, with typical face, embryotoxon posterior, peripheral pulmonary stenosis, butterfly vertebrae and intrahepatic paucity of bile ducts, may be less pronounced in young infants, so that diagnosis is difficult unless one of the parents shows typical features of this autosomal dominant-inherited disorder[7]. There are other disorders such as progressive familial intrahepatic cholestasis (PFIC), symptoms of which tend to start only after the neonatal period[8]. With regard to familial disorders, this PFIC syndrome is the most frequent indication for liver transplantation in many centres[6].

Idiopathic disorders

The most frequent idiopathic cholestasis syndrome in the neonatal period is extrahepatic biliary atresia (EBA). This benign disorder with malignant course is observed in between 1:10 000 and 1:21 000 livebirths. Due to the rapid progression to cholestatic cirrhosis within 4–6 weeks this disorder needs to be identified as soon as possible. The nature of EBA needs to be clarified; genetic or metabolic causes seem to be unlikely[9]. Associated malformations deriving from defects during organogenesis, such as preduodenal portal vein, polysplenia, aplasia of the inferior vena cava and azygos continuation, are seen in about 5–10% of patients with EBA. However, they do not indicate EBA as being a congenital malformation. The destruction process of the extrahepatic bile duct system begins shortly after birth[9]. Infections have not consistently been documented. This also holds true for many of the so-called neonatal hepatitis syndromes, in which only descriptive histology of liver specimens with parenchymal giant cells resulting from syncytial fusion, without serological proof of any infectious agent, is observed[10]. Even new sensitive methods such as polymerase chain reaction (PCR) do not help in better characterizing these diseases.

Structural disorders

Choledochal cysts, Caroli syndrome and congenital hypoplasia of parts of the choledochal duct normally present with cholestasis in later life. They may, however, be found as a cause of cholestasis in the neonatal period. Other disorders such as liver fibrosis and cystic degeneration of the kidneys may be listed as malformations or genetic defects; the same holds true for Caroli syndrome.

Toxic disorders

These disorders show the greatest overlap from infectious and metabolic to genetic background. Some of the toxic disorders have been discussed in the section on infectious disorders. A great deal of toxic cholestasis must be related to drug therapy. Hepatic drug reactions show a widespread spectrum, with cholestasis being only one aspect. Cholestasis may be induced by sex hormones, erythromycin, ceftriaxone, flucloxacillin, nitrofurantoin, azathioprine, cyclosporin, tacrolimus, antimycotic agents, cimetidine, ranitidine and chlorpromazine. Anticonvulsant agents induce liver enzyme activities, i.e. γ-GT. The excretion of metabolized drugs depends on polarity and molecular weight. Highly polar substances and drug metabolites with a molecular weight above 200 tend to be excreted in the bile. Non-polar substances and those with a molecular weight below 200 are excreted in the urine[11].

Endocrine disorders

Endocrine disorders may be associated with hepatitis syndrome. The most frequent disorder is hypothyroidism, so this must be excluded in every instance. Hypopituitarism may be associated with septo-optic dysplasia. The major symptoms are hypoglycaemia, unconjugated hyperbilirubinaemia and high or low serum sodium concentration[12].

DIAGNOSTIC APPROACH

The diagnostic approach in neonatal cholestasis must be easy, fast and efficient. The most important step is the identification of conjugated hyperbilirubinaemia. Any neonate with persistent or prolonged jaundice lasting more than 14 days after birth needs determination of conjugated and unconjugated bilirubin in serum (Fig. 2)[12]. In children with conjugated hyperbilirubinaemia the determination of serum catalytic concentration of γ-GT initiates a further stepwise diagnostic evaluation[2]. The cut-off value of 180 U/L is on the safe side, in order to identify patients with EBA as soon as possible; this means during the third week of life. A cut-off value of 300 U/L is suitable for children at the age of more than 4 weeks[13], since EBA is a dynamic disease which ends with complete obstruction of the extrahepatic bile ducts after an initial phase of incomplete biliary obstruction. A catalytic serum concentration above 300 U/L needs a further diagnostic work-up by liver biopsy and ultrasound. If there is a ductular proliferation in histology[10] and no gallbladder detectable in ultrasound, the next step must be a diagnostic laparotomy. In case of EBA a classical Kasai procedure is performed, the benefit of which is shown by the fact that about 50–70% of these children survive the first year of life, whereas non-operated children do not survive longer than 1 year[6].

Patients outside the high γ-GT category need a careful diagnostic work-up in order to identify the underlying nature of cholestasis. This work-up includes bacteriological, virological, metabolic, endocrine and structural evaluation[13–17].

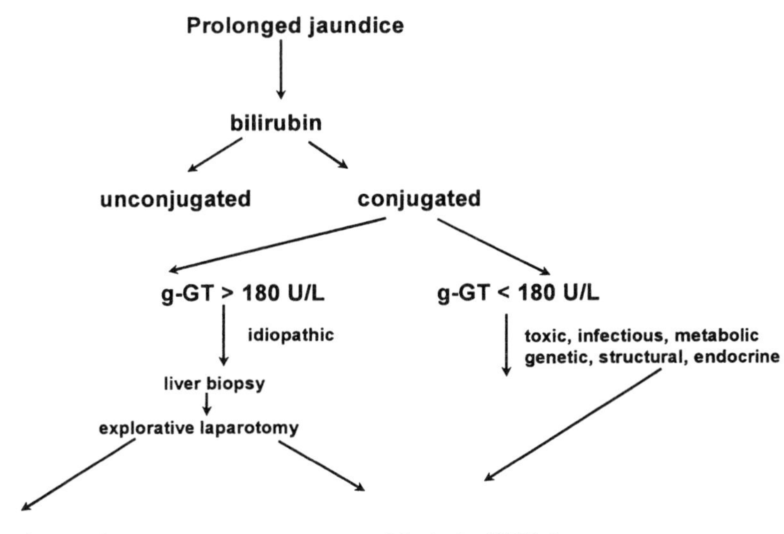

Fig. 2   Flow sheet of diagnostic work-up in patients with neonatal cholestasis. Modified according to (Bu)

SURGICAL THERAPY

Surgical therapy is needed in patients with EBA, progressive familial intrahepatic cholestasis (PFIC) and patients with malformation of the extrahepatic bile ducts (Table 1). In EBA the various modifications of the original Kasai procedure have proved to be less effective[18]. Primary transplantation at the age of less than half a year is difficult because of technical and donor-related problems[13]. Predictors affecting outcome following the repair of biliary atresia are: (1) time of operation, (2) length of the Roux-en-y loop and (3) use of postoperative antibiotic prophylaxis[18,19].

Table 1 Operative options in patients with extrahepatic bilary atresia, progressive familial intrahepatic cholestasis (PFIC) and extrahepatic bile duct malformation

Disorder	*Operation*
Biliary atresia	Hepato-porto-enterostomy
PFIC	Partial biliary diversion
Malformation	Hepatico-enterostomy

In patients with PFIC surgical therapy has been shown to be very effective. This therapy is a cholecysto-entero-cutaneostomy which diverts about 50% of the bile out of the enterohepatic circulation[20–22]. The benefit of this operation, however, is lost if performed too late, i.e. after the development of cirrhosis[15]. To date the mode of action of partial biliary diversion in these patients is not completely understood.

In patients with choledochal cysts, long common channel and Caroli syndrome conventional surgery with portoenterostomy or liver resection in unilateral manifestation of the Caroli syndrome is necessary as soon as the diagnosis is made, in order to prevent either cholangitis, spontaneous perforation or the development of cholangiocarcinoma[23].

MEDICAL THERAPY

Medical therapy in neonatal cholestasis is symptomatic in most cases. Only in patients with defects of bile acid synthesis may ursodeoxycholic acid (UDCA) be regarded as curative[24]. Since these patients represent only a minority of cholestatic infants, UDCA is mostly used as a symptomatic therapy acting: (1) on the enterohepatic circulation of endogenous bile acids, (2) by a cytoprotective effect towards hepatocytes and (3) by an effect on the immune system[25]. There are some patients with severe itching which does not respond to UDCA therapy, or may even get worse. In these children the use of cholestyramine may be tried. Patients not responding to cholestyramine may benefit from rifampicin (Table 2).

Cholestasis means impaired bile flow from the hepatocyte to the duodenum or into the Roux-en-y loop. This predisposes to cholangitis either by ascending

Table 2 Symptomatic medical therapy in neonatal cholestasis

Symptom	First drug	Second drug	Third drug
Itching	UDCA 10 mg/kg	Cholestyramine 2–4 g/day	Rifampicin 4 mg/kg
Infection	Cephalosporins	Trimethoprim	Sultamicillin
Malnutrition	MCT	Oligosaccharides	Branched-chain amino acids
Osteopathy	Cholecalciferol	Calcitriol	

bacterial agents or by haematogenic spread from the gut. The reticuloendothelial system being compromised, at least in late stages of liver diseases, cholangitis causes significant morbidity in these patients. The antibiotics preferably used are cephalosporins, for instance cephalotoxin, trimethoprim and sultamicillin (Table 2).

Malnutrition is one of the major factors contributing to morbidity and even mortality in cholestatic liver disorders. It is observed in almost 50% of transplant candidates[26] and needs to be prevented, since improvement of nutritional status in chronic end-stage liver disease is almost impossible. The most important issue in preventing malnutrition is replacement of normal fats by medium-chain triglycerides (MCT) as soon as significant cholestasis is recognized. The next step in optimizing the nutritional regimen in these children is the additional supplementation of fat-soluble vitamins[27]. Vitamin K and D depletion is responsible for bleeding episodes and osteopathy. In the context of portal hypertension and restricted motor activities these aspects of malnutrition need special attention. The metabolic imbalance of patients with cholestatic cirrhosis predisposes to hypoglycaemia, which may be prevented by adding oligosaccharides. The enrichment of proteins with branched-chain amino acids is restricted to patients in precoma or coma[28].

PROGNOSIS

The prognosis of neonatal cholestasis syndromes is characterized by high morbidity, mortality and only palliative medical therapy (Table 3). The character of the individual disorders, however, shows at least diagnosis-dependent

Table 3 Prognosis in neonatal cholestasis

Disorder	Mortality	Morbidity	Med. therapy	Conv. surg. therapy	Transplantation
EBA	100%	100%	Symptomatic	Kasai	70–80% survival
Neonatal hepatitis	25%	25–50%	Symptomatic	No	70–80% survival
PFIC	100%	100%	Symptomatic	Partial biliary diversion	80–90% survival
PFOC	40%	100%	Symptomatic	No	?
HMD	Variable	100%	Curative 10–20%	No	80–90% survival
Alagille syndrome	Variable	Variable	Symptomatic	No	70–80% survival

EBA = extrahepatic biliary atresia, PFIC = progressive familial intrahepatic cholestasis,
PFOC = progressive familial obstructive cholestasis, HMD = hepatic-based metabolic disorder

modifications, so exact diagnosis is mandatory. Conventional surgical therapy is essential, especially in EBA and PFIC. If it fails, liver transplantation has been shown to be very effective, with survival rates in the European Liver Transplant Registry being satisfactory at between 70% and 90%. In order to optimize these results the early presentation of any patient with neonatal cholestasis to a transplant centre is essential.

References

1. Sokol RJ. Lipid peroxidation in cholestasis. In: Lentze MJ, Reichen J, editors. Paediatric cholestasis: novel approaches to treatment. Dordrecht: Kluwer;1992:75–80.
2. Burdelski M. Current concepts in diagnosis and therapy of pediatric liver diseases. J Hepatol. 1995;23 (Suppl.):45–8.
3. Balistreri WF, Bucuvalas JC, Farrel MK, Bove KE. Total parenteral nutrition associated cholestasis: factors responsible for the decreasing evidence. In: Lentze MJ, Reichen J, editors. Paediatric cholestasis: novel approaches to treatment. Dordrecht: Kluwer; 1992:191–206.
4. Häussinger D. The role of cellular hydration in the regulation of cell function Biochem J. 1996;313:697–710.
5. Trivedi P, Mieli-Vergani G, Mowat AP. Cholestasis in infancy and childhood: an overview. In: Lentze MJ, Reichen J, editors. Paediatric cholestasis: novel approaches to treatment. Dordrecht: Kluwer; 1992:129–38.
6. Burdelski M. Clinical relevance of familial cholestatic disorders in infancy and childhood (In press).
7. Odievre M. Congenital ductopenia. In: Lentze MJ, Reichen J, editors. Paediatric cholestasis: novel approaches to treatment. Dordrecht: Kluwer; 1992:139–46.
8. Whitington PF, Freese DK, Alonso EM, Schwarzenberg SJ, Sharp HL. Clinical and biochemical findings in progressive intrahepatic cholestasis. J Pediatr Gastroenterol Nutr. 1994;18:134–41.
9. Lai, MW, Chang MH, Hsu HC, Kao CL, Lee CY. Differential diagnosis of extrahepatic biliary atresia from neonatal hepatitis, a prospective study. J Pediatr Gastroenterol Nutr. 1994;18:121–7.
10. Desmet VJ. Pathology of paediatric cholestasis In: Lentze MJ, Reichen J, editors. Paediatric cholestasis: novel approaches to treatment. Dordrecht: Kluwer; 1992:55–76.
11. Sherlock D, Dooley J. Drugs and the liver. In: Sherlock S, Dooley J, editors. Diseases of the liver and biliary system, 9th edn. London: Blackwell; 1993:322–56.
12. Mowat A. Hepatitis and cholestasis in infancy. In Mowat A, editor. Liver disorders in childhood, 3rd edn. Oxford: Butterworth Heineman; 1994:43–78.
13. Latta A, Burdelski M. Diagnostic procedures in neonatal cholestasis. Verdauungskrankheiten. 1995;14:2–9.
14. Drews D. Inborn errors of metabolism as a differential diagnosis of neonatal liver diseases. Verdauungskrankheiten. 1996;14:10–16.
15. Sturm E, Latta A, Rogiers X, Malago M, Burdelski M. Byler's disease (progressive familial intrahepatic cholestasis, PFIC) – Clinical findings, diagnostic strategies and therapy. Verdauungskrankheiten. 1996;14:17–21.
16. Helmke K. Imaging methods in pediatric hepatology. Verdauungskrankheiten. 1996;14:28–35.
17. Ikeda S, Sera Y, Akagi M. Serial ultrasonic examination to differentiate biliary atresia from neonatal hepatitis-special reference to changes in size of the gallbladder. Eur J Pediatr. 1989;148:396–400.
18. Lally KP, Kanegaye J, Matsamura M, Rosenthal P, Sinatra F, Atkonson JB. Perioperative factors affecting the outcome following repair of biliary atresia. Pediatrics. 1989;83:723–6.
19. Lilly JR, Karrer FM, Hall RJ, Stellin GP, Vasquez-Estevez JJ, Greenholz SK. The surgery of biliary atresia. Ann Surg. 1989;210:289–94.
20. Whitington PF, Freese DK, Alonso EN, Fishbein MH, Emond JC. Progressive familial intrahepatic cholestasis (Byler's disease) In: Lentze MJ, Reichen J, editors. Paediatric cholestasis: novel approaches to treatment. Dordrecht: Kluwer; 1992:165–79.
21. Whitington PF, Freese DK, Alonso EN, Schwarzenberg SJ, Sharp HL. Clinical and biochemical findings in progressive intrahepatic cholestasis. J Pediatr Gastroenterol Nutr. 1994;18:134–41.

22. Whitington PF, Whitington GL. Partial external diversion of bile for the treatment of intractable pruritus associated with intrahepatic cholestasis. Gastroenterology. 1988;95:130–6.
23. Komi N, Takehara H, Kunimoto K. Choledochal cyst: anomalous arrangement of the pancreatico biliary ductal system and biliary malignancy. J Gastroenterol Hepatol. 1989;4:63–74.
24. Setchell KDR, Piccoli D, Heubi J, Ballistreri WF. Inborn errors of bile acid metabolism. In Lentze MJ, Reichen J, editors. Paediatric cholestasis: novel approaches to treatment. Dordrecht: Kluwer; 1992:153–8.
25. Poupon R, Calmus Y, Poupon RE. Mechanisms of hepatoprotection by ursodeoxycholic acid. In: Lentze MJ, Reichen J, editors. Paediatric cholestasis: novel approaches to treatment. Dordrecht: Kluwer; 1992:319–24.
26. Burdelski M. Liver transplantation in pediatric hepatology. Verdauungskrankheiten. 1996;14:36–42.
27. Sokol RJ. Vitamin deficiency and replacement in childhood cholestasis. In: Lentze MJ, Reichen J, editors. Paediatric cholestasis: novel approaches to treatment. Dordrecht: Kluwer; 1992:289–304.
28. Burdelski M. Lebererkrankungen und Lebetransplantation. In: Koletzko B, editor. Ernährung chronisch kranker Kinder und Jugendlicher. Berlin: Springer; 1993:141–50.

14
Treatment of chronic cholestatic liver diseases with ursodeoxycholic acid

U. LEUSCHNER, S. GÜLDÜTUNA and M. LEUSCHNER

INTRODUCTION

Since 1985 ursodeoxycholic acid (UDCA) has been used for the treatment of chronic active hepatitis, primary biliary cirrhosis (PBC), primary sclerosing cholangitis (PSC), Caroli's syndrome, cystic fibrosis, and some rare alterations of bile acid metabolism. Because most investigations with UDCA have been done in PBC, we will concentrate on this disease.

TRIALS WITH DRUGS OTHER THAN UDCA

The analysis of studies with D-penicillamine in patients with PBC has shown that the drug does not influence symptoms, laboratory data or liver histology, except in a few patients. Therefore use of D-penicillamine has been abandoned. There is one study with glucocorticoids which had a positive result, but the problem was an augmentation of bone loss, already common in untreated patients with PBC. A meta-analysis of studies with colchicine had a negative result, as did studies using chlorambucil. Methotrexate and cyclosporin A had some positive effects on various laboratory parameters and histology, but because of the side-effects these substances are no longer used.

THERAPY WITH UDCA: CLINICAL ASPECTS

In 10 controlled studies including more than 1000 patients it has been shown that UDCA improves the symptoms in about 50% of the patients, the laboratory tests (ALT, AST, GGT, AP, GLDH, IgM) and in some patients with early stages of the disease even liver histology (Table 1)[1]. In 1995 a combined analysis of a French, American and Canadian trial in 553 patients (276 UDCA, 277 placebo) was published[2]. The UDCA dosage with 13–15 mg/kg per day was somewhat higher than in the 10 studies mentioned above (10 mg/kg per day). At entry baseline characteristics of the patients were comparable in the three groups. In

Table 1 UDC treatment in primary biliary cirrhosis – controlled trials

Author, date	No. of patients	PBC stage	Dose (mg/kg per day)	Laboratory tests	Histology	Time until transplantation
Leuschner, 1989	20	I–III	10	+	(n.s. +)	0
Hadziyannis, 1989	45	II–IV	12–15	+/–	(+)/–	(n.s. +)
Oka, 1990	45	I–IV	8–12	+	0	0
Battezzati, 1993	88	I–III	8.7	+	0	0
Hwang, 1993	12	I–IV	10	+	0	0
Turner, 1993	64	I–IV	10	+	(n.s. +)	0
Poupon, 1994	145	I–IV	13–15	+	+	+
Heathcote, 1994	222	I–IV	14	+	(n.s. +)	(n.s. +)
Lindor, 1994	180	I–IV	13–15	+	–	(n.s. +)
Combes, 1995	153	I–IV	Bilirubin <2 mg%	+	+	0
			Bilirubin >2 mg%	(+)	–	0

(n.s. +): not significant, but positive trend.

+, Significant improvement; –, no therapeutic effect; 0, not investigated.

the UDCA group death or liver transplantation occurred in 47 patients, in the placebo group in 68 patients ($p < 0.001$). The prolongation of survival was 3.66 years in the UDCA group and 3.45 years in the placebo group ($p = 0.014$). UDCA reduced the relative risk of dying without liver transplantation by 47%, and the authors conclude that UDCA improves survival of patients with PBC (Table 2).

The question of how long UDCA therapy is necessary, and whether interruption of treatment is followed by a rebound effect, has been answered by the only real long-term trial over a period of 12 years[3]. This study revealed that UDCA slowed the histological progression of PBC (Fig. 1), but it did not cure the disease. When therapy is interrupted, even after 5–6 years of continuous therapy, there is a marked rebound effect which indicates that UDCA apparently has little or no influence on the as-yet-unknown disorders underlying this disease. During treatment UDCA became the predominant bile salt in the serum;

Table 2 Combined analysis of French, American and Canadian trials of UDC versus placebo in primary biliary cirrhosis

Patient number: 553 (276 UDC, 277 placebo)
UDC dosage: 13–15 mg/kg per day
Two studies: 2 years double-blind, 2 years open UDC
One study: 4 years double-blind
Baseline characteristics were comparable at entry

Dead or OLT / UDC group: 47
Placebo group: 68 ($p < 0.001$)
Extension of survival: Placebo 3.45 years
UDC 3.66 years ($p = 0.014$)

Relative risk of dying without OLT reduced by 47% in the UDC group

UDC improves survival of PBC patients

From ref. 2

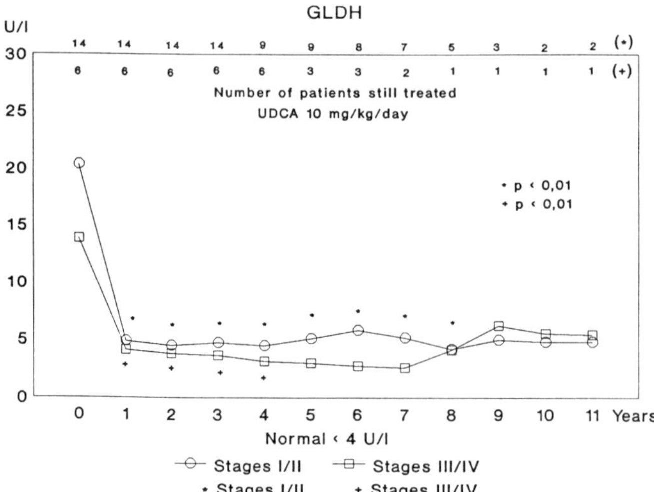

Fig. 1 Glutamate dehydrogenase (GLDH) before and during UDCA therapy. Values are mean values of all patients for one year. (From ref. 3)

lithocholic acid did not significantly increase, but did so in the stool. Since UDCA did not induce any adverse side-effects in patients with early and late stages (except diarrhoea in about 2%), UDCA therapy is believed to be safe. Obviously, UDCA therapy has to be a lifelong treatment.

Since UDCA is unable to cure the disease, eight trials with combination therapy have been performed[4-11]. In four studies UDCA was combined with colchicine (patient number 167). Only in one study was there a positive effect on laboratory data. In two studies in which liver biopsies have been taken, histology did not improve, and in two studies histology has not been investigated. A total of 36 patients had been treated with UDCA and methotrexate in three studies. In all three studies there was a positive effect on liver function tests; histology had been investigated in one study and was negative. In 1996 a study in 30 patients was published, 15 of which were treated with 10 mg/kg per day UDCA plus placebo, 15 with UDCA and 10 mg prednisolone per day[12]. In both groups laboratory data improved to the same extent, but liver histology improved significantly in the UDCA/prednisolone group ($p < 0.0032$). A trial with UDCA, prednisolone and azathioprine, which is performed in the Netherlands, is still in progress. Preliminary results presented at the Basel Liver Week in October 1995 have shown that this triple therapy also improves liver histology, which has not been shown clearly by previous studies with UDCA monotherapy.

SCIENTIFIC ASPECTS OF UDCA THERAPY

Although UDCA at present is the therapy of choice for patients with primary biliary liver diseases, the mechanisms by which UDCA exerts its beneficial effects are still unknown. Even the question of whether apolar bile acids are responsible for the outbreak of the disease, or at least for the deterioration of a primarily immunological disease, is unanswered. The increased serum concentrations of apolar bile acids found in patients with PBC and their decrease during UDCA therapy could be purely a chance finding, and could have nothing to do with the course of the disease. In a previous study we have shown that the administration of cholic acid (CA) in a dosage of 10 mg/kg per day to patients with PBC increased the symptoms (especially pruritus) and the concentrations of α-dihydroxy bile acids (chenodeoxycholic acid, deoxycholic acid) in the serum[13]. There was a strong correlation between liver damage (increase of GLDH) and serum α-dihydroxy bile acids ($r = 0.92$). Subsequent UDCA therapy decreased GLDH and α-dihydroxy bile acids in the serum; the correlation between the two figures was $r = -0.99$. The correlation between cholic acid and GLDH was only $r = 0.60$ (Figs 2 and 3). Since in these short-term studies nothing had changed except the bile acid pattern (α-dihydroxy bile acids especially had increased) these investigations corroborate the assumption that apolar bile acids are responsible at least for the deterioration of PBC.

In several studies it had been shown that treatment with UDCA lowered endogenous bile acid concentrations (CA, CDCA, DCA, LCA) in serum, urine and bile (Table 3)[14]. UDCA increased, and with more than 50% in the serum it became the predominant bile salt during therapy. If apolar bile acids are in part responsible for the deterioration of cholestatic liver diseases, and the more polar UDCA improves the disease, the questions arise in which compartment of the enterohepatic circulation UDCA intervenes and where the targets on a cellular level are.

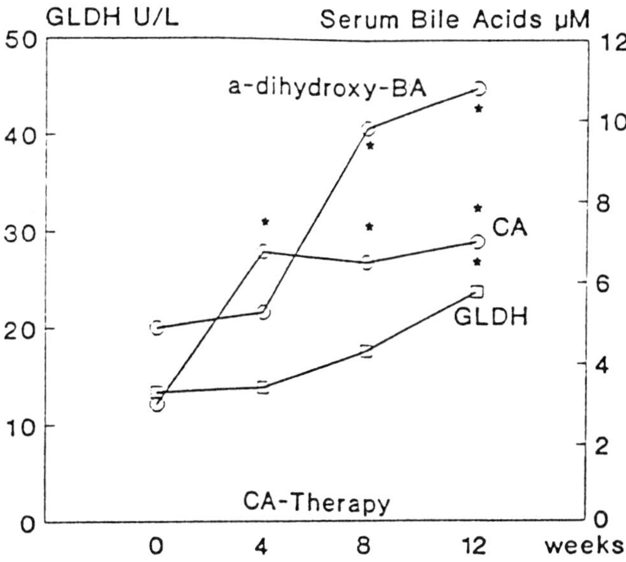

Fig. 2 Mean levels of GLDH (glutamate dehydrogenase) activity and bile salt concentrations in the serum of patients with primary biliary cirrhosis during CA (cholic acid) therapy (10 mg/kg per day). Correlation coefficients for α-dihydroxy bile acids/GLDH $r = 0.92$, and for CA/GLDH $r = 0.60$. * $p < 0.05$ versus commencement of therapy. (From ref. 13)

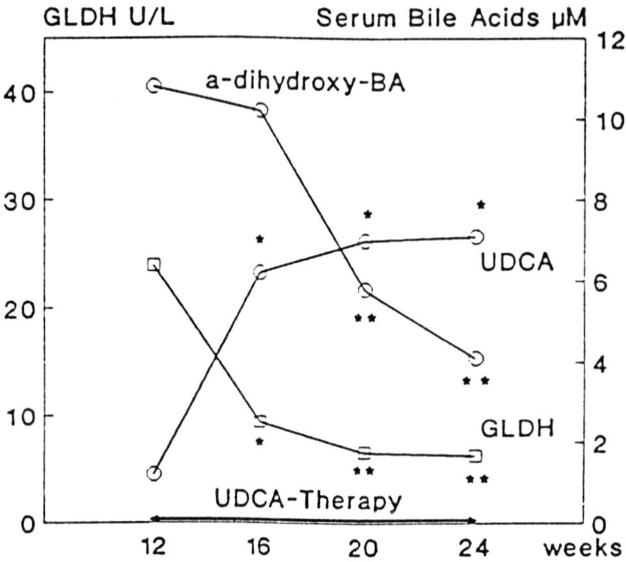

Fig. 3   Mean levels of GLDH (glutamate dehydrogenase) activity and bile salt concentrations in the serum of patients with primary biliary cirrhosis during subsequent treatment with UDCA (ursodeoxycholic acid: 10 mg/kg per day). Correlation coefficients for α-dihydroxy bile acids/GLDH $r = 0.74$, and for UDCA/GLDH $r = -0.99$.

* $p < 0.01$ and *$p < 0.05$ versus commencement of UDCA therapy. (From ref. 13)

Table 3   Effect of UDCA therapy on bile acid concentrations in patients with primary biliary cirrhosis

	Endogenous*	Hydroxylated	UDCA	Total†
Serum (μmol/L)				
Pre	46 ± 15	2 ± 0.4	1 ± 0.4	52 ± 13
UDC	23 ± 4	4 ± 0.4	31 ± 8	60 ± 10
Urine (μmol/g creatinine)				
Pre	37 ± 17	14 ± 10	3 ± 0.5	62 ± 22
UDC	18 ± 4	12 ± 5	97 ± 24	162 ± 34
Bile (μmol/L)				
Pre	25 ± 4		0.3 ± 0.2	
UDC	17 ± 4		31 ± 12	

* C, CDC, DC, LC.
† 'Others' deleted from the originals.
Data from ref. 14.

The following hypotheses have been discussed:

1. UDCA inhibits the absorption of toxic, apolar, endogenous bile salts from the intestine.
2. UDCA inhibits the secretion of toxic bile salts into the bile capillaries and interlobular ducts, thus preventing toxic interactions with epithelial cells.

3. UDCA dilutes toxic bile salts via a choleretic action.
4. UDCA prevents an increase of cytosolic ionized calcium, which is believed to induce cell death.
5. UDCA stabilizes hepatocyte membranes against toxic bile salts.
6. UDCA protects or repairs membrane function.

In 1990 it had been shown that UDCA in a dosage of 500 and 1000 mg/day increased the ileal excretion of CA and CDCA in three patients with ileostomy dose-dependently, which means that the reabsorption of these bile acids was reduced (Fig. 4)[15]. Bile acid binding resins also stimulate the excretion of toxic bile acids, but do not have any influence on the liver disease. Therefore, bile acid excretion via the stool may be one of the possible mechanisms by which UDCA works, but further aspects may be more important. The same arguments apply to the choleretic properties of UDCA. While CDCA in concentrations of 300–400 μmol/L inhibits bile flow in animal experiments statistically significantly, UDCA stimulates bile flow, and thus excretion and dilution of endogenous bile acids (Fig. 5). But since there are other choleretic agents available without influencing the disease, dilution of toxic bile salts is obviously not a predominant mechanism of UDCA. In contrast to the assumption that UDCA prevents the influx of toxic calcium into the hepatocyte, it had been shown that TUDCA increased intracellular calcium concentrations mobilizing both intra-

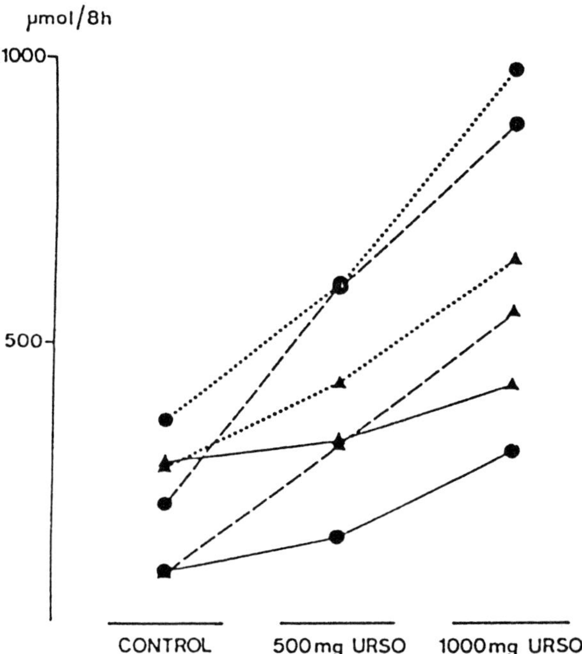

Fig. 4 Effect of UDCA on ileal excretion of (●) C and (▲) CDCA in three patients with ileostomy. URSO = ursodeoxycholic acid. (From ref. 15)

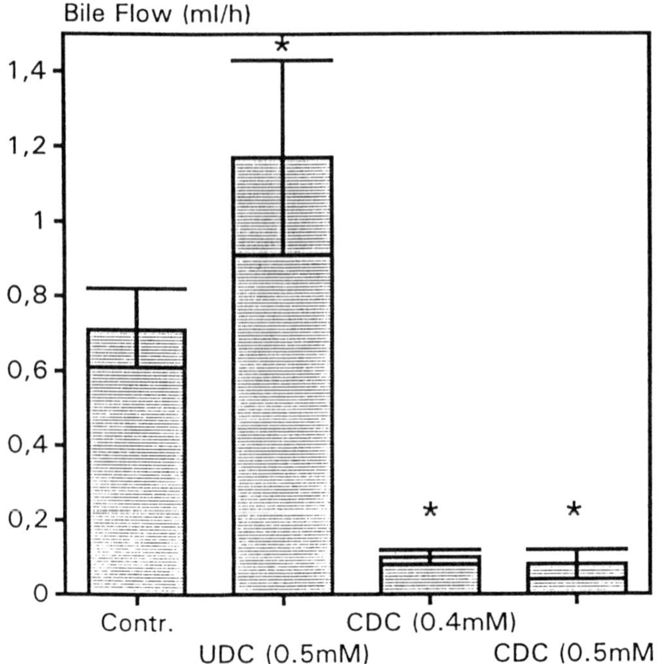

Fig. 5 Bile flow in the isolated perfused rat liver during different bile acid regimens * $p < 0.005$ versus control

and extracellular sources[16]. The TUDCA-induced calcium entry was associated with the stimulation of vesicular exocytosis, which is impaired in cholestasis. Therefore one of the beneficial effects of UDCA therapy could be related to the calcium-dependent stimulation of exocytosis, but others were unable to corroborate these data. Further, it had been shown that UDCA, in contrast to CA and CDCA, is intercalated into the apolar domain of hepatocyte membranes as a paired molecule[17]. Within the membrane it occupies a similar position to cholesterol. UDCA mimics the effects of cholesterol with respect to the membrane polarity and the enthalpy of the phase transition, as shown by EPR and differential calorimetry. Therefore it has been assumed that UDCA could adopt the stabilizing effect of cholesterol, which has recently been demonstrated with large unilamellar vesicles (100 nm, measured by laser light scattering) from egg yolk lecithin with increasing cholesterol concentrations from 0% to 40%[18]. When cholesterol was exchanged stepwise by UDCA, and the vesicles were incubated in apolar bile acid containing buffer (pH 7.4), UDCA had a stabilizing effect on membrane structure comparable to cholesterol, measured by the release of carboxyfluorescein from the vesicles and the phospholipid concentration in the supernatant (Fig. 6). This increase of membrane stability was accompanied by a decrease of membrane polarity and fluidity, as shown by EPR investigations in erythrocyte and basolateral hepatocyte membranes.

If UDCA is able to prevent structural membrane damage, the question arises whether this influences membrane function. With isolated erythrocyte mem-

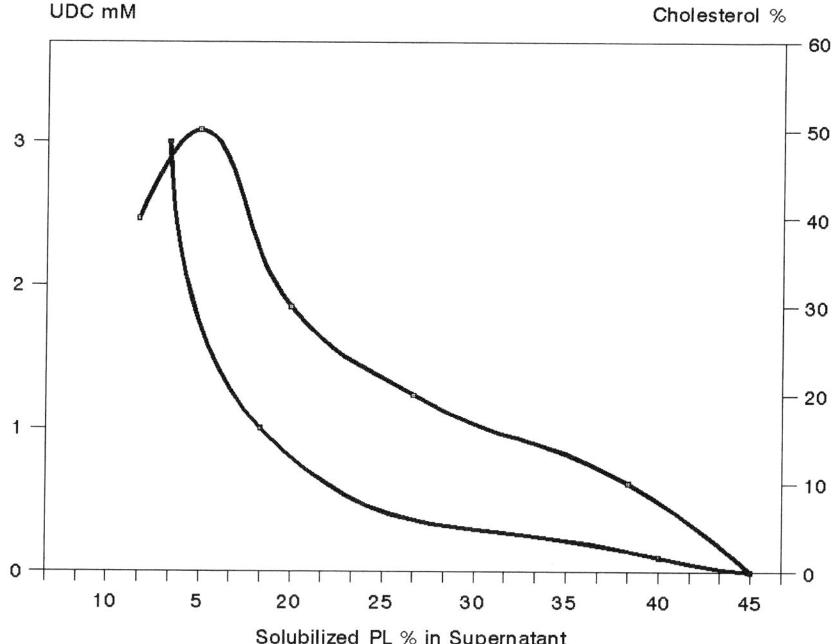

Fig. 6 Stabilizing effects of different concentrations of UDCA or cholesterol on vesicles of egg yolk lecithin. The upper curve represents the cholesterol concentration in the vesicle membrane, the lower curve the concentration of UDCA. Vesicles were incubated in 0.3 mmol/L CDCA containing buffer. PL = phospholipids

branes it has been shown that TCDCA increased the polarity and fluidity of bio-membranes, simultaneously decreasing Na-K/ATPase activity. UDCA had no influence on membrane structure or enzyme activity. Whether the disappearance of HLA class I antigen is also a marker of an improved membrane function, or whether this is the result of any other reaction in the immune system, remains open.

Most investigations concerning interactions of UDCA on a cellular level have been performed with outer cell membranes. Other targets, such as the membranes of the endoplasmic reticulum, of the Golgi apparatus or mitochondria, have been discussed only rarely. In these experiments it had been shown that UDCA prevented mitochondrial damage by toxic bile acids measured by the release of GLDH or swelling of the organelles, while CDCA in concentrations of 0.1 mmol/L increased membrane permeability, induced swelling and inhibited mitochondrial state 3 oxidation and complex I and III of the electron transport chain[19]. In a still-unpublished study we have shown that the above-mentioned protective effect of UDCA is rather short-lived and ends after 20–30 minutes. The explanation of this phenomenon could be attributed to the different composition and structure of mitochondrial membranes which contain a higher amount of proteins than the lipid-rich outer cell membrane. Thus the inner mitochondrial membranes contain virtually no cholesterol, far less lecithin than outer cell membranes, but 75% consist of proteins. Further investigations on cell organelles have to be expected.

Finally it has been discussed whether UDCA is able to influence immunological reactions, especially whether UDCA is immunosuppressive. The results of these investigations are still rather difficult to interpret, but it emerges that chenodeoxycholic acid is rather more immunosuppressive than UDCA. CDCA inhibited the proliferation of a mixed lymphocyte culture, it inhibited the activation of monocytes and the expression of IL-2, IL-10, IL-1, IL-6 and of TNF-α (Table 4)[20]. UDCA reduced aberrant HLA-I on the cell surface and ICAM-I, it reduced circulating IgM, inhibited the expression of IL-4 but stimulated IL-2, IFN-γ, TNF-β, and especially the proliferation of TH1 lymphocytes (Table 5)[21]. AMA concentrations in the serum are not affected. UDCA obviously has a more immunomodulatory effect.

HYPOTHETICAL MECHANISMS OF UDCA

Although UDCA therapy at present is the therapy of choice in primary biliary liver diseases, the mechanisms of action are still unknown. A cautious and very hypothetical interpretation of the data presented here led to the assumption that UDCA subdues the non-specific immune system (decrease of IgM, influence on B lymphocytes and macrophages), but does not 'switch it off' (persistence of AMA). Further, UDCA shifts the more apolar to a more polar bile acid pool (decrease of apolar bile acids in serum, bile and urine, increase of polar UDCA) and replaces toxic bile salts. Thereby it protects and repairs cell structures (increase of outer cell membrane stability by incorporation of UDCA, prevent-

Table 4 Effects of chenodeoxycholic acid on immune markers (more immunosuppressive)

1. Inhibits MLC proliferation
2. Inhibits monocyte activation
3. Inhibits IL-2 — Th1-related
   IL-10 — Th2-related
   IL-1, 6, TNF-α — monocyte-related

Table 5 Effects of ursodeoxycholic acid on immune markers (immunomodulatory)

In vivo
1. Reduction of aberrant HLA-I, ICAM-I
2. Reduces circulating IgM (IgG, IgA)
3. Reduces number of activated lymphocytes

In vitro
Modifies the production of cytokines
   inhibits IL-4 (IL-2)
   stimulates IL-2, IFN-γ, TNF-β
Stimulates lymphocyte proliferation
   T0 (T1, 2)

ing decrease of membranous enzyme activity, stabilization of mitochondrial membranes) which secondarily could influence the more specific (T-cell-related) immune system. Since 'antigenic structures' altered cell proteins caused by increased toxic bile acids augmenting epitope spreading and HLA antigens disappear from cell membranes, inflammation is reduced. But UDCA obviously has no effect on the currently unknown trigger for primary biliary liver disease (bacteria, viruses, enterotoxins?), since interruption of therapy induces severe rebound effects.

References

1. Leuschner U, Güldütuna S. Possible mode of action of ursodeoxycholic acid in the treatment of cholestatic liver disease. In: Reyes H, Leuschner U, Arias IM, editors. Pregnancy, sex hormones and the liver. Dordrecht: Kluwer; 1996:217–22.
2. Heathcote EJ, Lindor KD, Poupon ER *et al.* Combined analysis of French, American and Canadian randomized controlled trials of ursodeoxycholic acid therapy in primary biliary cirrhosis. Gastroenterology: 1995;108:A1082.
3. Leuschner U, Güldütuna S, Imhof M, Hübner K, Benjaminov A, Leuschner M. Effects of ursodeoxycholic acid after 4 to 12 years therapy in early and late stages of primary biliary cirrhosis. J Hepatol. 1994;21:624–33.
4. Schaffner F. Ursodeoxycholic acid (U) + colchicine (C) for treatment of primary biliary cirrhosis (PBC). Hepatology. 1991;14:62A (abstract).
5. Shibata J, Fujiyama S, Honda Y, Sato T. Combination therapy with ursodeoxycholic acid and colchicine for primary biliary cirrhosis. J Gastroenterol Hepatol. 1992;7:277–82.
6. Raedsch R, Stiehl A, Walker S *et al.* Controlled study on the effects of a combined ursodeoxycholic acid plus colchicine treatment in primary biliary cirrhosis. In: Paumgartner G, Stiehl A, Gerok W, editors. Bile acids and the hepatobiliary system. Dordrecht: Kluwer; 1993:303–9.
7. Podda M, Almasio P, Battezzati PM, Crosignani A and the Italian multicentre group for the study of UDC in PBC. Long-term effect of the administration of ursodeoxycholic acid alone or with colchicine in patients with primary biliary cirrhosis. A double-blind multicenter study. In: Paumgartner G, Stiehl A, Gerok W, editors. Bile acids and the hepatobiliary system. Dordrecht: Kluwer; 1993:310–15.
8. Kaplan MM. The therapeutic effects of ursodiol and methotrexate are additive and well tolerated in primary biliary cirrhosis. Hepatology. 1992;16:92A (abstract).
9. Buscher H-P, Zietzschmann Y, Gerok W. Positive responses to methotrexate and ursodeoxycholic acid in patients with primary biliary cirrhosis responding insufficiently to ursodeoxycholic acid alone. J Hepatol. 1993;18:9–14.
10. Van Steenbergen W, Sciot R, van Eyken P, Desmet V, Fevery J. Methotrexate alone or in combination with ursodeoxycholic acid as possible treatment in primary biliary cirrhosis. In: Van Berge Henegouwen GP, van Hoek B, de Groote J, Matern S, editors. Cholestatic liver diseases. New strategies for prevention and treatment of hepatobiliary and cholestatic liver diseases. Dordrecht: Kluwer; 1994:246–54.
11. Wolfhagen FHJ, van Buuren HR, Schalm SW. Combined treatment with ursodeoxycholic acid and prednisolone in primary biliary cirrhosis. Neth J Med. 1994;44:84–90.
12. Leuschner M, Güldütuna S, You T, Hübner K, Bhatti S, Leuschner U. Ursodeoxycholic acid and prednisolone versus ursodeoxycholic acid and placebo in the treatment of early stages of primary biliary cirrhosis. J Hepatol. 1996;25:48–57.
13. Güldütuna S, Leuschner M, Wunderlich N *et al.* Cholic acid and ursodeoxycholic acid therapy in primary biliary cirrhosis. Eur J Clin Pharmacol. 1993;45:221–5.
14. Salen G, Batta AK. Bile acid metabolism in primary biliary cirrhosis. In: Fromm H, Leuschner U, editors. Bile acids, cholestasis, gallstones. Dordrecht: Kluwer; 1996:275–82.
15. Stiehl A, Raedsch R, Rudolph G. Acute effects of ursodeoxycholic and chenodeoxycholic acid on the small intestinal absorption of bile acids. Gastroenterology. 1990;98:424–8.
16. Beuers U, Paumgartner G, Boyer JL. Effects of bile acids on signalling mechanisms in the hepatocyte. In: Hofmann AF, Paumgartner G, Stiehl A, editors. Bile acids in gastroenterology. Basic and clinical advances. Dordrecht: Kluwer; 1995:162–6.

17. Güldütuna S, Zimmer G, Imhof M, Bhatti S, You T, Leuschner U. Molecular aspects of membrane stabilization by ursodeoxycholate. Gastroenterology. 1993;104:1736–44.
18. Güldütuna S, Zimmer G, Leuschner U. Effect of bile salts on biomembranes. In: Paumgartner G, Beuers U, editors. Bile acids in liver diseases. Dordrecht: Kluwer; 1996:77–87.
19. Krähenbühl S, Talos C, Fischer S, Reichen J. Toxicity of bile acids on the electron transport chain of isolated rat liver mitochondria. Hepatology. 1994;19:471–9.
20. Poupon R, Calmus Y, Podevin R, Poupon RE. Immunomodulation by bile acids. In: Meyer zum Büschenfelde K-H, Paumgartner G, Schölmerich J, editors. Perspectives in gastroenterology. Current facts and future trends. Munich: Urban & Schwarzenberg; 1995:172–8.
21. Yoshikawa M, Tsujii T, Matsumura K *et al.* Immunomodulatory effects of UDCA on immune responses. Hepatology. 1992;16:358–64.

Section IV
Liver cirrhosis

15
Medical treatment of portal hypertension

D. LEBREC

INTRODUCTION

For the last 10 years various vasoactive substances have been tested to reduce or prevent portal hypertension in patients and animals[1]. Most of these drugs decrease portal pressure and portal tributary blood flow; others reduce intrahepatic vascular resistance or vascular resistance in the portosystemic collateral vessels. Certain substances have short-term haemodynamic effects and are used for acute variceal bleeding (see Table 1) while others have long-term haemodynamic effects and may be used to prevent gastrointestinal bleeding (see Table 2). More recently it has been shown in different models of portal hypertension that early administration of vasoactive substances limits the development of portal hypertension and portosystemic shunts[2–4] and thus should reduce the incidence of variceal bleeding. At the present time β-adrenergic antagonists are used for the prevention of the first bleeding and recurrent haemorrhage. Nitrates associated with β-blockers were also recently evaluated for this purpose. For acute variceal bleeding it has been established that administration of both terlipressin and somatostatin, or its analogues, is more effective than placebo and as effective as endoscopic sclerotherapy. Pharmacological treatment must be started as soon as possible before endoscopy, and may be administered for 5 days before β-adrenergic antagonist administration.

This chapter presents a summary of the results of clinical trials and a discussion of the indications for medical treatment for the prevention of variceal bleeding. The final section presents the possible future pharmacological treatments of portal hypertension.

Table 1 Drugs that decrease portal hypertension for a short period

Growth hormone inhibiting factor	Octreodide, somatostatin
Vasoconstrictor	Angiotensin, octapressin, terlipressin, vasopressin

Table 2 Drugs that decrease portal hypertension for a short and long period

Category	Drugs
α_1-Adrenergic agonist	Methoxamine
α-Adrenergic antagonist	Phenoxybenzamine, prazosin[*]
α_2-Adrenergic antagonist	Clonidine[*†]
Angiotensin-converting enzyme inhibitor	Enapril[*]
Angiotensin II blocker	Salarasin
Anti-glucagon	Anti-glucagon
β_2-Adrenergic agonist	Terbutaline
β-Adrenergic antagonist	
Nonselective	Long-acting propranolol[*], mepindolol, nadolol[*], penbutolol, propranolol[*], sotalol, tertatolol, timolol
Cardioselective	Atenolol[*], betaxolol, levomoprolol, metoprolol
β_2-antagonist	ICI 118,551
Blocker of ATP-sensitive K^+ channels	Glibenclamide
Diuretics	Chlorothiazide[*], furosemide, mersalyl, spironolactone[*†]
ET_A and ET_B receptor antagonist	Bosentan
5-Hydroxytryptamine receptor antagonist	Ketanserin[*†], ritanserin[*†]
Inhibitor of nitric oxide release	Naftazone, N^G-monomethyl-L-arginine
Nitrovasodilator	Isosorbide 5-mononitrate[*†], isosorbide dinitrate[*], linsidomine, molsidomine[*], nitroglycerin
Platelet-activating factor antagonist	BN 52021
Vasodilator	Parathyroid hormone (6 PTH (1-34)), pentifylline
Combination of drugs	
α–β-adrenergic antagonist	Labetalol
β-antagonist with nitroxy-base	Nipradilol[*]

[*] Substances with short- and long-term portal haemodynamic effects.

[†] Substances which had been combined with propanolol.

PREVENTION OF THE OCCURRENCE OF LARGE OESOPHAGEAL VARICES

A randomized blind study was performed to test the effects of long-acting propranolol on the occurrence of large oesophageal varices in patients with or without small oesophageal varices[5]. Two-hundred and six patients were randomized in two groups; 104 received a placebo and 102 propranolol. One-third had small oesophageal varices and two-thirds small oesophageal varices. Most of the patients were in good condition (Child Pugh grade A–B). The follow-up was 2 years. Preliminary results of this study showed that propranolol had no beneficial effects on the occurrence of large oesophageal varices since 34% of the patients developed oesophageal varices in the propranolol group and only 9% in the placebo group. The survival rate was not significantly different between the two groups.

Two controlled studies have been published to evaluate the efficacy of β-blockers on mortality in unselected patients with chronic liver disease[6,7]. Both studies failed to demonstrate a significant effect of propranolol on first variceal bleeding or in prolonging survival in these patients.

PREVENTION OF THE FIRST GASTROINTESTINAL BLEEDING

Various controlled studies have been performed comparing β-adrenergic antagonists to placebo, other vasoactive substances, endoscopic sclerotherapy and surgery.

β-Blockers vs placebo

Nine controlled studies have been published[8–16]. A total of 508 patients were treated with β-blockers and 491 received a placebo or vitamin K. In the patients with cirrhosis and oesophageal varices, half were not selected because of hepatocellular carcinoma, other severe chronic diseases or contraindications to β-blockers (absolute: severe heart disease, uncompensated heart failure, severe bradycardia; relative: diabetes, chronic obstructive airways disease, bronchial asthma). Most of the patients included had cirrhosis related to alcoholic intoxication and approximately 75% of them were Pugh's grade A or B. All had oesophageal varices (small and large or large only) seen at endoscopy. Propranolol (40–480 mg/day), long-acting propranolol (40–320 mg/day) or nadolol (40–160 mg/day) were administered orally once or twice a day (propranolol) at a dose which reduced the resting heart rate by approximately 20%. One study was double-blind while in the others the physicians, but not the patients, knew who was receiving β-blockers or placebo.

At 2 years, 6–31% of the patients bled in the β-blocker groups; these percentages ranged from 5% to 61% in the control groups. Most of the patients bled from ruptured oesophageal varices in both groups. The survival rate ranged from 65% to 94% at 2 years in the β-blocker groups and from 51% to 70% in the control groups. One study found a significant difference in the survival rate between the two groups[13]. In both groups of one study the risk of bleeding was eliminated in patients who showed a decreased hepatic venous pressure gradient to 12 mmHg or less[17]. These haemodynamic results were, however, not confirmed in a recent study[18].

Three meta-analyses confirmed that β-blockers significantly decrease the risk of the first episode of bleeding without heterogeneity in patients with cirrhosis and oesophageal varices[19–21] and that the risk of bleeding decreased by approximately 45%. These results were observed whatever the cause or severity of cirrhosis, in patients with or without ascites, in patients with moderate or large oesophageal varices and in patients using propranolol or nadolol. In both groups, however, the risks of bleeding and death due to bleeding were higher in patients with severe liver disease than in those in good condition or without ascites[21]. At 2 years the survival rate was significantly higher in patients treated with β-blockers than in those receiving a placebo.

Side-effects occurred in approximately 16% of 286 patients who received β-blockers[22]. In these trials hepatic encephalopathy occurred in less than 0.05% of the patients; similar complications occurred in controls.

β-Blockers vs isosorbide-5-mononitrate

One controlled study compared propranolol and isosorbide-5-mononitrate in the prevention of first bleeding in patients with cirrhosis[23]. The risks of bleeding were not significantly different. At 2 years the percentage of patients free of bleeding was 82% in the isosorbide-5-mononitrate-treated group and 86% in the propranolol-treated group. The 2-year survival rate did not differ between the two groups (92% and 85%, respectively). The conclusion of this study was that oral administration of isosorbide-5-mononitrate is a safe and effective alternative to propranolol in the prophylaxis of bleeding in patients with cirrhosis. This study needs to be confirmed.

β-Blockers vs isosorbide-5-mononitrate plus β-blockers

The efficacy of nadolol plus isosorbide-5-mononitrate has been compared to nadolol alone in the prevention of first gastrointestinal bleeding in patients with cirrhosis[24]. With a follow-up ranging from 1 to 44 months, cumulative probability of variceal bleeding was 18% in the nadolol group and significantly lower (8%) in the nadolol plus isosorbide-5-mononitrate group. There was no significant difference in survival rate between the two groups (21% and 19%, respectively). It was concluded that the addition of isosorbide-5-mononitrate significantly improves the efficacy of β-blockers in the primary prophylaxis of variceal bleeding. A final report of this study, and other controlled studies, are, however, needed.

β-Blockers vs endoscopic sclerotherapy

Two controlled studies compared propranolol and endoscopic sclerotherapy in the prevention of first bleeding in patients with cirrhosis[8,14]. In one study the risk of bleeding was significantly lower in the propranolol group than in the sclerotherapy group at 2 years (6% and 31%, respectively)[8]. No significant difference was observed in the second trial (18% in both groups at 2 years)[14]. No significant difference was observed in survival rate.

β-Blockers vs β-blockers plus endoscopic sclerotherapy

In one controlled trial, propranolol plus endoscopic sclerotherapy was compared to propranolol alone in the prevention of first bleeding in patients with cirrhosis[14]. Combined treatment was not significantly different compared with pharmacological treatment alone (16% and 18%, respectively). Moreover, this trial showed that the survival rate was significantly higher (85%) in the propranolol group than in the combined treatment group (41%).

Conclusion of the pharmacological prevention of the first bleeding

The results of these trials show that oesophageal endoscopy must be performed in patients with cirrhosis. When oesophageal varices are present, β-blockers must be prescribed. In case of failure or contraindications to β-blockers, isosorbide-5-mononitrate may be used. Prospective studies which measure the hepatic venous pressure gradient should be performed to try to select good responders. Endoscopic sclerotherapy should not be combined with β-blockers in patients who have not bled.

PREVENTION OF RECURRENT GASTROINTESTINAL BLEEDING

β-Blockers were first used to prevent recurrent haemorrhage[25]. Then various controlled studies confirmed the first results[9,26–37]. Controlled trials comparing endoscopic sclerotherapy with or without β-blockers vs β-blockers have also been performed.

β-Blockers vs placebo

Thirteen controlled studies have been published[9,26–37]. Morcover, one trial only studied early recurrent bleeding, since propranolol or placebo was given for 2 weeks[38]. This latter study showed that the risk of rebleeding was significantly lower in the propranolol group (20%) than in the placebo group (90%), indicating that β-blockers might prevent early recurrent bleeding and should be administered as soon as possible in patients with cirrhosis who have bled. Another study evaluated recurrent bleeding only in patients who bled from portal hypertensive gastropathy[39]. At 30 months the risk of rebleeding was 48% in the propranolol group and 93% in the control group; there was a significant difference between the two groups. The survival rate was slightly but not significantly higher in the propranolol group than in the placebo group.

A total of 428 patients were treated with β-blockers and 400 received a placebo. The criteria for non-inclusion were similar to those of the prevention of the first bleeding. Most of these patients had cirrhosis related to alcoholic intoxication and approximately 75% of them were Pugh's A or B. Propranolol (20–800 mg/day), long-acting propranolol (160 mg/day) and nadolol (40 mg/day) were administered orally, at a dose which reduced the resting heart rate by approximately 20%. These trials were not double-blind.

At 2 years 21–72% of the patients rebled in the β-blocker groups. These percentages ranged from 50% to 87% in the control groups. Most of the patients rebled from ruptured oesophageal varices and the survival rate ranged from 64% to 96% at 2 years in the β-blocker groups and from 44% to 95% in the control groups. One study found a significant difference in the survival rate between the two groups at 2 years.

Three meta-analyses confirmed that β-blockers significantly decreased the risk of recurrent gastrointestinal bleeding and improved survival rate without heterogeneity in patients with portal hypertension[19,40,41]. They showed that the risk of rebleeding decreased by approximately 40%, and total mortality by 20%. Certain factors were shown to be associated with the risk of rebleeding in patients with cirrhosis receiving propranolol[42]: occurrence of hepatocellular carcinoma, lack of compliance, lack of persistent decrease in heart rate, lack of alcohol abstinence and previous history of bleeding. Neither the dose of propranolol nor the cause or severity of cirrhosis was a factor associated with rebleeding.

One haemodynamic study did not show any significant difference in the initial hepatic venous pressure gradient or in the propranolol-induced changes of the hepatic venous pressure gradient between patients with and without rebleeding[43].

β-Blockers were well tolerated, as in patients treated for the prevention of first bleeding. The incidence of hepatic encephalopathy was 0.025% in both groups. A rebound phenomenon might explain certain rebleeding[44], suggesting that, in patients with cirrhosis, β-blockers should be discontinued progressively over a period of 1 week.

β-Blockers vs endoscopic sclerotherapy

Ten controlled studies compared β-blockers and endoscopic sclerotherapy in the prevention of recurrent gastrointestinal bleeding in patients with cirrhosis[33,37,45–52]. Ethanolamine, polidocanol and absolute alcohol were used, and eradication of varices was obtained between 4 months and 1 year. The risk of rebleeding was significantly lower in the sclerotherapy groups than in the propranolol groups in two studies[45,52], while in one study the risk was higher in patients treated by endoscopic sclerotherapy[46].

Two meta-analyses did not show any significant difference in the risk of recurrent bleeding and survival rate between the two groups[40,53].

Minor side-effects occurred in both groups, but certain severe complications were observed in some patients treated with endoscopic sclerotherapy.

β-Blockers plus endoscopic sclerotherapy vs endoscopic sclerotherapy

Eight controlled trials compared the combination of β-blockers and endoscopic sclerotherapy with endoscopic sclerotherapy alone in the prevention of recurrent gastrointestinal bleeding in patients with cirrhosis[54–61]. β-Blockers were started during the first sclerotherapy session. Among two studies which evaluated early rebleeding, one did not find any significant difference between the two groups, while one trial found that the combined treatment significantly reduced the risk of early rebleeding. Two trials also found that the combination of treatments was more effective than endoscopic sclerotherapy alone, but this finding was not observed in other trials.

One meta-analysis did not find any significant difference in the risk of rebleeding between the two groups[40], while a second meta-analysis showed that the combination of endoscopic sclerotherapy plus β-blockers was more effective on recurrent bleeding than endoscopic sclerotherapy alone[62]. In both meta-analyses the survival rate was not significantly different between the two groups. Moreover, the times for eradication of varices and the recurrence of oesophageal varices following eradication were not significantly different between the two groups. Side-effects were similar in the two groups.

β-Blockers vs β-blockers plus endoscopic sclerotherapy

In two controlled studies, propranolol plus endoscopic sclerotherapy were compared to propranolol alone in the prevention of recurrent gastrointestinal bleeding in patients with cirrhosis[63,64]. At 2 years the risks of rebleeding were 42% and 45% in the combined groups and 59% and 65% in the β-blocker group. A significant difference was observed in only one study. No significant difference was found in the survival rate (64% and 45% in the combined therapy and 74% and 75% in the β-blocker group).

β-Blockers vs β-blockers plus transhepatic sclerotherapy

In one study, propranolol alone was compared to the combination of propranolol and transhepatic sclerotherapy in the prevention of recurrent bleeding in patients with cirrhosis[64]. This study did not show any significant difference in the risk of rebleeding at 2 years (approximately 60% in both groups). Survival rates were also similar.

β-Blockers vs disconnection of the oesophagus

In one study, propranolol was compared to oesophagal clip in the prevention of rebleeding in patients with cirrhosis[65]. Although the risk of rebleeding was significantly higher in the propranolol group (73%) than in the surgical group (17%), no significant difference was observed in survival rate.

β-Blockers plus isosorbide-5-mononitrate vs surgical shunts or endoscopic sclerotherapy

The association of propranolol and isosorbide-5-mononitrate was compared to surgical shunt in patients with cirrhosis in good condition and endoscopic sclerotherapy in patients in bad conditions (Child grade C) in the prevention of the variceal rebleeding[66]. During a mean follow-up of 15 months, rebleeding occurred in 48% of patients in the drug group and in 39% of patients in the invasive treatment group. At 2 years the risk of rebleeding in Child A–B patients was 48% in the drug group and 42% in the shunt group; in Child C patients the risk was 69% in the drug group and 54% in the sclerotherapy group. There was no significant difference between the three groups. The mortality rate was also not significantly different between the three groups. The conclusion of these preliminary results suggests that the association of propranolol and isosorbide-5-mononitrate has to be considered as a first-line treatment in the prevention of the recurrent gastrointestinal bleeding in patients with cirrhosis.

Conclusions on the pharmacological prevention of recurrent gastrointestinal bleeding

The results of these trials showed that β-blockers must be prescribed in patients who have bled from either oesophageal varices or portal hypertensive gastropathy. This pharmacological treatment might be associated with endoscopic sclerotherapy. If this treatment fails, or if patients are non-compliant, they must be treated in some other way.

FUTURE PHARMACOLOGICAL TREATMENTS

Drugs with long-term portal hypotensive effects

Among the various portal hypotensive substances some may be used continuously in the same manner as β-blockers to treat portal hypertension (see Table 2).

Prazosin, an α-blocker, has been used in patients with cirrhosis[67,68]. Two studies showed that continuous administration of this substance to patients with cirrhosis significantly decreased the hepatic venous pressure gradient, and did not alter systemic circulation.

Clonidine, a centrally acting α_2-agonist which reduces sympathetic activity, continuously reduced portal hypertension in patients with cirrhosis[69–71]. The reduction of portal pressure depends on a decrease in blood flow in the superior portosystemic collateral circulation, but in these studies hepatic blood flow was not altered. Clonidine was well tolerated in these patients.

Different diuretics which reduce blood volume, and thus cardiac output, have been used to treat portal hypertension. For example, continuous administration of spironolactone reduces the hepatic venous pressure gradient by approximately 20% for more than 1 month[72,73].

Both ketanserin and ritanserin, two 5-hydroxytryptamine (5-HT$_2$) receptor antagonists, have been tested in patients with cirrhosis since certain results indicate a possible role of serotoninergic mechanisms in portal hypertension. A significant decrease in the hepatic venous pressure gradient was observed following 1 week or 1 month of treatment[74,75]. Hepatic encephalopathy, however, occurred in some patients with severe cirrhosis. This side-effect was mild and transient.

Some nitrates, such as isosorbide-5-mononitrate, isosorbide dinitrate and molsidomine, have been given to patients with cirrhosis for a period ranging from 2 weeks to 6 months[76–80]. These studies showed that nitrates continuously reduced the hepatic venous pressure gradient by 7–53% with a mild decrease in arterial pressure.

Combinations of drugs

β-Blockers have been combined with other substances to obtain a more marked decrease in portal pressure than one drug alone (see Table 2). For example, when nitrovasodilators[81–84], 5-HT$_2$ antagonists[85,86], α_2-adrenergic antagonist[87] or diuretic[73], were associated with propranolol, the hepatic venous pressure gradient or portal pressure decreased more than with one drug alone.

New pharmacological approaches

Various experimental studies have shown that either nitric oxide inhibitors[88] or ATP sensitive K$^+$ channel blockers[89] may reduce portal pressure in portal hypertensive rats. These new approaches should also help us to understand and treat portal hypertension.

The limitation or reduction of hepatic fibrosis could also limit or reduce hepatic vascular resistance, and thus reduce the development of portal hypertension[90].

GENERAL CONCLUSION

At present, non-selective β-blockers and certain nitrates reduce the risk of bleeding in patients with portal hypertension, and must be given to these patients. New vasoactive substances must be tested and more experimental and clinical studies are needed to improve the pharmacological treatment of portal hypertension.

References

1. Lebrec D. Pharmacological treatment of portal hypertension: hemodynamic effects and prevention of bleeding. Pharmacol Ther. 1994;61:65–107.
2. Lin HC, Soubrane O, Cailmail S, Lebrec D. Early chronic administration of propranolol reduces the severity of portal hypertension and portal-systemic shunts in conscious portal vein stenosed rats. J Hepatol. 1991;13:213–19.
3. Lin HC, Soubrane O, Lebrec D. Prevention of portal hypertension and portosystemic shunts by early chronic administration of clonidine in conscious portal vein-stenosed rats. Hepatology. 1091;14:325–30.
4. Sarin SK, Groszmann RJ, Mosca PG *et al.* Propranolol ameliorates the development of portal-systemic shunting in a chronic murine schistosomiasis model of portal hypertension. J Clin Invest. 1991;87:1032–6.
5. Groupe Français de la Prévention Pré-Primaire. Propranolol does not decrease the development of large esophageal varices in patients with cirrhosis. A controlled study. Hepatology. 1995;22:155A.
6. Hayes PC, Crichton S, Shipherd AN, Bouchier IAD. Propranolol in chronic liver disease: a controlled trial of its effect and safety over twelve months. Q J Med. 1987;65:823–34.
7. Plevris JN, Elliot R, Mills PR *et al.* Effect of propranolol on prevention of first variceal bleed and survival in patients with chronic liver disease. Aliment Pharmacol Ther. 1994;8:63–70.
8. Andréani T, Poupon RE, Balkau BJ *et al.* Preventive therapy of first gastrointestinal bleeding in patients with cirrhosis: results of a controlled trial comparing propranolol, endoscopic sclerotherapy and placebo. Hepatology. 1990;12:1413–19.
9. Colman J, Jones P, Finch C, Dudley F. Propranolol in the prevention of variceal haemorrhage in alcoholic cirrhotic patients. Hepatology. 1990;12:851.
10. Conn HO, Grace ND, Bosch J and members of the Boston–New Haven–Barcelona Portal Hypertension Study Group. Propranolol in the prevention of the first hemorrhage from esophagogastric varices: a multicenter, randomized clinical trial. Hepatology. 1991;13:902–12.
11. Idéo G, Bellati G, Fesce E, Grimoldi D. Nadolol can prevent the first gastrointestinal bleeding in cirrhotics: a prospective, randomized study. Hepatology. 1988;6:6–9.
12. Lebrec D, Poynard T, Capron JP *et al.* Nadolol for prophylaxis of gastrointestinal bleeding in patients with cirrhosis. A randomized trial. J Hepatol. 1988;7:118–25.
13. Pascal JP, Calès P and a Multicenter Study Group. Propranolol in the prevention of first upper gastrointestinal tract hemorrhage in patients with cirrhosis of the liver and esophageal varices. N Engl J Med. 1987;317:856–61.
14. The PROVA Study Group. Prophylaxis of first hemorrhage from esophageal varices by sclerotherapy, propranolol or both in cirrhotic patients: a randomized multicenter trial. Hepatology. 1991;14:1016–24.
15. Strauss E, de Sa MFG, Albano A, Lacet CMC, Leite MO, Maffei RA. A randomized controlled trial for the prevention of the first upper gastrointestinal bleeding due to portal hypertension in cirrhosis: sclerotherapy or propranolol versus control groups. Hepatology. 1988;8:1395.
16. Italian Multicenter Project for Propranolol in Prevention of Bleeding. Propranolol prevents first gastrointestinal bleeding in non-ascitic cirrhotic patients. Final report of a multicenter randomized trial. J Hepatol. 1989;9:75–83.
17. Groszmann RJ, Bosch J, Grace ND *et al.* Hemodynamic events in a prospective randomized trial of propranolol versus placebo in the prevention of a first variceal hemorrhage. Gastroenterology. 1990;99:1401–7.
18. McCornick PA, Patch D, Greenslade L, Chin J, McIntyre N, Burroughs AK. Clinical vs hemodynamic response to drugs in portal hypertension. Hepatology. 1995;22:255A.
19. Hayes PC, Davis JM, Lewis JA, Bouchier IA. Meta-analysis of value of propranolol in prevention of variceal haemorrhage. Lancet. 1990;336:153–6.
20. Pagliaro L, D'Amico G, Sörensen TIA *et al.* Prevention of first bleeding in cirrhosis. A meta-analysis of randomized trials of nonsurgical treatment. Ann Intern Med. 1992;117:59–70.
21. Poynard T, Calès P, Pasta L *et al.* and the Franco-Italian Multicenter Study Group. Beta-adrenergic-antagonist drugs in the prevention of gastrointestinal bleeding in patients with cirrhosis and esophageal varices: an analysis of data and prognostic factors in 589 patients from four randomized clinical trails. N Engl J Med. 1991;324:1532–8.
22. Poynard T. Calès P, Pasta L, Ideo G, Pascal JP, Lebrec D. Prevention of gastrointestinal bleeding in cirrhosis. N Engl J Med. 1991;325:1517.

23. Angelico M, Carli L, Piat C *et al.* Isosorbide-5-mononitrate versus propranolol in the prevention of first bleeding in cirrhosis. Gastroenterology. 1993;104:1460–5.
24. Merkel C, Gatta A, Amodio P *et al.* Nadolol or nadolol plus isosorbide-5-mononitrate in the prophylaxis of first variceal bleeding in patients with cirrhosis. Interim analysis of a multicenter study. J Hepatol. 1993 (Suppl. 1);8:S147–8.
25. Lebrec D, Poynard T, Hillon P, Benhamou JP. Propranolol for prevention of gastrointestinal bleeding in patients with cirrhosis. A controlled study. N Engl J Med. 1981;305:1371–4.
26. Burroughs AK, Jenkins WJ, Sherlock S *et al.* Controlled trial of propranolol for the prevention of recurrent variceal hemorrhage in patients with cirrhosis. N Engl J Med. 1983;309:1539–42.
27. Cerbelaud P, Lavignolle A, Perrin D *et al.* Propranolol et prévention des récidives des ruptures de varice oesophagienne du cirrhotique. Gastroenterol Clin Biol. 1986;10:18A.
28. Colombo M, De Franchis R, Tommasini M, Sangiovanni A, Dioguardi N. β-Blockade prevents recurrent gastrointestinal bleeding in well-compensated patients with alcoholic cirrhosis: a multicenter randomized controlled trial. Hepatology. 1989;9:433–8.
29. Garden OJ, Mills PR, Birnie GG, Murray GD, Carter DC. Propranolol in the prevention of recurrent variceal hemorrhage in cirrhotic patients. A controlled trial. Gastroenterology. 1990;98:185–90.
30. Gatta A, Merkel C, Sacerdoti D *et al.* Nadolol for prevention of variceal rebleeding in cirrhosis: a controlled clinical trial. Digestion. 1987;37:22–8.
31. Lebrec D, Poynard T, Bernuau J *et al.* A randomized controlled study of propranolol for prevention of recurrent gastrointestinal bleeding in patients with cirrhosis: a final report. Hepatology. 1984;4:355–8.
32. Queuniet, AM, Czernichow P, Lerebours E, Ducrotte P, Tranvouez JL, Colin R. Etude contrôlée du propranolol dans la prévention des récidives hémorragiques chez les patients cirrhotiques. Gastroenterol Clin Biol. 1987;11:41–7.
33. Rossi VV, Cales P, Burtin P *et al.* Prevention of recurrent variceal bleeding in alcoholic cirrhotic patients: prospective controlled trial of propranolol and sclerotherapy. J Hepatol. 1991;12:283–9.
34. Sheen IS, Chen Y, Liaw YF. Randomized controlled study of propranolol for prevention of recurrent esophageal varices bleeding in patients with cirrhosis. Liver. 1989;9:1–5.
35. Villeneuve JP, Pomier-Layrargues G, Infante-Rivard C *et al.* Propranolol for the prevention of recurrent variceal hemorrhage: a controlled trial. Hepatology. 1986;6:1239–43.
36. Kiire CF. Controlled trial of propranolol to prevent recurrent variceal bleeding in patients with non-cirrhotic portal fibrosis. Br Med J 1989;298:1363–5.
37. Qureshi H, Zuberi SJ, Alam E. Efficacy of oral propranolol and injection sclerotherapy in the long-term management of variceal bleeding. Digestion. 1990;46:193–8.
38. Jensen LS, Krarup N. Propranolol may prevent recurrence of oesophageal varices after obliteration by endoscopic sclerotherapy. Scand J Gastroenterol. 1990;25:352–6.
39. Perez-Ayuso RM, Piqué JM, Bosch J *et al.* Propranolol in prevention of recurrent bleeding from severe portal hypertensive gastropathy in cirrhosis. Lancet. 1991;337:1431–4.
40. Pagliaro L, Burroughs AK, Sorensen TIA *et al.* Therapeutic controversies and randomised controlled trials (RCTs): prevention of bleeding and rebleeding in cirrhosis. Gastroenterol Int. 1989;2:71–84.
41. Bernard B, Lebrec D, Mathurin P, Opolon P, Poynard T. Meta-analysis of β-blockers in the prevention of recurrent variceal bleeding in patients with cirrhosis. Hepatology. 1994;20:106A.
42. Poynard T, Lebrec D, Hillon P *et al.* Propranolol for prevention of recurrent gastrointestinal bleeding in patients with cirrhosis: a prospective study of factors associated with rebleeding. Hepatology. 1987;7:447–51.
43. Valla D, Jiron MI, Poynard T, Braillon A, Lebrec D. Failure of haemodynamic measurements to predict recurrent gastrointestinal bleeding in cirrhotic patients receiving propranolol. J Hepatol. 1987;5:144–8.
44. Lebrec D, Bernuau J, Rueff B, Benhamou JP. Gastrointestinal bleeding after abrupt cessation of propranolol administration in cirrhosis. N Engl J Med. 1982;307:560.
45. Alexandrino PT, Alves MM, Pinto Correia J. Propranolol or endoscopic sclerotherapy in the prevention of recurrence of variceal bleeding. A prospective, randomized controlled trial. J Hepatol. 1988;7:175–85.
46. Andréani T, Poupon RE, Baldau B *et al.* Efficacité comparée du propranolol et de sclérose endoscopique de varices oesophagiennes dans la prévention des récidives d'hémorragies digestives au cours des cirrhoses. Etude contrôlée. Gastroenterol Clin Biol. 1991;15 (Suppl. 2):A215.

47. Dasarathy S, Dwivedi M, Bhargava DK, Sundaram KR, Ramachandran K. A prospective randomized trial comparing repeated endoscopic sclerotheraphy and propranolol in decompensated (Child class B and C) cirrhotic patients. Hepatology. 1992;16:89–94.

48. Dollet JM, Champigneulle B, Patris MA, Gaucher P. Sclérothérapie endoscopique contre propranolol après hémorragie par rupture de varices oesophagiennes chez le cirrhotique. Résultats à 4 ans d'une étude randomisée. Gastroenterol Clin Biol. 1988;12:234–9.

49. Fleig WE, Stange EF, Hunecke R et al. Prevention of recurrent bleeding in cirrhotics with recent variceal hemorrhage: prospective, randomized comparison of propranolol and sclerotherapy. Hepatology. 1987;7:355–61.

50. Martin TH, Taupignon A, Lavignolle A, Perrin D, Le Bodic L. Prévention des récidives hémorragiques du cirrhotique: résultats d'une étude contrôlée comparant propranolol et sclérose endoscopique. Gastroenterol Clin Biol. 1991;15:833–7.

51. Terés J, Bosch J, Bordas JM et al. Propranolol versus sclerotherapy in preventing variceal rebleeding: A randomized controlled trial. Gastroenterology. 1993;105:1508–14.

52. Westaby D, Polson RJ, Gimson, AES, Hayes P, Hayllar K, Williams R. A controlled trial of oral propranolol compared with injection sclerotherapy for the long-term management of variceal bleeding. Hepatology. 1990;11:353–9.

53. Bernard B, Lebrec D, Mathurin P, Opolon P, Poynard T. Meta-analysis of propranolol and endoscopic sclerotherapy in the prevention of gastrointestinal rebleeding in patients with cirrhosis. Hepatology. 1994;20:106A.

54. Acharya SK, Dasarathy S, Saksena S, Pande JN. A prospective randomized study to evaluate propranolol in patients undergoing long-term endoscopic sclerotherapy. J Hepatol. 1993;19:291–300.

55. Argerinos A, Rekoumis G, Klonis C et al. Propranolol in the prevention of recurrent upper gastrointestinal bleeding in patients with cirrhosis undergoing endoscopic sclerotherapy. J Hepatol. 1993;19:301–11.

56. Gerunda GE, Neri D, Zangrandi F et al. Nadolol does not reduce early rebleeding in cirrhotics undergoing endoscopic variceal sclerotherapy: a multicenter randomized controlled trial. Hepatology. 1990;12:988.

57. Jensen LS, Krarup N. Propranolol in prevention of rebleeding from oesophageal varices during the course of endoscopic sclerotherapy. Scand J Gastroenterol. 1989;24:213–22.

58. Lundell L, Leth R, Lind T, Lönroth H, Sjövall M, Olbe L. Evaluation of propranolol for prevention of recurrent bleeding from esophageal varices between sclerotherapy sessions. Acta Chir Scand. 1990;156:711–15.

59. Vickers C, Rhodes J, Chesner I et al. Prevention of rebleeding from oesophageal varices: two-year follow up of a prospective controlled trial of propranolol in addition to sclerotherapy. J Hepatol. 1994;21:81–7.

60. Vinel JP, Lamouliatte H, Cales P et al. Propranolol reduced the rebleeding rate during endoscopic sclerotherapy before variceal obliteration. Gastroenterology. 1992;102:1760–3.

61. Westaby D, Melia W, Hegarty J, Gimson AES, Stellon AJ, Williams R. Use of propranolol to reduce the rebleeding rate during injection sclerotherapy prior to variceal obliteration. Hepatology. 1986;6:673–5.

62. Bernard B, Lebrec D, Mathurin P, Opolon P, Poynard T. Meta-analysis of propranolol plus endoscopic sclerotherapy and endoscopic sclerotherapy alone in the prevention of gastrointestinal rebleeding in patients with cirrhosis. Hepatology. 1995;22:252A.

63. Ink O, Martin T, Poynard T et al. Does elective sclerotherapy improve the efficacy of long-term propranolol for prevention of recurrent bleeding in patients with severe with cirrhosis? A prospective multicenter, randomized trial: Hepatology. 1992;16:912–19.

64. O'Connor KW, Lehman G, Yune H et al. Comparison of three nonsurgical treatments for bleeding esophageal varices. Gastroenterology. 1989;96:899–906.

65. Parelon G, Guiry P, Daures JP et al. Prévention de la récidive hémorragique par rupture de varices oesophagiennes chez le cirrhotique. Etude contrôlée comparant le propranolol et la ligature de l'oesophage sur clip. Presse Med. 1989;18:1743–7.

66. Feu F, McCormick PA, Planas R, Burroughs AK, Bosch J and the Variceal Rebleeding Study Group. Randomized controlled trial comparing propranolol + isosorbide-5-mononitrate vs shunt surgery/sclerotherapy in the prevention of variceal rebleeding. J Hepatol. 1995;23 (Suppl. 1):69.

67. Mills PR, Rae AP, Farah DA, Russell RI, Lorimer AR, Carter DC. Comparison of three adrenoreceptor blocking agents in patients with cirrhosis and portal hypertension. Gut. 1984;25:73–8.

68. Albillos A, Lledo JL, Rossi I *et al.* Continuous prazosin administration in cirrhotic patients: effects on portal hemodynamics and on liver and renal function. Gastroenterology. 1995;109:1257–65.
69. Albillos A, Banares R, Barrios C *et al.* Oral administration of clonidine in patients with alcoholic cirrhosis. Hemodynamic and liver function effects. Gastroenterology. 1992;102:248–54.
70. Esler P, Dudley F, Hennings F *et al.* Increased sympathetic nervous activity and the effects of its inhibition with clonidine in alcoholic cirrhosis. Ann Intern Med. 1992;16:446–55.
71. Roulot D, Moreau R, Gaudin C *et al.* Long-term sympathetic and hemodynamic responses to clonidine in patients with cirrhosis and ascites. Gastroenterology. 1992;102:1309–18.
72. Okumura H, Aramaki T, Katsuta Y *et al.* Reduction in hepatic venous pressure gradient as a consequence of volume contraction due to chronic administration of spironolactone in patients with cirrhosis and no ascites. Am J Gastroenterol. 1991;86:46–52.
73. Garcia-Pagan JC, Salmeron JM, Feu F *et al.* Spironolactone decreases portal pressure in patients with compensated cirrhosis. J Hepatol. 1992;13 (Suppl. 2):S30.
74. Huet PM, Pomier-Layrargues G, Semret MM. Effects of ritanserin, a serotonin antagonist, in cirrhotic patients with portal hypertension. Hepatology. 1988;8:1422.
75. Vorobioff J, Garcia-Tsao G, Groszmann RJ *et al.* Long-term hemodynamic effects of ketanserin, a 5-hydroxytryptamine blocker, in portal hypertensive patients. Hepatology. 1989;8:88–91.
76. Freeman JG, Barton JR, Record CO. Effect of isosorbide dinitrate, verapamil, and labetalol on portal pressure in cirrhosis. Br Med J. 1985;291:561–2.
77. Cervinka J, Kordac V, Kalab M. Effect of per oral administration of isosorbide dinitrate on portal pressure and blood flow in patients with cirrhosis of the liver. J Int Med Res. 1989;17:560–4.
78. Garcia-Pagan JC, Feu F, Navasa M *et al.* Long-term haemodynamic effects of isosorbide-5-mononitrate in patients with cirrhosis and portal hypertension. J Hepatol. 1990;1:189–95.
79. Hüppe D, Jäger D, Tromm A, Tunn S, Barmeyer J, May B. Acute and long-term effects of molsidomine on portal and cardiac haemodynamis in patients with cirrhosis of the liver. Eur J Gastroenterol Hepatol. 1992;4:849–55.
80. Vorobioff J, Picabea E, Gamen M, Villavicencio R. Isosorbide dinitrate in portal hypertensive patients. J Hepatol. 1992;16:387.
81. Garcia-Pagan JC, Navasa M, Bosch J, Bru C, Pizcueta P, Rodés J. Enhancement of portal pressure reduction by the association of isosorbide-5-mononitrate to propranolol administration in patients with cirrhosis. Hepatology. 1990;11:230–8.
82. Kroeger RJ, Groszmann RJ. The effect of the combination of nitroglycerin and propranolol on splanchnic and systemic hemodynamics in a portal hypertensive rat model. Hepatology. 1985;5:425–430.
83. Monnin JL, Vinel JP, Le Quellec A *et al.* Etude par échographie Doppler pulsé des effets de la molsidomine et de l'association propranolol-molsidomine sur l'hémodynamique portale. Gastroenterol Clin Biol. 1992;16:745–50.
84. Oshuga M, Cailmail S, Lebrec D. Hemodynamic effects of nipradiol, a new β-adrenergic antagonist combined with a nitroxy-base, in rats with intra- or extra-hepatic portal hypertension. J Hepatol. 1993;17:236–40.
85. Hadengue A, Moreau R, Cerini R, Koshy A, Lee SS, Lebrec D. Combination of ketanserin and verapamil or propranolol in patients with alcoholic cirrhosis: research for an additive effect. Hepatology. 1989;9:83–7.
86. Pomier-Layrargues G, Giroux L, Rocheleau B, Huet PM. Combined treatment of portal hypertension with ritanserin and propranolol in conscious and unrestrained cirrhotic rats. Hepatology. 1992;15:878–82.
87. Roulot D, Gaudin C, Braillon A, Sekiyama T, Bacq Y, Lebrec D. Hemodynamic effects of combination of clonidine and propranolol in conscious cirrhotic rats. Can J Physiol Pharmacol. 1989;67:1369–72.
88. Vallance P, Moncada S. Hyperdynamic circulation in cirrhosis: a role for nitric oxide. Lancet. 1991;337:776–8.
89. Moreau R, Komeichi H, Cailmail S, Lebrec D. Blockade of ATP-sensitive K^+ channels by glibenclamide reduces portal pressure and hyperkinetic circulation in portal hypertensive rats. J Hepatol. 1992;16:215–18.
90. Brenner DA, Alcorn JM. Therapy for hepatic fibrosis. Sem Liver Dis. 1990;10:75–83.

16
Interventional treatment for portal hypertension

T. SAUERBRUCH, K. -A. BRENSING and P. RAAB

INTRODUCTION

Interventional treatments for portal hypertension can be divided into procedures which reduce the bleeding risk locally (e.g. sclerotherapy, injection of glue, endoscopic ligation, transection) and procedures that lead to a systemic reduction of portal hypertension (various shunts including transjugular intrahepatic portosystemic stent shunt – TIPS). The latter procedures are accompanied by systemic effects on mental status, renal sodium handling, ascites formation and systemic haemodynamics.

This chapter focuses mainly on endoscopic measures and shunt procedures for the therapy and prophylaxis of variceal bleeding.

PROPHYLAXIS OF FIRST BLEEDING

About 50–60% of patients with liver cirrhosis have oesophageal varices at the time they are examined for liver disease. About 30% of those patients with varices and no history of previous bleeding will eventually bleed within the next 2 years[1,2]. Endoscopic parameters are probably the best risk indicators for bleeding, such as large varices, concomitant fundic varices or varices with the so-called red-colour-sign[2,3]. All these signs reflect high transmural variceal pressure. Besides long-term medical decompression of portal hypertension with propranolol[4], two interventional methods have been evaluated for the prevention of first bleeding, namely portacaval shunt operation and endoscopic sclerotherapy (see ref. 5).

Three of the four important controlled studies in the late 1960s showed that the first bleeding risk can be reduced from 30–40% to 10% or less by a prophylactic shunt. One trial found no difference. However, there was an excess mortality rate in the shunt group, ranging between 42% and 80% as against 27% to 55% in the controls[5]. Prophylactic surgery obviously proved more dangerous for these patients than a wait-and-see attitude. Later, in the 1970s and 1980s, quite a large number of patients – predominantly with large varices – were randomized to sclerotherapy or non-active observation. Overall there was a positive trend in favour of sclerotherapy[5]. However, the results are too heterogeneous to advocate sclerotherapy, especially since two trials found an excess bleeding rate in the sclerotherapy group[6,7]. Sclerotherapy, at least in some hands, still bears too high a potential for complications. Thus, today, propranolol is believed to be the method of choice to prevent first bleeding. According to a large meta-analysis the risk of bleeding within 2 years can be reduced from 35% to 22%[4]. However, the death rate is not influenced to any major extent[4,5]. Further studies are necessary to determine whether ligation is a valuable alternative to propranolol or a combined medical treatment, e.g. propranolol and nitrates.

TREATMENT OF ACUTE VARICEAL BLEEDING

Injection sclerotherapy, emergency shunt or emergency TIPS are the three interventional options for treating variceal bleeding. In some centres these measures arc accompanicd by balloon tamponade in case of heavy bleeding.

Emergency injection sclerotherapy – according to randomized trials[5] – controls bleeding in 70–95% of patients. However, early rebleeding is the major problem of injection sclerotherapy, especially when sclerosing substances such as polidocanol are used[8]. Early rebleeding may be caused by insufficient variceal thrombosis and/or fibrosis after the first session, or by bleeding from mucosal ulcerations. The first situation can be improved by bucrylate injection, which immediately blocks the vessels[9,10]. Ulcerations may be prevented by using fibrin glue[11] or ligation[12]. Early rebleeding is also reduced by adjuvant medical treatment with octreotide over a period of 5 days[13].

EMERGENCY SHUNT

Emergency shunt – defined as a portacaval shunt operation within 8 hours – has been advocated by some specialized centres for more than 30 years. Although these groups presented excellent results[14,15] with up to 80% 30-day survival in Child C patients, their data have been questioned by others[16]. Nowadays, endoscopy with ligation and/or injections of sclerosants or glue – possibly with adjuvant medical decompressive therapy[13,17] – offers a less invasive approach for arresting bleeding in the majority of patients. Thus, the shunt has its use as a rescue procedure[18] for patients with refractory recurrent bleeding. Many of these patients belong to Child's group C and – according to most randomized trials – have a high operative risk (mortality 50% or more[16,19]).

The role of emergency TIPS is ill-defined. We found that the degree of multi-organ failure, high bilirubin, low prothrombin time, and emergency TIPS insertion are the most important risk factors for mortalities (see Table 1).

When we used emergency TIPS, we had a 30-day mortality rate of 53%, although procedure-related mortality was only 6%, and no rebleeding occurred. Thus, the emergency shunt procedure should mainly be considered in Child's A and B patients with recurrent bleeding. In these patients it guarantees definite

Table 1   Risk factors of 60-day mortality after TIPS ($n = 60$)

	Survival (n = 48)	Death (n = 12)	p-Value
Bilirubin (mg/dl)	1.9 (± 1.4)	5.1 (± 4.5)	$p<0.05$
Prothrombin time (Quick %)	77 (± 18)	60 (± 23)	$p<0.01$
Serum albumin	3.3 (± 0.6)	3.1 (± 0.7)	n.s.
Serum creatinine	1.1 (± 0.9)	1.6 (± 1.2)	n.s.
Child–Pugh score	7.8 (± 1.9)	10.5 (± 2.7)	$p<0.001$
APACHE II score	9.9 (± 4)	17.9 (± 7.8)	$p<0.01$
Elective TIPS ($n = 43$)	40 (93%)	3 (7%)	$p<0.01$
Emergency TIPS ($n = 17$)	8 (47%)	9 (53%)	

control of haemorrhage. In most Child C patients, impending liver failure, and not the therapeutic procedure, dictates the outcome. Intermittent TIPS insertion with transplant rescue may be a solution for those candidates whose bleeding cannot be arrested by other means.

RECURRENT BLEEDING

Patients who survive their first variceal bleed have a rebleeding risk of about 70%[1]. These patients therefore require a rebleeding prophylaxis. Interventional treatment probably has the greatest impact on this situation.

Endoscopic therapy and shunt procedures have been evaluated thoroughly in randomized controlled trials[5]. The classic shunt trials in the 1970s, including a total of 412 patients, demonstrated the dramatic decrease in bleeding risk after successful operations. Rebleeding ranged between 65% and 98% in the control groups and between 9% and 20% in the shunt groups. The death rate, however, was only marginally affected (47–68% in the controls vs 44–58% after shunt operation). Furthermore, the occurrence of severe portosystemic encephalopathy rose by a factor of 4 to 5 (from 4% to around 20%).

The advantage of distal splenorenal shunt over the total portacaval shunt is probably minor with respect to rebleeding, survival or chronic portosystemic encephalopathy[5].

The lack of improvement in survival and the further development of better endoscopes was one major reason for the advent of endoscopic measures such as rebleeding prophylaxis. Although rebleeding events remained relatively high under long-term sclerotherapy (around 50%), they were significantly reduced[8] compared with the control populations (ranging between 54% and 84%). The impact on survival was marginal and very similar to the effect of shunt operations. Therefore, it is not surprising that the direct comparison of shunt operation and sclerotherapy found significantly less rebleeding events in the shunt groups as compared to the sclerotherapy groups, while the death rate was practically the same with a two-fold higher risk of portosystemic encephalopathy in the shunted patients[5]. The patient may thus opt for an increased risk of bleeding or an increased risk of encephalopathy, as regards the interventional prophylaxis of rebleeding. One study indicates that sequential therapy may be the solution, e.g. starting with an endoscopic measure and using surgery to rescue sclerotherapy failures[18].

In this context two major improvements must be taken into consideration: the transjugular intrahepatic portosystemic stent shunt (TIPS) and the ligation of varices to replace injection sclerotherapy.

There is now no doubt that ligation is superior to sclerotherapy[12]. As documented by randomized trials, patients experience less rebleeding, fewer complications such as strictures, bleeding ulceration, pneumonia or spontaneous bacterial peritonitis. This probably also translates into a slight improvement in survival time.

Comparison of TIPS vs sclerotherapy showed, as expected, less bleeding in the TIPS group as compared to sclerotherapy[20–23] and a higher encephalopathy rate[24]. A direct comparison with TIPS showed fewer bleeding events in the TIPS group (11% vs 52%) with a higher encephalopathy rate in the shunt group, and both with a similar survival rate[25] (see also Figs 1 and 2).

Beta-blockers in combination with sclerotherapy further reduce the bleeding risk[5]. Their adjuvant effect for ligation has not yet been defined.

In patients receiving rebleeding prophylaxis, three situations need special attention: concomitant severe ascites, hepatorenal dysfunction or bleeding from portal-hypertensive gastropathy.

It has been clearly shown that – after shunt surgery – the risk of ascites formation is lower than after therapies that do not lead to portavenous decompression[26]. This also holds true for TIPS insertion. TIPS leads to an

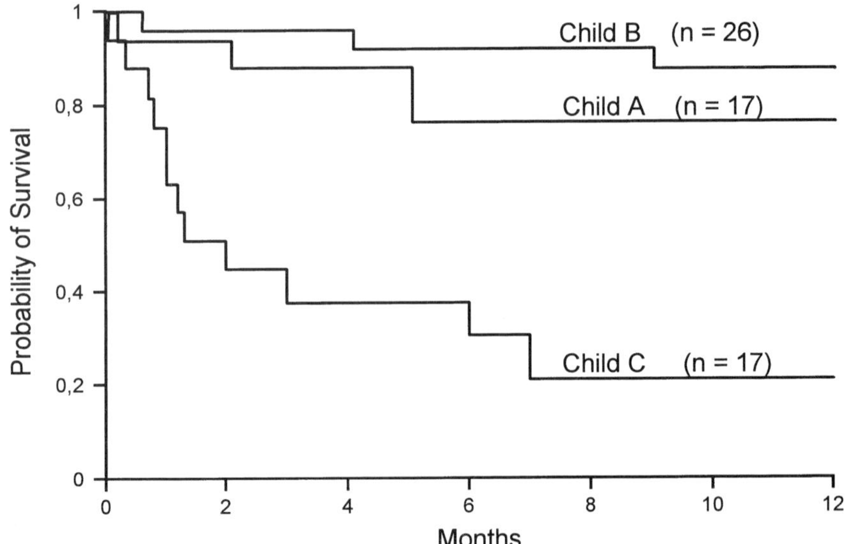

Fig. 1   Survival of 60 consecutive patients receiving TIPS for recurrent variceal haemorrhage (*n* = 53) or refractory ascites (*n* = 7) between 1992 and 1995 at the Medical and Radiological Department of the University of Bonn (Kaplan–Meier)

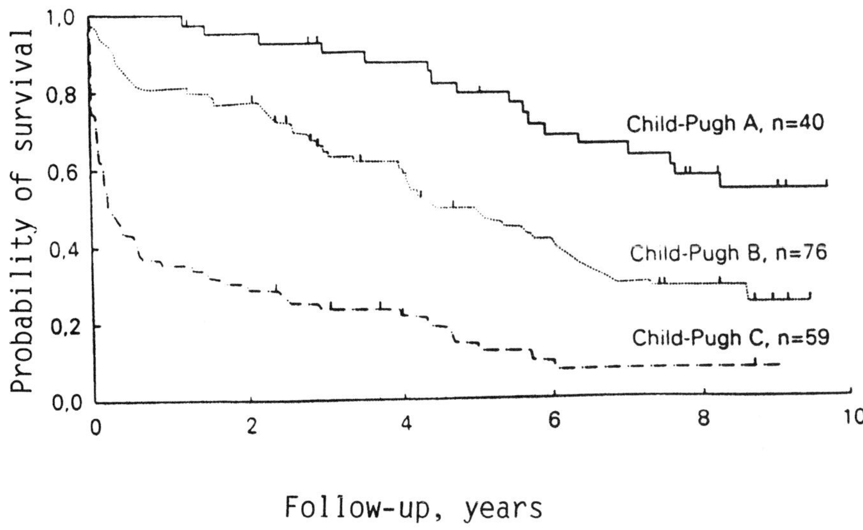

Follow-up, years

Fig. 2 Survival of 175 consecutive patients receiving sclerotherapy for initial haemostasis and subsequent rebleeding prophylaxis at the Department of Internal Medicine II in Munich (Head G. Paumgartner) between 1980 and 1992. Data from ref. 34 are extended to a 10-year follow-up

increase in sodium excretion which allows the mobilization of ascites – previously refractory to therapy – in most patients[27–29]. Therefore, patients with bleeding and severe ascites may be good candidates for a rebleeding prophylaxis with a shunt procedure, especially if they belong to Child's group B.

Acute bleeding hypertensive gastropathy is rare (less than 5% in patients with liver disease admitted for gastrointestinal bleeding[30]). These patients are candidates for medical decompression with propranolol[31]. However, this often fails and even TIPS, which reduces portal pressure less pronouncedly than a total shunt, may be insufficient. Some of these patients, therefore, require an open shunt operation[32].

SUMMARY

Interventional treatment of portal hypertension has led to several options, namely different shunt procedures, i.e. transection, sclerotherapy and ligation. The role of these different therapeutic modalities has been defined in a considerable number of randomized controlled trials. Shunts offer the best prophylaxis for primary and recurrent bleeding. Furthermore, the sodium balance is positively influenced. However, they do not improve survival and they have the disadvantage of increasing the risk of encephalopathy. Ligation is superior to sclerotherapy[12]. For most patients it should be the first choice for preventing recurrent bleeding, possibly together with propranolol. If these patients rebleed, they should be considered for a shunt procedure. The prophylaxis of first bleeding, to date, is not an indication for interventional treatment[33]. This, however, may change if ligation is used.

Thus, randomized controlled trials have defined the efficacy of different treatment modalities. With this knowledge, sequential treatment should probably be offered to the patients. Medical decompressive therapy should be begun immediately when a patient with liver disease shows signs of intestinal bleeding. On admission the patient should go on to endoscopy (sclerotherapy, injection of glue or ligation) for active haemostasis. As concerns rebleeding prophylaxis, the patient should be introduced to a ligation programme – possibly with concomitant beta-blockers – to prevent rebleeding. In case of rebleeding a shunt rescue (TIPS, open surgery) should be considered, especially in patients with refractory ascites. If liver function continues to decline despite abstinence from alcohol or despite other effective causal treatments, a liver transplantation is the next consideration.

Acknowledgement

We thank Mrs S. Körner for superb secretarial help.

References

1. Calès P, Pascal JP. Histoire naturelle des varices oesophagiennes au cours de la cirrhose (de la naissance à la rupture). Gastroenterol Clin Biol. 1988;12:245–54.
2. Kleber G, Sauerbruch T, Ansari H, Paumgartner G. Prediction of variceal hemorrhage in cirrhosis: a prospective follow-up study. Gastroenterology. 1991;100:1332–7.
3. Sauerbruch T, Kleber G. Upper gastrointestinal endoscopy in patients with portal hypertension. Endoscopy. 1992;24:45–51.
4. Poynard T, Calès P, Pasta L *et al.* and the Franco-Italian Multicenter Study Group. Beta-adrenergic-antagonist drugs in the prevention of gastrointestinal bleeding in patients with cirrhosis and esophageal varices. N Engl J Med. 1991;324:1532–8.
5. D'Amico G, Pagliaro L, Bosch J. The treatment of portal hypertension: a meta-analytic review. Hepatology. 1995;22:332–54.
6. Santangelo WC, Dueno MI, Estes BL, Krejs GJ. Prophylactic sclerotherapy of large esophageal varices. N Engl J Med. 1988;318:814–18.
7. Veterans Affairs Cooperative Variceal Sclerotherapy Group. Prophylactic sclerotherapy for esophageal varices in alcoholic liver disease: a randomized, single-blind, multicenter clinical trial. N Engl J Med. 1991;324:1779–84.
8. Sauerbruch T, Fischer G, Ansari H. Variceal injection sclerotherapy. Baillière's Clin Gastroenterol. 1991;5:131–53.
9. Soehendra N, Grimm H, Nam VCh, Berger B. N-Butyl-2-cyanoacrylate: a supplement to endoscopic sclerotherapy. Endoscopy. 1987;19:221–4.
10. Feretis C, Tabakopoulos D, Benakis P, Xenofontos M, Golematis B. Endoscopic hemostasis of esophageal and gastric variceal bleeding with histoacryl. Endoscopy. 1990;22:282–4.
11. Zimmer T, Rucktäschel F, Stölzel U *et al.* Endoscopic sclerotherapy with polidocanol as compared with fibrin glue to prevent esophageal variceal rebleeding. (Submitted).
12. Laine L, Cook D. Endoscopic ligation compared with sclerotherapy for treatment of esophageal variceal bleeding. Ann Intern Med. 1995;123:280–7.
13. Sung JJY, Chung SCS, Yung MY *et al.* Prospective randomised study of effect of octreotide on rebleeding from esophageal varices after endoscopic ligation. Lancet. 1995;346:1666–9.
14. Orloff MJ, Orloff MS, Ranbotti M, Girard B. Is portal systemic shunt worthwhile in Child's Class C cirrhosis? Long-term results of emergency shunt in 94 patients with bleeding varices. Ann Surg. 1992;216:256–68.
15. Orloff MJ, Bell RH, Orloff MS, Hardison WGM, Greenburg AG. Prospective randomized trial of emergency portacaval shunt and emergency medical therapy in unselected cirrhotic patients with bleeding varices. Hepatology. 1994;20:863–72.

16. Henderson JM, Grace ND. Editorial: A perspective on emergency portacaval shunt. Hepatology. 1994;20:1090–1.
17. Levacher S, Letoumelin P, Pateron D, Blaise M, Lapandry C, Pourriat J-L. Early administration of terlipressin plus glyceryl trinitrate to control active upper gastrointestinal bleeding in cirrhotic patients. Lancet. 1995;346:865–8.
18. Henderson JM, Kutner MH, Millikan WJ *et al.* Endoscopic variceal sclerosis compared with distal splenorenal shunt to prevent recurrent variceal bleeding in cirrhosis. A prospective, randomized trial. Ann Intern Med. 1990;112:262–9.
19. Cello JP, Grendall JH, Crass RA *et al.* Endoscopic sclerotherapy versus portacaval shunt in patients with severe cirrhosis and acute variceal hemorrhage. N Engl J Med. 1987;316:11–15.
20. Sanyal AJ, Freedman AM, Purdum PP *et al.* Transjugular intrahepatic portosystemic shunt (TIPS) vs sclerotherapy for prevention of recurrent variceal hemorrhage: a randomized prospective trial. Gastroenterology. 1994;106:A975.
21. Cabrera J, Maynar M, Granados R *et al.* Transjugular intrahepatic portosystemic shunt (TIPS) vs sclerotherapy in the elective treatment of variceal bleeding. Hepatology. 1994;20:203A (no. 425).
22. Rössle M, Deibert P, Haag K, Ochs A, Siegerstetter V, Langer M. TIPS versus sclerotherapy and β-blockade: preliminary results of a randomized study in patients with recurrent variceal hemorrhage. Hepatology. 1994;20:107A (no. 44).
23. Merli M, Riggio O, Capocaccia L *et al.* and GIST. Transjugular intrahepatic portosystemic shunt (TIPS) vs endoscopic sclerotherapy (ES) in preventing variceal rebleeding. Preliminary results of a randomized controlled trial. Hepatology. 1994;20:107A (no. 43).
24. Sanyal AJ, Freedom AM, Shiffman ML, Purdum III PP, Luketic VA, Cheatham AK. Portosystemic encephalopathy after transjugular intrahepatic portosystemic shunt: results of a prospective controlled study. Hepatology. 1994;20:46–55.
25. Jalan R, Forrest EH, Redhead DN *et al.* TIPSS vs variceal band ligation in the secondary prevention of variceal haemorrhage in cirrhosis: preliminary results of a randomised, controlled study. Hepatology. 1995;22:251A (no. 578).
26. Quiroga J, Sangro B, Núñez M *et al.* Transjugular transhepatic portal-systemic shunt in the treatment of refractory ascites: effect on clinical, renal, humoral, and hemodynamic parameters. Hepatology. 1995;21:986–94.
27. Wong F, Sniderman K, Liu P, Allidina Y, Sherman M, Blendis L. Transjugular intrahepatic portosystemic stent shunt: effects on hemodynamics and sodium homeostasis in cirrhosis and refractory ascites. Ann Intern Med. 1995;122:816–22 (no. 3168).
28. Wong F, Blendis L. Transjugular intrahepatic portosystemic shunt for refractory ascites: tipping the sodium balance. Hepatology. 1995;22:358–64.
29. Brensing KA, Raab P, Textor J *et al.* Besserung von Aszites und Nierenfunktion nach TIPS-Anlage wegen refraktärer Varizenblutung, Diuretika-refraktärem Aszites oder hepatorenalem Syndrom. Z Gastroenterol. 1996;34:101 (no. 5.167).
30. Gostout CJ, Viggiano TR, Balm RK. Acute gastrointestinal bleeding from portal hypertensive gastropathy: prevalence and clinical features. Am J Gastroenterol. 1993;88:2030–3.
31. Triger DR. Portal hypertensive gastropathy. Baillière's Clin Gastroenterol. 1992;6:481–95.
32. Orloff MJ, Orloff MS, Orloff SL, Haynes KS. Treatment of bleeding from portal hypertensive gastropathy by portacaval shunt. Hepatology. 1995;21:1011–17.
33. Sauerbruch T. Prophylaxis of first variceal bleeding: where does the truth lie? Endoscopy. 1994;26:748–9.
34. Sauerbruch T, Weinzierl M, Ansari H, Paumgartner G. Injection sclerotherapy of esophageal variceal haemorrhage. A prospective long-term follow-up study. Endoscopy. 1987;19:181–4.

17
Treatment of ascites

A. L. GERBES and G. PAUMGARTNER

INTRODUCTION

Consideration of the important features of pathophysiology of ascites formation helps towards a rational therapy and to avoid complications[1–6]. The pathophysiology of sodium retention and ascites formation in cirrhosis is governed by portal hypertension and two seemingly contradictory phenomena (Fig. 1): renal vasoconstriction despite peripheral vasodilatation and contraction of centrally effective blood volume concomitant with expanded total blood volume. Therapeutic activities should take these pathophysiological changes into consideration, and should aim at correcting them or at least not causing a deterioration of them.

The following therapeutic options are available for ascites in cirrhosis of the liver: bed rest, sodium-restricted diet, diuretics, vasoactive substances (such as the vasopressin analogue ornipressin), large-volume paracentesis, peritoneovenous shunting, portacaval shunting (surgical or non-surgical, such as TIPS (transjugular intrahepatic portosystemic shunt)), and ultimately liver transplantation.

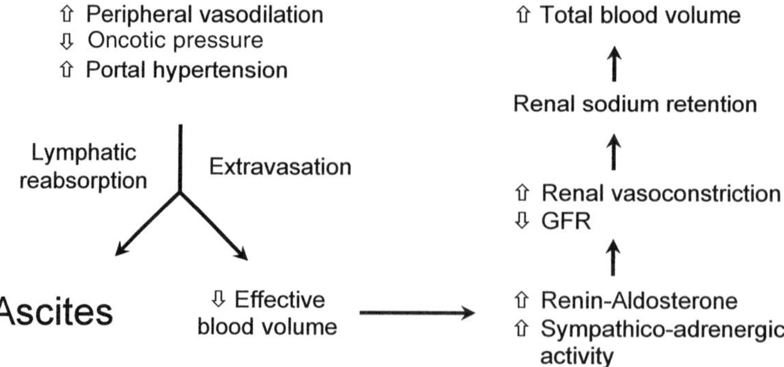

Fig. 1 Important pathophysiological factors for ascites formation in liver disease

POSTURE AND SODIUM RESTRICTION

Changes of posture can affect volume receptors and baroreceptors and induce neurohumoral changes[7–9], even in healthy subjects. While the change from supine to sitting position usually activates the sympathico-adrenergic system, and increases plasma renin activity and aldosterone concentration, healthy subjects do not respond with a decrease of urinary sodium excretion. In contrast, patients with decompensated cirrhosis show more marked alterations and react with a significant reduction in renal sodium excretion. Therefore, the supine posture of bed rest, by preventing a further decrease of centrally effective blood volume, can promote natriuresis in decompensated cirrhosis and augment natriuretic effects of diuretics. However, only a minority of patients can mobilize ascites sufficiently following prolonged bed rest.

There is a largely accepted contention that dietary sodium restriction helps to mobilize ascites. However, this is not well supported by published data. Interestingly, a recent study found virtually no difference in the success of treatment of ascites between a group with a 40 mmol sodium diet and another group with a 120 mmol sodium diet[10]. Other studies comparing 10 or 20 mmol sodium to a non-restricted diet obtained similar results[11–13]. Decrease of serum sodium and impairment of renal function accompanying diuretic therapy seem more prominent with a severely sodium-restricted diet. Thus, in patients who respond well to diuretic treatment very severe sodium restriction seems not to be justified. This may be different in patients with a borderline response to diuretic treatment, who could benefit from sodium restriction.

DIURETICS

Patients who do not respond sufficiently to bed rest, and eventually dietary sodium restriction, will be treated sequentially with aldosterone antagonists and loop diuretics. The definition of response to treatment is quite variable, and in several studies ranges between 200 and 400 g loss of body weight per day determined in an interval of between 3 and 7 days. Removal of ascites can be achieved by spironolactone or K^+-canrenoate alone in about 65–80% of patients. The maximum doses applied in controlled studies were between 300 mg/day and 600 mg/day. The addition of loop diuretics can increase the response to 85–90%[14,15] (Fig. 2). Regarding loop diuretics, most data exist for furosemide and maximum doses employed again are highly variable (between 80 and 240 mg/day). For clinical practice we would recommend a stepwise increase to a maximum of 300 mg spironolactone and 120 mg furosemide daily.

Obviously, there are complications of vigorous diuretic therapy, mainly encephalopathy, impairment of renal function and derangement of serum electrolytes. As has been summarized earlier[16–19] complications seem to increase in parallel with the dose of diuretics employed, and with the response rate achieved. Cautious management of patients, comprising thorough initial evaluation and close monitoring for side-effects as well as observation of therapeutic guidelines, can help to minimize the side-effects[14,16].

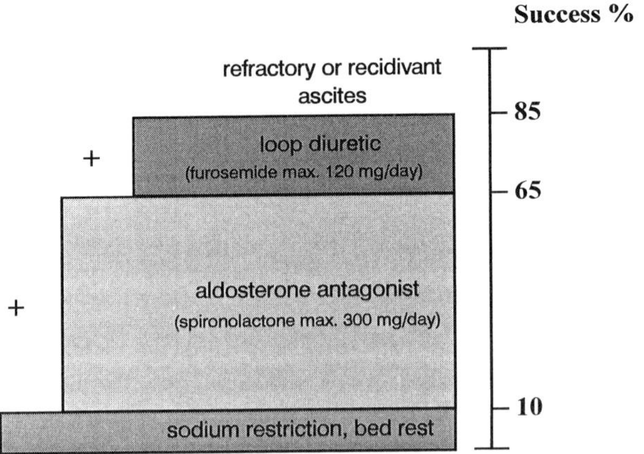

Fig. 2 Conventional sequential therapy of ascites

Amiloride has been recommended as a substitute for spironolactone[20]. A recent investigation, however, has shown that amiloride is clearly less effective than spironolactone, and probably can substitute for spironolactone only in patients without marked hyperaldosteronism[21].

There is evidence that the loop diuretic torasemide could excel over furosemide in patients with cirrhotic ascites[22-24]. This might possibly be due to its longer half-life and smoother, more prolonged action. Of particular interest, patients with very poor response to furosemide exhibited significantly greater natriuresis after receiving torasemide[23]. Similarly the combination of spirono-lactone and torasemide yielded more natriuresis and diuresis than the combination of spironolactone and furosemide[24]. These studies were single-dose and 3-day observations, respectively; therefore further investigations are needed to establish the clinical value of torasemide in these patients.

There are thus the following problems requiring special therapeutic efforts:

1. Rapid relief of massive ascites.
2. Refractory or recidivant ascites.

Massive ascites

Therapeutic paracentesis used to be the only therapy for ascites prior to the development of modern diuretic drugs in the 1960s. Thereafter it had been abandoned due to side-effects such as infections, renal insufficiency or encephalopathy (following a further decrease in effective plasma volume after paracentesis). A few years ago, however, it was shown that daily paracenteses of 4–6 litres could be safely performed provided they were accompanied by intravenous substitution of 40–60 g albumin[25]. *Therapeutic paracentesis* was shown to be no more dangerous than conventional diuretic treatment, but relief of ascites was obviously achieved much faster[26,27]. It was also shown that total paracentesis had no more side-effects than repeated puncture of 4–6 litres[28]. Regarding the high costs of albumin, the use of less expensive plasma expanders was investigated[29,30]. Following administration of dextran or hemaccel plasma renin activity as a parameter of decreased effective blood volume was further increased, which was not the case after the administration of albumin. However, there were no differences in the frequency of serious complications, rehospitalization due to massive ascites, renal insufficiency or survival.

Altogether, for practical purposes daily paracenteses of up to 6 litres with intravenous albumin substitution can be recommended, provided that contraindications are respected (serum bilirubin >10 mg/dl, prothrombin time <40%, thrombocytes <40 g/L, serum creatinine >3 mg/100 ml, marked encephalopathy).

Refractory or recidivant ascites

So far there is no generally accepted definition of refractory or recidivant ascites. Attempts have been made by an international expert panel to reach a consensus[31]. The term 'refractory ascites' is applied if sufficient mobilization of ascites cannot be reached despite maximum diuretic treatment, or when diuretics have to be discontinued due to side-effects. 'Recidivant ascites' is used for patients who, following initial successful ascites therapy, repeatedly present with massive ascites (three times or more within 1 year).

For treatment of patients with refractory ascites *peritoneovenous shunts (PVS)* (Fig. 3) were developed in the 1970s[32]. The PVS consists of a silicon rubber tube with a peritoneal limb in the ascitic fluid and a venous end which, following subcutaneous tunnelling, is fixed in the jugular vein. A chamber with a mitre valve prevents regurgitation of blood into the shunt system. The pressure gradient between peritoneal cavity and jugular vein leads to an infusion of ascites into the central venous circulation. Thus, ascitic fluid could be used to refill the diminished centrally effective blood volume. Unfortunately these beneficial

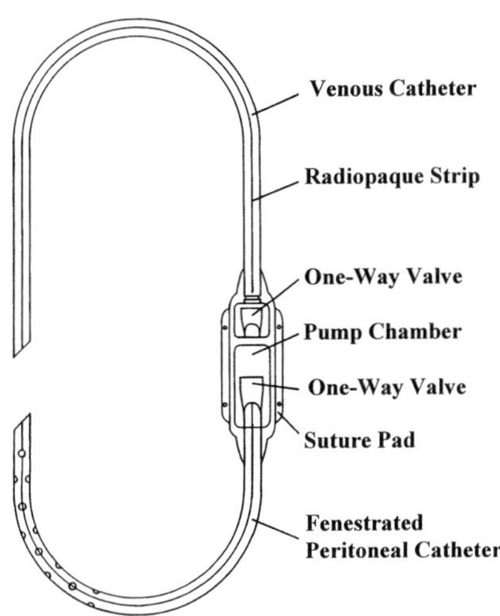

Fig. 3 Schematic illustration of a peritoneovenous shunt (PVS)

effects of PVS, mitigating the activation of the renin–aldosterone and sympathico-adrenergic systems, and promoting diuresis and natriuresis, are accompanied by complications. Among these, coagulopathy, infection, sepsis and clotting of the shunt have prevented general use of this device in these patients.

Therefore, following the good results of paracentesis and albumin substitution in patients with massive ascites, paracentesis was compared to PVS in patients with refractory or recidivant ascites[33,34]. In a prospective randomized trial[33] with more than 80 patients ascites could be mobilized with both procedures in approximately 90% of patients. Frequency of side-effects and 1-year survival were comparable. Following paracentesis each patient was rehospitalized an average of three times a year because of massive ascites, but just once a year in the group with PVS. However, while patients following paracentesis needed more diuretics, a shunt occlusion in half of the patients of the other group required reintervention. Results of this study demonstrate that therapeutic paracentesis yields results comparable to the implantation of a PVS. However, both approaches are unsatisfactory for the treatment of these patients.

Portosystemic shunts reduce the hepatic–venous pressure gradient. The development of a non-surgical portosystemic shunt, the *transjuglar intrahepatic portosystemic shunt (TIPS)* allows a graded decrease of the portosystemic pressure gradient[35,36]. Initially TIPS (Fig. 4) was mainly used for acute variceal bleeding or prophylaxis of recidivant oesophageal variceal bleeding[37]. Many of these patients had ascites which was relieved following TIPS insertion. Therefore,

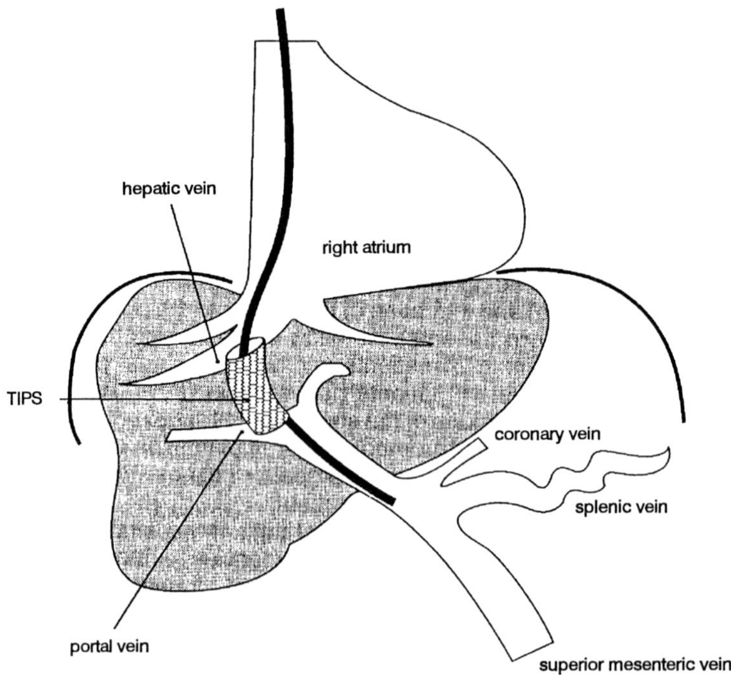

Fig. 4 Schematic illustration of a transjugular intrahepatic portosystemic shunt (TIPS)

refractory and recidivant ascites was selected as the indication for TIPS in a study comprising 50 patients[38]. Following TIPS insertion ascites was fully mobilized in 66% and partially in 26% of patients; there was no effect in only 8%. The 1-year survival rate of 50% was to be expected in these severely ill patients. Thus, TIPS seems to be a promising novel therapeutic approach for patients with refractory or recidivant ascites. Its value, however, needs to be investigated in prospective randomized trials.

LIVER TRANSPLANTATION

Refractory ascites will only rarely be the sole indication for liver transplantation. Often patients with refractory ascites show severe cirrhosis (Child C) with muscle wasting and their nutritional status is not sufficient for transplantation. With Child B patients, however, appearance of refractory ascites could indicate the appropriate time for liver transplant. Success of liver transplantation in patients with massive ascites is comparable to that in patients with small ascites[39]. The presence of massive ascites should prompt consideration of liver transplantation in order not to miss the best time for transplantation.

SUMMARY

Important factors involved in ascites formation of liver cirrhosis are portal hypertension, peripheral vasodilatation and renal vasoconstriction, and a decrease of centrally effective blood volume. Therapeutic approaches should take these changes, which lead to renal sodium retention, into consideration. Therapeutic options for ascites in liver disease comprise bed rest, dietary sodium restriction, diuretic drugs, therapeutic paracentesis, peritoneovenous shunts, portosystemic shunts, treatment with vasoactive substances and ultimately liver transplantation. Conventional sequential therapy of ascites with sodium restriction, bed rest and diuretic treatment with aldosterone antagonists, and eventually loop diuretics, controls ascites in about 85% of patients.

The following clinical situations require special consideration: (a) presence of massive ascites; (b) refractory or recidivant ascites.

1. It has been clearly demonstrated that patients with tense ascites benefit from large-volume paracentesis provided there is a concomitant infusion of plasma expanders, preferably albumin.
2. For patients with refractory or recidivant ascites therapeutic paracentesis has been shown to be of similar benefit as the insertion of a peritoneovenous shunt. Both treatments, however, are unsatisfactory; therefore new therapeutic approaches are being investigated; the transjugular intrahepatic portosystemic shunt (TIPS) seems to be a promising novel approach for the treatment of refractory or recidivant ascites.

References

1. Gerbes AL. Pathophysiology of ascites formation in cirrhosis of the liver. Hepatogastroenterology. 1991;38:360–4.

2. Bichet DG, Van Putten VJ, Schrier RW. Potential role of increased sympathetic activity in impaired sodium and water excretion in cirrhosis. N Engl J Med. 1982;307:1552–7.
3. Bosch J, Arroyo V, Betriu A *et al.* Hepatic hemodynamics and the renin–angiotensin–aldosterone system in cirrhosis. Gastroenterology. 1980;78:92–9.
4. Henriksen JH, Ring-Larsen H, Christensen NJ. Circulating noradrenaline and central haemodynamics in patients with cirrhosis. Scand J Gastroenterol. 1985;20:1185–90.
5. Schrier RW, Arroyo V, Bernardi M, Epstein M, Henriksen JH, Rodes J. Peripheral arterial vasodilatation hypothesis: a proposal for the initiation of renal sodium and water retention in cirrhosis. Hepatology. 1988;8:1151–7.
6. Gerbes AL. Portale Hypertension. In: Henne-Bruns D, Dürig M, Kremer B, editors. Lehrbuch Chirurgie. Duale Reihe: Hippokrates Verlag (In press).
7. Karnad DR, Tembulkar P, Abraham P, Desai NK. Head-down tilt as a physiological diuretic in normal controls and in patients with fluid-retaining states. Lancet. 1987;2:525–8.
8. Bernardi M, Santini C, Trevisani F, Baraldini M, Ligabue A, Gasbarrini G. Renal function impairment induced by change in posture in patients with cirrhosis and ascites. Gut. 1985;26:629–35.
9. Ring-Larsen H, Henriksen JH, Wilken C, Clausen J, Pals H, Christensen NJ. Diuretic treatment in decompensated cirrhosis and congestive heart failure: effect of posture. Br Med J. 1986;292:1351–3.
10. Bernardi M, Laffi G, Salvagnini M *et al.* Efficacy and safety of the stepped care medical treatment of ascites in liver cirrhosis: a randomised controlled clinical trial comparing two diets with different sodium content. Liver. 1993;13:156–62.
11. Descos L, Gauthier A, Levy VG *et al.* Comparison of six treatments of ascites in patients with liver cirrhosis. A clinical trial. Hepatogastroenterology. 1983;30:15–20.
12. Reynolds TB, Lieberman FL, Goodman AR. Advantages of treatment of ascites without sodium restriction and without complete removal of excess fluid. Gut. 1978;19:549–53.
13. Gauthier A, Levy VG, Quinton A *et al.* Salt or no salt in the treatment of cirrhotic ascites: a randomised study. Gut. 1986;27:705–9.
14. Gerbes AL, Paumgartner G. Therapie des Aszites bei Lebererkrankungen. Dtsch Med Wochenschr. 1994;119:1549–54.
15. Gentilini P, La Villa G, Laffi G *et al.* Sodium retention in cirrhosis: aspects of pathophysiology and treatment. Front Gastrointest Res. 1986;9:203–18.
16. Schölmerich J. Aszites. Berlin: Springer; 1991.
17. Conn HO. Diuresis of ascites: fraught with or free from hazard. Gastroenterology. 1977;73:619–21.
18. Sherlock S, Shaldon S. The aetiology and management of ascites in patients with hepatic cirrhosis: a review. Gut. 1963;4:95–105.
19. Gerok W, Rössle M, Schölmerich J. Leberzirrhose. In: Gerok W, Blum HE, editors. Hepatologie. Munich: Urban & Schwarzenberg; 1995:323–75.
20. Runyon BA. Care of patients with ascites. N Engl J Med. 1994;330:337–42.
21. Angeli P, Pria MD, De Bei E *et al.* Randomised clinical study of the efficacy of amiloride and potassium canrenoate in nonazotemic cirrhotic patients with ascites. Hepatology. 1994;19:72–9.
22. Broekhuysen J, Deger F, Douchamps J, Ducarne H, Herchuelz A. Torasemide, a new potent diuretic. Double-blind comparison with furosemide. Eur J Pharmacol. 1986;31(Suppl.):29–34.
23. Gerbes AL, Bertheau-Reith U, Falkner C, Jüngst D, Paumgartner G. Advantages of the new loop diuretic torasemide over furosemide in patients with cirrhosis and ascites. A randomized, double blind cross-over trial. J Hepatol. 1993;17:353–8.
24. Laffi G, Marra F, Buzzelli G *et al.* Comparison of the effects of torasemide and furosemide in nonazotemic cirrhotic patients with ascites: a randomized, double-blind study. Hepatology. 1991;13:1101–5.
25. Gines P, Tito L, Arroyo V *et al.* Randomized comparative study of therapeutic paracentesis with and without albumin in cirrhosis. Gastroenterology. 1988;94:1493–502.
26. Gines P, Arroyo V, Quintero E *et al.* Comparison between paracentesis and diuretics in the treatment of cirrhotics with tense ascites. Results of a randomized study. Gastroenterology. 1987;93:234–41.
27. Salerno F, Badalamenti S, Incerti P *et al.* Repeated paracentesis and i.v. albumin infusion to treat 'tense' ascites in cirrhotic patients: a safe alternative therapy. J Hepatol. 1987;5:102–8.

28. Tito L, Gines P, Arroyo V *et al.* Total paracentesis associated with intravenous albumin management of patients with cirrhosis and ascites. Gastroenterology. 1990;98:146–51.
29. Planas R, Gines P, Arroyo V *et al.* Dextran-70 versus albumin as plasma expanders in cirrhotic patients with tense ascites treated with total paracentesis: results of a randomized study. Gastroenterology. 1990;99:1736–44.
30. Salerno F, Badalamenti S, Lorenzano E, Moser P, Incerti P. Randomized comparative study of hemaccel vs. albumin infusion after total paracentesis in cirrhotic patients with refractory ascites. Hepatology. 1991;13:707–13.
31. Arroyo V, Gines P, Gerbes AL *et al.* Definition and diagnostic criteria of refractory ascites and hepatorenal syndrome in cirrhosis. Hepatology. 1996;23:164–76.
32. Le Veen HH, Christoudias G, Moon IP, Luft R, Falk G, Grosberg S. Peritoneo-venous shunting for ascites. Ann Surg. 1974;180:580–91.
33. Gines P, Arroyo V, Vargas V *et al.* Paracentesis with intravenous infusion of albumin as compared with peritoneovenous shunting in cirrhosis with refractory ascites. N Engl J Med. 1991;325:829–35.
34. Stanley MM, Ochi S, Lee KK *et al.* Peritoneovenous shunting as compared with medical treatment in patients with alcoholic cirrhosis and massive ascites. N Engl J Med. 1989;321:1632–8.
35. Conn HO. Transjugular intrahepatic portal-systemic shunts: the state of the art. Hepatology. 1993;17:148–58.
36. Rössle M, Haag K, Ochs A *et al.* The transjugular intrahepatic portosystemic stent-shunt procedure for variceal bleeding. N Engl J Med. 1994;330:165–71.
37. Rössle M. The transjugular intrahepatic portosystemic shunt: indications and results. J Hepatol. 1996;25:224–31.
38. Ochs A, Rössle M, Haag K *et al.* The transjugular intrahepatic portosystemic stent shunt procedure for refractory ascites. N Engl J Med. 1995;332:1192–7.
39. Neuhaus P, Bechstein WO. Aszites und Lebertransplantation. Chirurg. 1993;64:16–20.

18
Hepatic encephalopathy

D. HÄUSSINGER, U. WARSKULAT, R. FISCHER, R. SINNING and F. SCHLIESS

INTRODUCTION

Hepatic encephalopathy is a neuropsychiatric syndrome which develops during the course of acute or chronic liver disease. Symptoms are highly variable and range from mild personality changes to deep coma, but are, at each level of severity, potentially reversible. Although there is general agreement that hepatic encephalopathy (HE) is functional in nature, its pathogenesis has not yet been elucidated. A variety of mechanisms have been implicated, such as the action of ammonia and other neurotoxins, disturbances of the blood–brain barrier and alterations of various neurotransmitter systems and their receptors (for review see refs 1 and 2). However, previous hypotheses on the pathogenesis of HE were finally disappointing, because they could explain only some, but not all, aspects of HE. Such hypotheses discussed in the past include the hypothesis on false neurotransmitters, the γ-aminobutyric acid (GABA)-hypothesis, the hypothesis on endogenous benzodiazepines, and the ammonia or neurotoxin hypothesis. It is highly likely that HE is causally related to disturbances of hepatocellular function and/or haemodynamic abnormalities accompanying liver disease; both will result in an impairment of hepatic detoxication processes and will augment access of neurotoxins, such as ammonia, to the brain. Undoubtedly, ammonia plays a decisive role in the pathogenesis of HE; however, to view HE merely as ammonia intoxication would be an oversimplification. Hypotheses on the pathogenesis of HE have to explain why hepatic encephalopathy is precipitated by quite different factors, such as bleeding, infections, sedatives, diuretics, electrolyte disturbances and trauma. The difficulties in unravelling the pathogenesis of HE are mainly due to the lack of reliable animal models, problems in studying the human brain and problems in extrapolating findings in animal studies to humans.

In HE no morphological abnormalities of the neurons are detectable, but astrocytes exhibit signs of Alzheimer type II degeneration. Such Alzheimer type II changes can be induced even in cultured astrocytes *in vitro* by addition of ammonia[3]. In view of the increasing evidence for an important role of astrocytes in maintaining proper neuronal function[4,5], it was hypothesized that HE may be a primary disorder of the astrocytes with neuronal dysfunction being a secondary event[3]. This chapter focuses on some new aspects on the pathogenesis of HE and its treatment. The account is in no way exhaustive, and the reader is referred to recent reviews[1–3].

ASTROCYTE SWELLING AS AN EARLY EVENT IN THE PATHOGENESIS OF HE

Astrocytes are the only cellular compartment in the brain capable of glutamine synthesis[6], which is the major pathway for cerebral ammonia detoxication. Brain oedema in HE of acute liver failure is common, and eventually determines the patient's final outcome. Under these conditions astrocyte swelling due to an intracellular accumulation of glutamine is the most prominent neuropathological abnormality[7]. Although grade I–III portosystemic encephalopathy (PSE) in chronic liver disease was not considered in the past to involve cell swelling in the brain, recent *in-vivo* evidence suggests that disturbances of astrocyte cell volume homeostasis (without clinically overt increase of intracranial pressure) may be an early event in HE in cirrhosis[8]. This suggestion is largely based on proton-magnetic resonance (MR) spectroscopic ([1H]MRS) studies.

[1H]MRS can be used to study metabolic abnormalities in the human brain *in vivo*, and allows a myo-inositol signal to be picked up, which was recently identified to reflect an osmosensitive cerebral myo-inositol pool[8]. *In-vitro* studies have shown that astrocytes contain high amounts of myo-inositol in contrast to neurons[9], suggesting that the myo-inositol signal in MRS studies derived from whole brain is largely of glial origin. In astrocytes, myo-inositol acts as an organic osmolyte[4,10,11]. Organic osmolytes are compounds which are specifically accumulated inside the cells, or released from the cells in response to osmotic cell shrinkage or swelling, respectively (for review see ref. 12). In line with this, hypo-osmotic astrocyte swelling in culture induces myo-inositol release, whereas hyperosmotic shrinkage stimulates its uptake[4,13–15]. Myo-inositol is taken up by astrocytes and glioma cells via a cumulative, specific Na^+-dependent transporter. The expression of the gene (SMIT) coding for the myo-inositol transporter in the plasma membrane is regulated by osmolarity, whereby hypo-osmolarity down-regulates, and hyperosmolarity up-regulates, SMIT mRNA levels (Fig. 1).

There is a strong depletion of brain myo-inositol in humans with hepatic encephalopathy, as shown by *in-vivo* [1H]MR spectroscopy (Fig. 2)[8,16–18]. The loss of myo-inositol is accompanied by an increase in the glutamine/glutamate signal (Fig. 2). Such alterations are also induced in the rat following portacaval shunting[18] and in humans following institution of a transjugular portosystemic intrahepatic stent shunt (TIPS)[8]. The loss of cerebral myo-inositol, as detected by [1H]MR-spectroscopy, is not necessarily a feature accompanying cirrhosis in general, but is apparently related to the presence of hepatic encephalopathy[8]. In line with this, a high sensitivity and specificity of the myo-inositol signal for the diagnosis of hepatic encephalopathy in cirrhotics has been reported[16]. In fact, a decrease of the spectroscopic myo-inositol signal is already found in subclinical, latent HE[8] (Fig. 2). In view of the role of myo-inositol as an osmolyte in astro-cytes, the MRS findings suggest that the markedly decreased myo-inositol signal

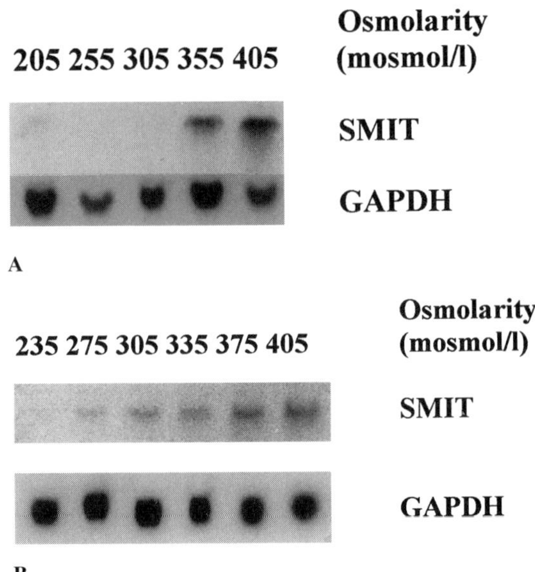

Fig. 1 Effect of hyperosmotic exposure on SMIT (myo-inositol transporter) mRNA levels in cultivated rat astrocytes (**A**) and C6 glioma cells (**B**). Cells were exposed for 12 h to aniso-osmolarity. Thereafter mRNA was extracted and subjected to Northern blot analysis. Glyceraldehyde phosphate dehydrogenase (GAPDH) mRNA levels are used as standards. In both cell types SMIT mRNA levels are regulated by osmolarity with the basal mRNA levels under normo-osmotic (305 mOsmol/L) conditions being much higher in glioma cells than in primary astrocytes

in patients with PSE (Fig. 2) reflect a disturbance of cell volume homeostasis in brain, which may occur at preclinical stages of PSE *in vivo*. This disturbance of brain cell volume homeostasis in PSE may at least in part be attributed to an intracellular accumulation of glutamine in response to hyperammonaemia, which tends to swell the cells. Indeed, cultured astrocytes swell under the influence of ammonia[19] and the [^{1}H]MR signal for glutamine is increased in parallel with the decrease of myo-inositol in both latent and manifest PSE, with the alterations being less pronounced in the latent stage (Fig. 2). Apparently a volume-regulatory myo-inositol release occurs in response to ammonia-induced glutamine accumulation in astrocytes, indicating that astrocyte swelling may be an early event in HE in chronic liver disease. However, ammonia may not be the only mechanism by which astrocyte swelling is triggered in hepatic encephalopathy, because *in-vitro* experiments indicate that astrocyte swelling also occurs under the influence of hyponatraemia, some neurotransmitters[11], tumour necrosis factor-α[20] and benzodiazepines[21].

FUNCTIONAL CONSEQUENCES OF ASTROCYTE SWELLING

It should be noted that a 'deficiency' of cerebral myo-inositol *per se* does not necessarily predict significant encephalopathy symptoms[8]. The myo-inositol

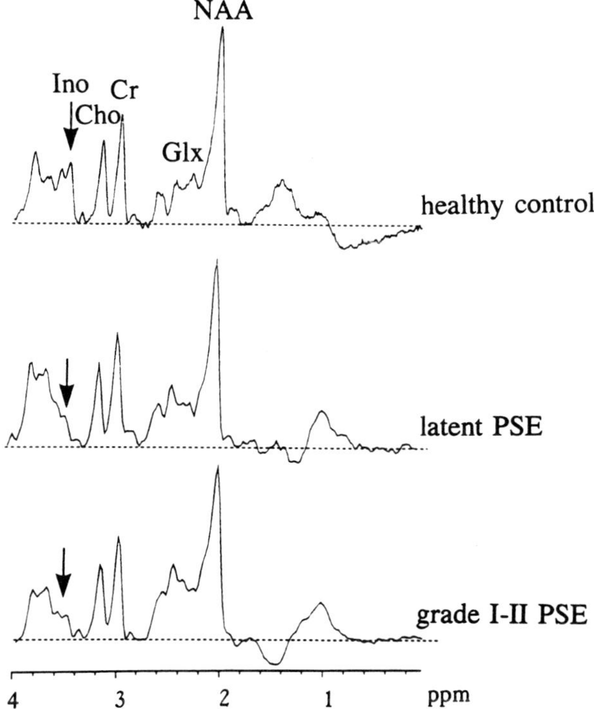

Fig. 2 Parietal [^{1}H]MR spectra from a healthy subject, patients with posthepatic cirrhosis and latent PSE or manifest grade I–II PSE. Representative spectra are given. Note the decrease in the myo-inositol (Ino) signal and the increase in the glutamine/glutamate (Glx) signal. Other peaks refer to choline (Cho), creatine (Cr) and *N*-acetylaspartate (NAA) (From ref. 8)

loss, however, which indicates glial swelling, may – when persistent – lead to sustained disturbances of cell function, with as yet unknown consequences for glial–neuronal communication. In other cell types (e.g. hepatocytes and macrophages), cell swelling, even when less than 10%, leads to marked alterations of carbohydrate and protein metabolism, gene expression, intracellular membrane flow, plasma membrane transport, protein phosphorylation, pH in subcellular compartments, intracellular signalling and of the cytoskeletal organization (for reviews see refs 22–25). Thus, astrocyte swelling in PSE as indicated by inositol release could have important functional consequences despite the absence of clinically overt increases of intracranial pressure. In hepatocytes and hepatoma cells, osmosignalling towards cell function involves at least in part a swelling-induced, G-protein-and tyrosine kinase-dependent, but Ca^{2+}-independent activation of the mitogen-activated protein (MAP) kinases Erk-1 and Erk-2[26,27]. Similar to the findings in rat hepatocytes, astrocyte swelling also leads to an activation of these MAP kinases (Fig. 3) which, however, is Ca^{2+}- and PI_3-kinase-dependent, but G-protein- and tyrosine kinase-independent[28]) (Fig. 4). MAP kinases are known to be central elements of

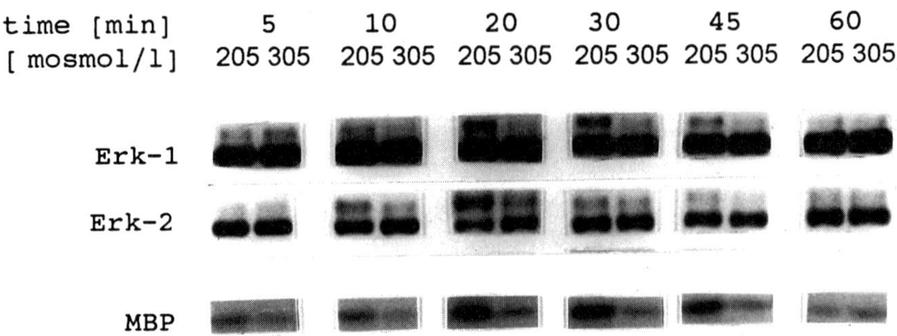

Fig. 3 Activation of MAP kinases following hypo-osmotic swelling of primary rat astrocytes as determined by band shift assay and immune-complex assay. Cells were incubated in normo-osmotic (305 mOmol/L) or hypo-osmotic (205 mOsmol/L) media for the time periods indicated. Erk-1 and Erk-2 are activated within 5 min of hypo-osmotic swelling as revealed by the appearance of a second, phosphorylated protein band. In these band shift assays, total protein extracts were analysed in Western blots using specific antibodies against Erk-1 and Erk-2, respectively. MAP-kinase activation is also shown directly by immune complex assays using the myelin basic protein (MBP) as phosphorylation substrate and the antibody against Erk-2 as described in ref. 26

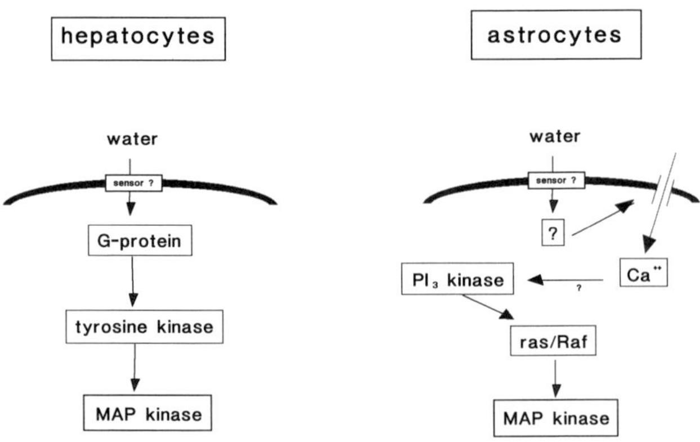

Fig. 4 Cell volume signalling in hepatocytes and astrocytes. The scheme focuses on the upstream events involved in the swelling-induced MAP kinase activation as revealed by inhibitor studies

growth factor signalling, and have multiple protein substrates, such as S6 kinase, cytoskeletal proteins and transcription factors, thereby affecting a variety of cellular functions. Indeed, astrocyte swelling leads to an up-regulation of peripheral type benzodiazepine receptors[29], affects protein phosphorylation and Ca^{2+} homeostasis[30], amino acid transport[11], intracellular pH and the acidification of intracellular vesicular compartments[31]. These alterations of astrocyte function may be relevant for the development of HE.

THE 'ASTROCYTE SWELLING HYPOTHESIS'

In view of the above it is hypothesized that HE is at least in part the result of astrocyte swelling, with subsequent alterations of glial function and glioneuronal communication (Fig. 5). This working model could explain why heterogeneous factors can precipitate HE (Fig. 6), because all these factors (e.g. ammonia, TNF, benzodiazepines, hyponatraemia, etc.) augment cell swelling, and may thus act synergistically to trigger a common end-path, i.e. glial swelling with its functional consequences. Further, astrocyte swelling can trigger functional disturbances, which resemble several established phenomena in PSE, such as alterations of cerebral glucose metabolism, selective alterations of blood–brain permeability (which is equivalent to changes in astrocyte membrane transport), cytoskeletal changes and the up-regulation of benzodiazepine receptors. However, further studies are required to establish the validity of this 'swelling hypothesis'.

LIVER DISEASE AND HEPATIC AMMONIA DETOXICATION

Although HE is not identical to ammonia intoxication, clinical observations suggest that ammonia is one major factor in the pathogenesis of HE. This is derived from the observation that clinical conditions which are accompanied by increased ammonia formation (bleeding, protein catabolic states, uraemia, dietary protein intake) or impaired ammonia detoxication (liver failure) precipitate HE, and measures to improve ammonia detoxication, or to lower ammonia generation, are effective in the treatment of HE. Hyperammonaemia in chronic liver disease is due to both increased portosystemic shunting of ammonia-rich portal blood and an impairment of ammonia detoxication in the diseased liver.

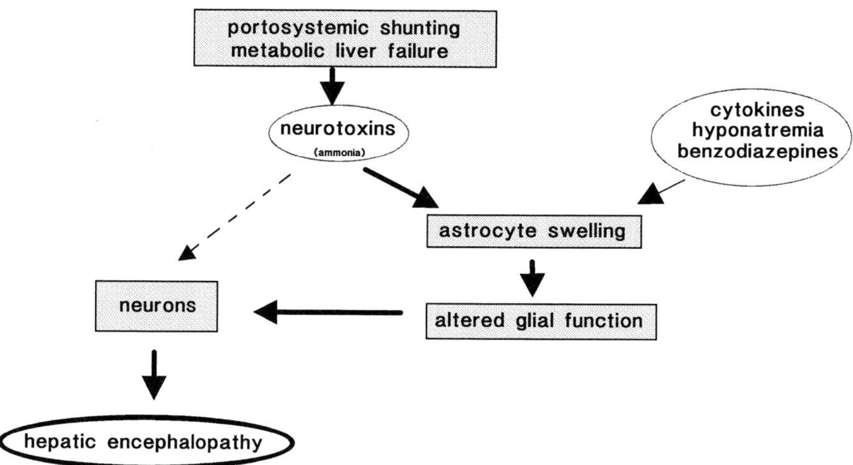

Fig. 5 Glial swelling hypothesis. Astrocyte swelling is induced by ammonia, tumour necrosis factor, benzodiazepines and hyponatraemia. Glial swelling activates intracellular signalling pathways and produces alterations of glial function. This results in a disturbance of the glia–neuronal communication, triggering the clinical picture of HE

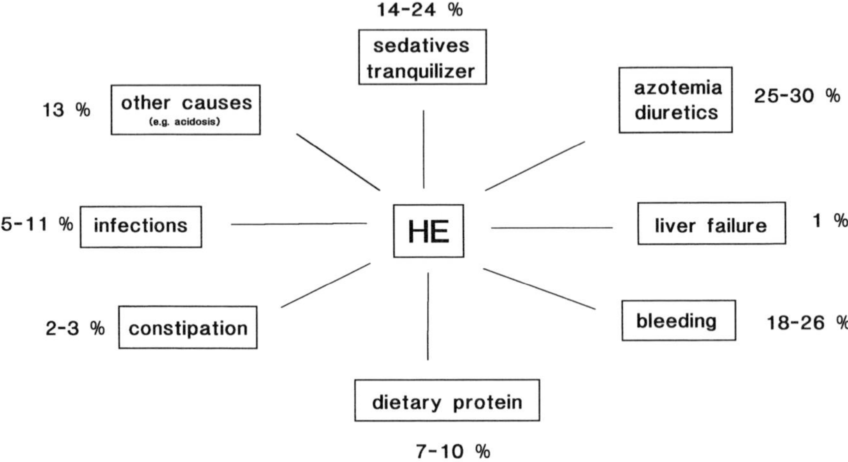

Fig. 6 Precipitating factors of hepatic encephalopathy

A better pathophysiological understanding of the latter process has to consider the structural and functional organization of ammonia detoxication in the liver acinus, which is the functional unit of the liver (for review see refs 32 and 33). In the intact liver acinus the two major ammonia-detoxicating systems, urea and glutamine synthesis, are anatomically switched behind each other: urea synthesis is found in a large periportal compartment, whereas glutamine synthesis is restricted to a small perivenous cell population at the end of the acinus, which surrounds the terminal hepatic venule[32–35] (Fig. 7). Accordingly, the portal blood

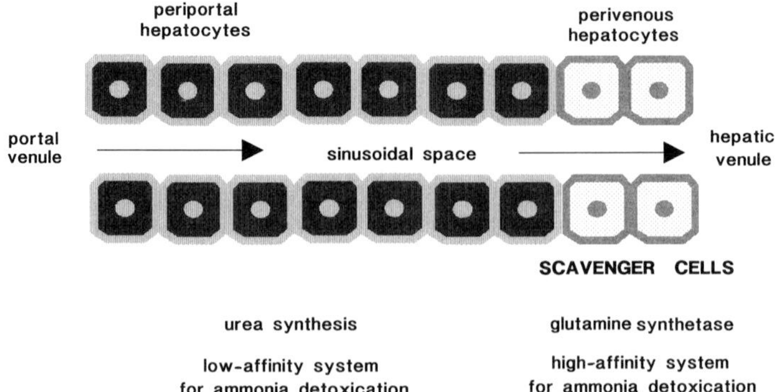

Fig. 7 Structural and functional organization of ammonia detoxication in the liver acinus. In the liver lobule the pathways of urea and glutamine synthesis are anatomically switched behind each other, and represent the sequence of a periportal low-affinity system (urea synthesis) and a perivenous high-affinity system (glutamine synthesis) for ammonia detoxication. Glutamine synthase in perivenous cells acts as scavenger for the ammonia escaping periportal urea synthesis ('high-affinity system for ammonia detoxication'). A scavenger cell defect on liver cirrhosis contributes to the development of hyperammonaemia

will first come into contact with hepatocytes capable of urea synthesis, before glutamine-synthesizing cells ('scavenger cells') at the end of the acinar bed are reached. In functional terms this organization represents the sequence of a periportal low-affinity, but high-capacity system (ureogenesis) and a perivenous high-affinity system for ammonia detoxication (glutamine synthesis)[34]. In isolated perfused rat liver, efficient ammonia extraction with physiologically low portal ammonia concentrations requires an intact glutamine synthase activity ('high-affinity system') and ammonia at physiological portal concentrations of 0.2–0.3 mol/L is converted by about two-thirds into urea and by about one-third into glutamine, although these pathways are anatomically organized in sequence. *In vitro* and *in vivo* a considerable fraction of the ammonia delivered via the portal vein from the intestine reaches the perivenous end of the liver acinus. Here, perivenous glutamine synthase acts as a high-affinity scavenger for the ammonia which escaped periportal detoxication by urea synthesis[32–34]. The important scavenger role of perivenous glutamine synthesis for the maintenance of physiologically low ammonia concentrations in the hepatic vein becomes rapidly evident after inhibition of glutamine synthase by methionine sulphoximine[34] or after destruction of perivenous cells by CCl_4 treatment[36]. In the latter case hyperammonaemia ensues due to an almost complete scavenger cell failure to synthesize glutamine, although periportal urea synthesis is not affected[36].

Human liver cirrhosis is characterized by a severe scavenger cell defect: the capacity to synthesize glutamine from ammonia is decreased by about 80% and defective perivenous ammonia scavenging may contribute to the development of hyperammonaemia in liver cirrhosis[37,38]. Interestingly, after portacaval anastomosis in the rat, the number and immunohistochemical staining intensity of perivenous scavenger cells for glutamine synthase is markedly decreased compared to sham-operated controls (Fig. 8), although urea cycle enzyme activities were reported not to be decreased following portacaval shunting[39]. This indicates that portacaval shunting *per se* may augment the scavenger cell defect. Accordingly the discussion on what is more important for the development of hyperammonaemia (portosystemic blood shunting or the the metabolic defect inside the liver), becomes less relevant. Recent data suggest that perivenous hepatocytes also play an important role in the inactivation of signal molecules such as extracellular nucleotides and eicosanoids, thereby extending their well-documented scavenger role for ammonia to a variety of other compounds[40] and opening new perspectives on the pathophysiology of extrahepatic manifestations in chronic liver diseases.

Liver cirrhosis is also characterized by an 80% decrease in the capacity to synthesize urea[37,38,41]. This urea cycle defect is, however, compensated by a marked increase in glutaminase activity in cirrhosis. Liver glutaminase is found in periportal hepatocytes[34] and has a joint mitochondrial localization together with carbamoylphosphate synthase. Liver glutaminase is activated by its product ammonia in the physiological concentration range and in alkalosis (for review see ref. 32). Its function is now seen as a pH-controlled ammonia-amplifying system in the mitochondria, whose activity determines the actual flux through the urea cycle and mediates a strong pH sensitivity of urea synthesis. This is because urea synthesis is controlled by flux through carbamoylphosphate synthase, which largely depends on the actual ammonia concentration inside the

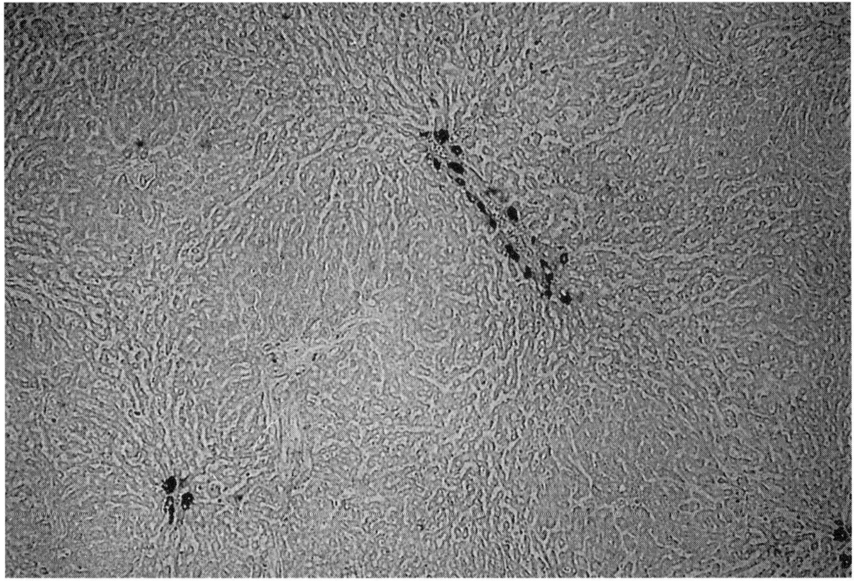

A

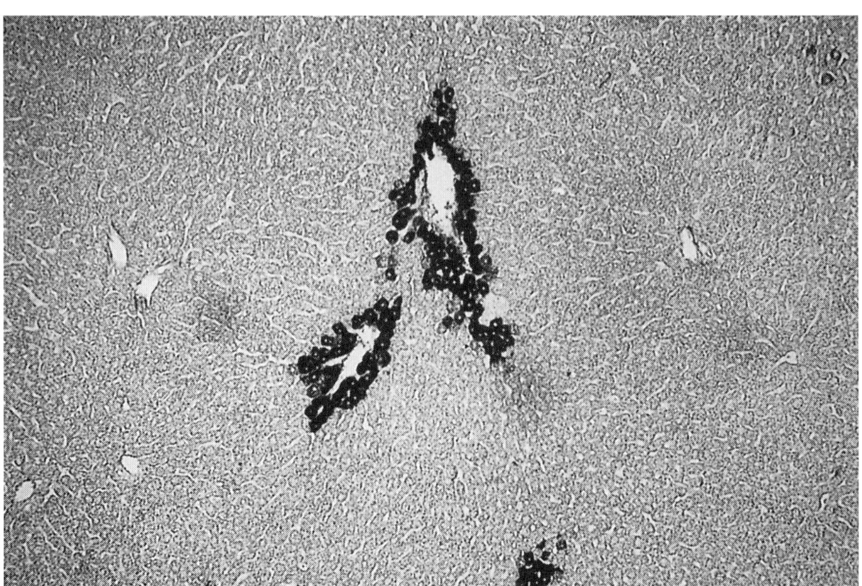

B

Fig. 8 Immunohistochemical staining for glutamine synthetase in rat liver 6 weeks after porta-caval shunting **(A)** or sham-operated control **(B)**. Note the marked reduction of number and staining intensity of scavenger cells following portacaval anastomosis (from ref. 33)

mitochondria. Amplification of mitochondrial ammonia via glutaminase action becomes an important determinant of urea cycle flux in the presence of physiologically low ammonia concentrations. The latter are about one order of magnitude below the K_m(ammonia) of carbamoyl phosphate synthase. This interplay between pH-sensitive glutaminase regulation and urea synthesis provides the basis for an important role of the liver in the maintenance of acid–base homeostasis (for reviews see refs 32, 33, and 42–44). Suffice to say that urea synthesis is a major pathway for the irreversible removal of bicarbonate in the body, and a sensitive feedback control loop between the actual acid–base status and bicarbonate-consuming ureogenesis has been established[32,42–44]. For example, metabolic alkalosis activates glutaminase and thereby augments bicarbonate-consuming ureogenesis. This physiological relationship is preserved in cirrhosis: here, the urea cycle defect results in an impaired disposal of bicarbonate and consequently metabolic alkalosis[37,38,41], a frequent finding in cirrhosis. Alkalosis in turn activates glutaminase. In human liver cirrhosis, flux through glutaminase is increased about 5-fold, thereby allowing the maintenance of a near-normal urea cycle flux despite a decrease of the capacity to synthesize urea by about 80% in these patients[37,38]. Simply explained, creation of a high periportal ammonia concentration (via amplification) allows the cirrhotic patient to synthesize normal amounts of urea despite a decreased urea cycle capacity. This pathogenetic sequence is depicted in Fig. 9. This implies that maintenance of

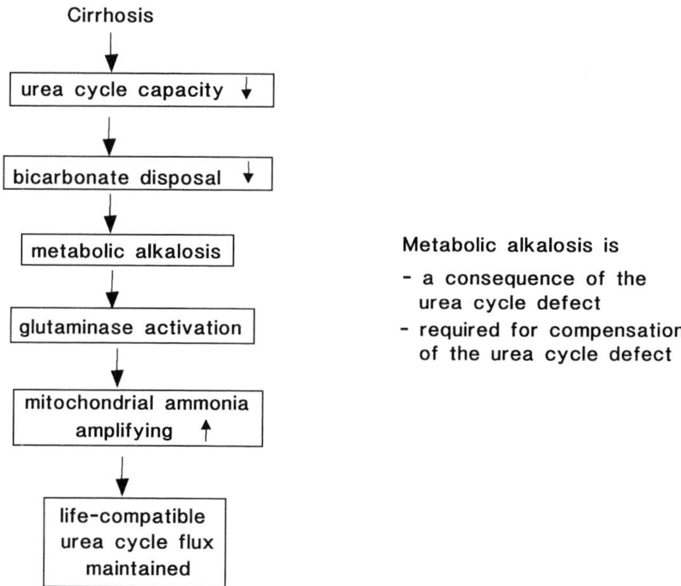

Fig. 9 Pathobiochemistry in liver cirrhosis. The decreased urea cycle capacity in cirrhosis results in a diminished bicarbonate disposal via the urea cycle and consequently in metabolic alkalosis. Alkalosis in turn activates glutaminase, which augments 'mitochondrial ammonia amplifying'. The increase in mitochondrial ammonia allows maintenance of a near-normal urea cycle flux despite a 80% decrease of urea cycle capacity

near-normal urea cycle flux requires metabolic alkalosis in order to keep the amplification system glutaminase highly active. When acidosis develops, however, the amplifier is shut off and urea synthesis ceases. This may explain the rapid development of hyperammonaemia in the cirrhotic patient, when acidosis develops. The compensatory mechanism depicted in Fig. 9 also implies a high periportal ammonia concentration. Periportal hyperammonaemia, however, may become systemic, when the capacity of the defective perivenous scavenger cells for ammonia detoxication is exhausted. Thus, one rationale for treatment should involve augmentation of scavenger cell function in cirrhosis. Indeed, treatment options, such as benzoate, ornithine-aspartate and ornithine-ketoglutarate, as well as branched-chain ketoacids, may augment ammonia fixation in perivenous scavenger cells by interfering with scavenger cell-specific transport systems in the plasma membrane.

The scavenger cell defect in cirrhosis also explains why loop diuretics are well tolerated in patients with normal liver function, but may precipitate hyper-ammonaemia in patients with liver disease. The diuretics, such as mefruside, thiazides and xipamide, inhibit hepatic mitochondrial carbonic anhydrase, which is required for urea synthesis[45]. Accordingly, these compounds inhibit urea synthesis even at therapeutic concentrations[45], and the ammonia load to perivenous scavenger cells increases. This is of little relevance as long as these scavenger cells are intact; however, hyperammonaemia develops in cirrhosis when the capacity of these defective cells to synthesize glutamine is exhausted (Fig. 10).

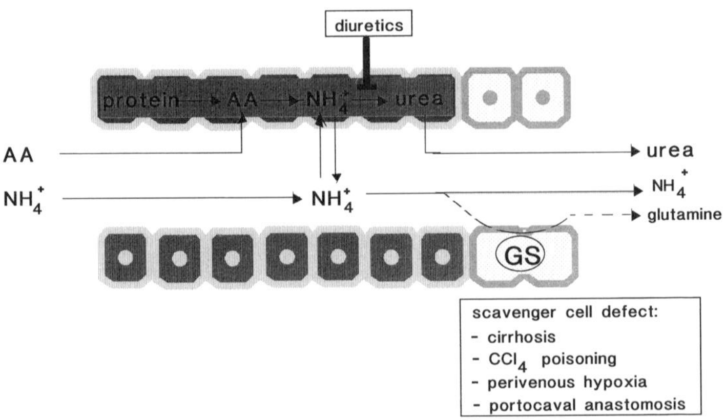

Fig. 10 Pathogenesis of diuretics-induced hyperammonaemia in cirrhosis. Loop diuretics inhibit urea synthesis due to inhibition of mitochondrial carbonic anhydrase V. This results in an increased ammonia load to downstream scavenger cells, which contain glutamine synthase and normally prevent overflow of ammonia into the systemic circulation (high-affinity system of ammonia detoxication). In liver cirrhosis, however, scavenger cells are defective and cannot cope with the increased ammonia load: systemic hyperammonaemia develops. The scavenger cell defect can also be unmasked following perivenous hypoxia, and by poisons mainly damaging the perivenous hepatocytes, such as CCl_4

TREATMENT OF HEPATIC ENCEPHALOPATHY

In view of the complex pathogenesis of HE, no single medical treatment can be expected to improve HE under all conditions. Treatment should rather focus on the major pathogenetic events present in the patient, if these can be disclosed. Indeed, identification and treatment of these underlying events (so-called precipitating factors) is the most important and most effective therapeutic approach. Most other therapeutic measures interfere with ammonia generation/disposal; however, the efficacy of these measures was only rarely demonstrated in placebo-controlled studies and conflicting data exist in the literature. The major problems in assessing the efficacy of such treatment devices are low case numbers, variable co-medication and the heterogeneity of the patients studied. Figure 11 shows these therapeutic options depending on the severity of HE.

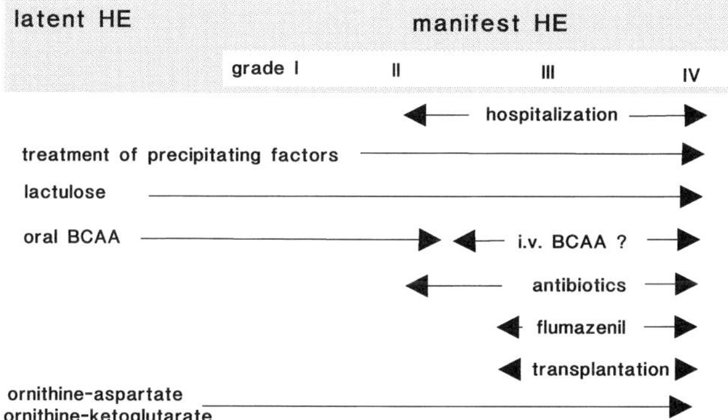

Fig. 11   Treatment of HE depending on severity (for further details see text)

Precipitating factors

The most important therapeutic measure is the identification and treatment of precipitating factors (Fig. 6). Their elimination alone usually improves, or even abolishes, HE episodes. Frequently several precipitating factors are identified simultaneously. Careful attention should be paid to the medication (diuretics, tranquillizers, sedatives). Infection and bleeding should be controlled vigorously. In ascitic patients attention should be given to spontaneous bacterial peritonitis, the only clinical manifestation of which is frequently precipitation or worsening of HE. Metabolic acidosis should be treated early, in the mild stages, because acidosis shuts off the ammonia amplifier glutaminase and thereby ureogenesis (Fig. 9). Metabolic alkalosis may no longer be seen as a precipitating factor; it is an epiphenomenon and indicator of the urea cycle defect[38] and develops in parallel with hyperammonaemia, because urea synthesis consumes both NH_4^+ and HCO_3^- in equimolar amounts.

Bowel cleaning

This can be performed by MgSO$_4$ enemas or lactulose. The removal of nitrogenous compounds (e.g. blood in the case of upper gastrointestinal bleeding) from the bowel is undoubtedly beneficial by reducing the ammonia load to the liver, although controlled studies are lacking.

Lactulose and lactitol

Both these are non-resorbable disaccharides, which are converted under the influence of the intestinal flora into organic acids. The accompanying acidification of the bowel content produces a laxative effect[46]. This may be important because recent evidence suggests that HE is accompanied by delayed oral–caecal transit, which may favour enteric production of ammonia and other putative encephalogenic material of dietary origin[47]. In addition, lactulose may promote nitrogen fixation by colonic bacteria, and may thus reduce the ammonia burden to the diseased liver. However, further mechanisms of action may exist. The efficacy of oral lactulose in the treatment of HE was shown in three double-blind controlled trials including a total of 45 subjects, in addition to many less well-controlled studies. Although this number is small, and there are no studies with comparison against placebo, lactulose became a standard for the treatment of HE. Lactulose is given orally at a dose which results in the delivery of two or three soft stools. It can also be given as enema. The efficacies of lactulose and lactitol are comparable, although better tolerance of the latter compound was suggested. In patients with intestinal lactase deficiency, lactose will fulfil the same purpose as lactulose.

Protein diet

Vegetable protein is better tolerated than animal-derived protein in patients with HE. The reason for this is not clear, but may relate to the high fibre content and the amino acid composition of vegetable protein. In a recent randomized crossover trial, psychometric test results, plasma ammonia and nitrogen balance were significantly better on vegetable protein diet compared to an iso-nitrogenous animal protein diet[48]. However, acceptance may be impaired due to flatulence. Protein restriction is recommended during severe episodes of HE. However, protein and amino acid starvation for more than 3 days triggers a protein catabolic state which will not only increase the nitrogen load to the liver, but simultaneously impair ammonia detoxication in skeletal muscle and liver. Thus, in response to prolonged protein restriction HE may even deteriorate. It is therefore recommended to institute protein restriction for 3 days only, and to increase protein supply by 10 g/day every 3 days in order to achieve a final minimal protein intake of 1 g/kg body weight per day. If this is not tolerated by the patient (i.e. when HE worsens at protein intakes below 1 g/kg body weight per day), protein diets enriched with branched amino acids should be used.

Non-resorbable antibiotics

Neomycin was shown to be as effective as lactulose in the treatment of HE. Similar efficacy is ascribed to paromomycin, metronidazole and vancomycin. Although generally assumed to be effective and used like lactulose as a 'gold standard', there is only one placebo-controlled trial on neomycin, which showed little effectivity[49]. Neomycin is highly nephrotoxic and ototoxic, and about 1–4% of the orally administered dose is absorbed, providing a risk of side-effects. Therefore treatment periods should not exceed 2–3 weeks. Some patient benefit was reported from the combined use of lactulose and neomycin, although this may be unexpected from a mechanistic point of view (requirement of intestinal bacteria for lactulose action, but damage of the flora by neomycin).

Urea cycle intermediates

The efficacy of ornithine aspartate and ornithine ketoglutarate is currently subject to controlled trials, and the ammonia-lowering potency was shown in animal experiments. These compounds may interfere with scavenger cell function, because oxaloacetate and α-ketoglutarate are selectively taken up by this cell population and may augment glutamine synthesis from ammonia[50].

Benzoate

Although having an unpleasant taste, this compound was seen to augment ammonia detoxication by hippurate formation. Recent evidence suggests that benzoate may augment ammonia detoxication by interfering with an anion exchange system in the plasma membrane in perivenous scavenger cells in liver[51]. Benzoate has been successfully used in the treatment of hyperammonaemic states due to inborn errors of metabolism, and in chronic HE[52].

Branched-chain amino acids

Branched-chain amino acids (BCAA) are available orally or in parenteral formulations. Most studies on oral BCAA showed clinical improvement of latent or low-grade HE[53]. Diets enriched in BCAA are better tolerated than conventional protein. These diets should be given in the highly protein-intolerant patient. Nine controlled studies on the efficacy of parenteral BCAA have been presented, with inconclusive and conflicting results. When these compounds are used, energy should be provided in the form of carbohydrates.

Zinc

Zinc is the co-factor of many enzymes, including carbonic anhydrase and ornithine transcarbamylase, i.e. enzymes involved in hepatic ammonia detoxication. In addition, zinc binding sites are contained in the GABA/benzodiazepine receptor complex. Because zinc deficiency is common in cirrhosis, zinc supplements were used for the treatment of HE. Anecdotal observations suggest a role of zinc deficiency in the pathogenesis of HE and its improvement following supplementation. However, further studies are required to establish the efficacy of zinc supplementation as a treatment option in HE.

Benzodiazepine receptor antagonists

Based on the concept of increased levels of endogenous benzodiazepine ligands as a pathogenetic factor in HE[54,55], benzodiazepine receptor antagonists, such as flumazenil, were introduced in the treatment of HE. Its efficacy was convincingly demonstrated in a case report[56]. Since then, several controlled trials have been reported with modest success and response rates in about one-half of the patients only[57]. Thus, although flumazenil may be helpful in a subset of patients, the findings argue against a major role of endogenous benzodiazepines in the pathogenesis of HE. Clearly, flumazenil may be used for differential diagnosis of coma, and to antagonize benzodiazepine-precipitated HE.

Finally, liver transplantation should be considered in patients with severe HE as the only definite and causal treatment option.

References

1. Lockwood AH. Hepatic encephalopathy. Boston, MA: Butterworth–Heinemann; 1992.
2. Ferenci P, Püspök A, Steindl P. Current concepts in the pathogenesis of hepatic encephalopathy. Eur J Clin Invest. 1992;22:573–81.
3. Norenberg MD, Neary JT, Bender AS, Dombro RS. Hepatic encephalopathy: a disorder in glial–neuronal communication. In: Yu ACH, Hertz L, Norenberg MD, Sykova E, Waxman SG, editors. Progress in brain research. Amsterdam: Elsevier; 1992:261–9.
4. Murphy S, editor. Astrocytes – pharmacology and function. San Diego, CA: Academic Press; 1993.
5. Nedergaard M. Direct signalling from astrocytes to neurons in cultures of mammalian brain cells. Science. 1994;263:1768–71.
6. Martinez-Hernandez A, Bell KP, Norenberg MD. Glutamine synthetase: glial localization in brain. Science. 1977;195:1356–8.
7. Swain M, Butterworth RF, Blei AT. Ammonia and related amino acids in the pathogenesis of brain edema in acute ischemic liver failure in rats. Hepatology. 1992;15:449–53.
8. Häussinger D, Laubenberger J, vom Dahl S *et al.* Proton magnetic resonance spectroscopic studies on human brain myo-inositol in hypoosmolarity and hepatic encephalopathy. Gastroenterology. 1994;107:1475–80.
9. Brand A, Leibfritz D. Metabolic markers in glial cells for differentiation of brain tissue. Commun 11th Ann Meet Soc MR Med 1992;649 (abstract).
10. Lien YHH, Shapiro JL, Chan L. Effects of hypernatremia on organic brain osmoles. J Clin Invest. 1990;85:1427–35.
11. Kimelberg HK, O'Connor ER, Kettenmann H. Effects of swelling on glial cell function. In Lang F, Häussinger D, editors. Interactions cell volume and cell function Heidelberg: Springer Verlag; 1993:158–86.
12. Burg M. Molecular basis of osmotic regulation. Am J Physiol. 1995;268:F983–96.
13. Sterns RH, Baer J, Ebersol S, Thomas D, Lohr JW, Kamm DE. Organic osmolytes in acute hyponatremia. Am J Physiol. 1993;264:F833–6.
14. Isaacks RE, Bender AS, Kim CY, Prieto NM, Norenberg MD. Osmotic regulation of myo-inositol uptake in primary astrocyte cultures. Neurochem Res. 1994;19:331–8.
15. Paredes A, McManus M, Kwon HM, Strange K. Osmoregulation of Na^+-inositol cotransporter activity and mRNA levels in brain glial cells. Am J Physiol. 1992;263:C1282–8.
16. Kreis R, Farrow NA, Ross BD. Diagnosis of hepatic encephalopathy by proton magnetic resonance spectroscopy. Lancet. 1990;336:635–6.
17. Kreis R, Ross BD, Farrow NA, Ackerman Z. Metabolic disorders of the brain in chronic hepatic encephalopathy detected with [1]H-MR spectroscopy. Radiology. 1992; 182:19–27.
18. Moats RA, Lien, YHH, Filippi D, Ross BD. Decrease in cerebral inositols in rats and humans. Biochem J. 1993;295:15–18.
19. Norenberg MD, Baker L, Norenberg LOB, Blicharska J, Bruce-Gregorius JH, Neary JT. Ammonia-induced astrocyte swelling in primary culture. Neurochem Res. 1991;16:833–6.
20. Bender AS, Rivera IV, Norenberg MD. Tumor necrosis factor α induces astrocyte swelling. Trans Am Soc Neurochem. 1992;23:113.
21. Norenberg MD, Bender AS. Astrocyte swelling in liver failure: role of glutamine and benzodiazepines. In: Ito U, editor. Brain edema, vol. IX. Vienna: Springer Verlag; 1994:24–7.
22. Häussinger D, Lang F. Cell volume in the regulation of hepatic function: a mechanism for metabolic control. Biochem Biophys Acta. 1991;1071:331–50.

23. Häussinger D, Roth E, Lang F, Gerok W. The cellular hydration state: an important determinant for protein catabolism in health and disease. Lancet. 1993;341:1330–2.
24. Häussinger D, Lang F, Gerok W. Regulation of cell function by the cellular hydration state. Am J Physiol. 1994;267:E343–55.
25. Häussinger D. The role of cellular hydration in the regulation of cell function. Biochem J. 1996;313:697–710.
26. Schliess F, Schreiber R, Häussinger D. Activation of extracellular signal-related kinases Erk-1 and Erk-2 by cell swelling in H4IIE hepatoma cells. Biochem J. 1995;309:13–17.
27. Noé B, Schliess F, Wettstein M, Heinrich S, Häussinger D. Regulation of taurocholate excretion by a hyposmolarity-activated signal transduction pathway in rat liver. Gastroenterology. 1996;110:858–65.
28. Schliess F, Sinnig R, Fischer R, Schmalenbach C, Häussinger D. Calcium-dependent activation of Erk-1 and Erk-2 following hypoosmotic astrocyte swelling. Biochem J. 1996 (in press).
29. Itzhak Y, Bender AS, Norenberg MD. Effect of hypoosmotic stress on peripheral-type benzodiazepine receptors in cultured astrocytes. Brain Res. 1994;644:221–5.
30. Bender AS, Neary JT, Norenberg MD. Involvement of second messengers and protein phosphorylation in astrocyte swelling. Can J Physiol Pharmacol. 1992, 70(Suppl.):S362–6.
31. Lang F, Busch G, Völkl H, Häussinger D. Lysosomal pH – a link between cell volume and metabolism. Biochem Soc Trans. 1994;22:504–7.
32. Häussinger D. Nitrogen metabolism in liver: structural–functional organization and physiological implications. Biochem J. 1990;267:281–90.
33. Häussinger D, Lamers W, Moorman AFM. Metabolism of amino acids and ammonia. Enzyme. 1993;46:72–93.
34. Häussinger D. Hepatocyte heterogeneity in glutamine and ammonia metabolism and the role of an intercellular glutamine cycle during ureogenesis in perfused rat liver. Eur J Biochem. 1983;133:269–74.
35. Gebhardt R, Mecke D. Heterogeneous distribution of glutamine synthetase among rat liver parenchymal cells in situ and in primary cultures. EMBO J. 1983;2:567–70.
36. Häussinger D, Gerok W. Hepatocyte heterogeneity in ammonia metabolism: impairment of glutamine synthesis in CCl_4-induced liver cell necrosis with no effect on urea synthesis. Chem Biol Interact. 1984;48:191–4.
37. Häussinger D, Steeb W, Gerok W. Ammonium and bicarbonate homeostasis in chronic liver disease. Klin Wochenschr. 1990;68:175–82.
38. Häussinger D, Steeb R, Gerok W. Metabolic alkalosis as driving force for urea synthesis in liver disease: pathogenetic model and therapeutic implications. Klin Wochenschr. 1992;70:411–15.
39. Colombo JP, Berüter J, Bachmann C, Peheim E. Enzymes of ammonia detoxication after portocaval shunt in the rat. Enzyme. 1977;22:391–8.
40. Häussinger D, Stehle T. Hepatocyte heterogeneity in response to eicosanoids. The perivenous scavenger cell hypothesis. Eur J Biochem. 1988;175:395–403.
41. Kaiser S, Gerok W, Häussinger D. New aspects on the pathogenesis of hyperammonemia in chronic liver disease. Eur J Clin Invest. 1988;18:535–42.
42. Häussinger D, editor. pH Homeostasis – mechanisms and control. London: Academic Press; 1988.
43. Atkinson DE, Bourke E. The role of ureogenesis in pH homeostasis. Trends Biochem Sci. 1984;9:297–300.
44. Häussinger D, Gerok W, Sies H. Hepatic role in pH regulation: role of the intercellular glutamine cycle. Trends Biochem Sci. 1984;9:300–2.
45. Häussinger D, Kaiser S, Stehle T, Gerok W. Liver carbonic anhydrase and urea synthesis. The effect of diuretics. Biochem Pharmacol. 1986;35:3317–22.
46. Conn HO, Bircher J, editors. Hepatic encephalopathy: syndromes and therapy. Bloomington, DE: Medi-Ed Press; 1994.
47. Van Thiel DH, Fagiuoli S, Wright HI, Chien M-C, Gavaler JS. Gastrointestinal transit in cirrhotic patients: effect of hepatic encephalopathy and its treatment. Hepatology. 1994;19:67–71.
48. Bianchi GP, Marchesini G, Fabbri A. Vegetable versus animal protein diet in cirrhotic patients with chronic hepatic encephalopathy: a randomized cross over comparison. J Intern Med. 1993,233:385–92.

49. Strauss E, Tramote R, Silva EPS *et al.* Double-blind randomized clinical trial comparing neomycin and placebo in the treatment of exogenous hepatic encephalopathy. Hepatogastroenterology. 1992;39:542–5.
50. Stoll B, McNelly S, Buscher HP, Häussinger D. Functional hepatocyte heterogeneity in glutamate, aspartate and α-ketoglutarate metabolism: a histoautoradiographic study. Hepatology. 1991;12:247–53.
51. Häussinger D, Stehle T, Colombo JP. Benzoate stimulates glutamate release from perfused rat liver. Biochem J. 1989;264:837–43.
52. Mendenhall CL, Rouster S, Marshall L, Weesner R. A new therapy for portal systemic encephalopathy. Am J Gastroenterol. 1986;81:540–3.
53. Plauth M, Egberts EH, Hamster W *et al.* Long-term treatment of latent portosystemic encephalopathy with branched chain amino acids. A double-blind placebo-controlled trial. J Hepatol. 1993;17:308–14.
54. Basile AS, Jones EA, Skolnick P. The pathogenesis and treatment of hepatic encephalopathy: evidence for the involvement of benzodiazepine receptor ligands. Pharmacol Rev. 1991;43:27–71.
55. Basile AS, Harrison PM, Hughes RD *et al.* Relationship between plasma benzodiazepine receptor ligand concentrations and severity of hepatic encephalopathy. Hepatology. 1994;19:112–21.
56. Ferenci P, Grimm G, Meryn S, Gangl A. Successful long-term treatment of portal-systemic encephalopathy by the benzodiazepine antagonist flumenazil. Gastroenterology. 1989;96:240–3.
57. Pomier-Layrargues G, Giguere JF, Lavoie J *et al.* Flumazenil in cirrhotic patients in hepatic coma: a randomized double-blind placebo-controlled trial. Hepatology. 1994;19:32–7.

19
Treatment of liver fibrosis

B.-E. WANG and J.-D. JIA

INTRODUCTION

Liver fibrosis is a common path leading to liver cirrhosis in a variety of chronic liver diseases caused by diverse aetiologies[1]. Liver fibrosis and cirrhosis are two of the main causes of morbidity and mortality, creating a great social and economic burden worldwide, especially in developing countries where chronic viral hepatitis is prevalent[2]. In recent decades an enormous amount of knowledge has been accumulated in respect of cellular and molecular mechanisms of liver fibrosis. Up to now most researchers agree that lipocyte and its activated form, myofibroblast-like cells, are the most important cellular sources of extracellular matrix, while platelet-derived growth factor (PDGF) and transforming growth factor-β (TGF-β) are the key mediators driving the unfavourable process of enhanced lipocyte proliferation, activation, and fibrogenesis, as well as inhibited extracellular matrix degradation[3–5]. The knowledge that the pathogenesis of liver fibrosis shares a common pathobiological route irrespective of the underlying disorders gives us the opportunity and rational basis, to intervene in the process of fibrosis itself, besides treating the specific diseases such as viral hepatitis, alcoholism or parasitic liver diseases. There are many reports on the therapeutic approach to liver fibrosis, but most of them are from cell culture and animal experiments, with very few using clinical trials. Therefore, advances in the field of the treatment of liver fibrosis are great and exciting, but far from satisfactory. This chapter will review some of the interesting and promising reports, not only in Western medicine but also in Traditional Chinese Medicine, which is believed to be of great potential, and worth exploring.

CURRENT TRENDS IN THE TREATMENT OF LIVER FIBROSIS

Colchicine

Colchicine is a tubulin polymerization-blocking agent which can retard the secretion of newly synthesized procollagen[6]. *In vitro* it can inhibit collagen type I mRNA levels and stimulate collagenase activity[7]. It is effective against CCl_4-induced liver cirrhosis or fibrosis induced by bile duct ligation in the rat[8,9]. In

1988 Kershenobich *et al.* reported the results of a randomized, controlled clinical trial on 100 patients with cirrhosis of mainly alcoholic or viral aetiologies[10]. After a mean follow-up period of 4.7 years (up to 14 years), there were significant improvements in median survival time (11 years in the colchicine group versus 3.5 years in the placebo group; $p<0.001$), cumulative 5-year survival rate (75% versus 34%) and 10-year survival rate (56% versus 20%); more importantly, nine of 30 treated patients showed histological improvement of liver fibrosis, whereas none of the 14 placebo group patients showed improvement. However, this promising result has not been confirmed in primary biliary cirrhosis patients, in whom there was no significant regression in liver histopathology in spite of partial biochemical improvement[11,12]. Recently, Wang *et al.* published their data from 100 HBV-related cirrhotics and showed that after 15–51 months (median 26 months) follow-up, there was no significant difference between colchicine and placebo groups in cumulative survival rate, biochemical liver function tests, serum levels of propeptide of type III procollagen (PIIINP) or liver fibrosis scores[13]. They concluded that colchicine did not significantly influence the progression of cirrhosis[13].

Polyunsaturated lecithin (PUL)

In 1990 Lieber *et al.* reported that long-term administration of PUL extracted from soybean could attenuate liver fibrosis in ethanol-fed baboons[14]. Thereafter they demonstrated that only one component of PUL, dilinoleoylphosphatidylcholine (DLPC), could duplicate the antifibrotic effect of whole PUL[15]. A further *in-vitro* study by the same group showed that PUL did not affect the type I collagen mRNA level in lipocytes, but did increase their collagenase activity[16]. Recently these workers also found that PUL are also effective in CCl_4- or human serum albumin-induced rat liver fibrosis and cirrhosis, not only preventing the development of fibrosis but also promoting the regression of established fibrosis (Ma *et al.* personal communication, 1994). The clinical effect of this agent is under multicentre study.

Interferon-γ

Rockey *et al.* reported that *in-vitro* IFN-γ could prevent rat lipocyte activation by inhibiting its proliferation and expression of ECM components such as types I and IV collagen, fibronectin, and smooth muscle-specific α-actin, which is regarded as a marker of transformation of lipocytes to myofibroblast-like cells[17]. Similar results were also found by Mallat *et al.* on cultured human lipocyte in both baseline status and after stimulation by TGF-β and PDGF[18]. These antifibrogenic effects have been confirmed in CCl_4-induced, heterogeneous serum-induced rat cirrhosis and murine schistosomiasis models[19–21]. Furthermore, Shi *et al.* found IFN-γ gene-deficient mice are much more prone to hepatotoxin such as CCl_4- and dimethylnitrosamine-induced liver fibrosis and cirrhosis, and supplements of exogenous IFN-γ could down-regulate type I collagen mRNA in CCl_4-induced liver injury. All of these data suggest IFN-γ is a key mediator in the development of liver fibrosis[22]. Considering the multiple biological effects of IFN-γ, and the complex interactions between different cytokines *in vivo*, whether IFN-γ is effective for treatment of human cirrhosis, especially HBV- or HCV-related cirrhosis, remains unproven.

Interferon-α

IFN-α was a well-known antiviral agent for chronic hepatitis B and C. Castilla *et al.* reported that in chronic hepatitis C patients IFN-α can decrease the serum propeptide of PIIINP concentration, as well as liver tissue mRNA levels for collagen type I and TGF-β[23]. While some authors reported no changes in liver fibrosis score despite decrease of serum PIIIP level and liver necroinflammatory scores[24], Manabe *et al.*, by means of quantitative histological assessment, found a slight but significant regression in liver fibrosis after IFN-α treatment in chronic hepatitis C patients[25]. These results need to be proven by well-designed, controlled clinical trials.

Retinoids

In normal or quiescent lipocyte-abundant vitamin A maintains high-level expression of decorin which can bind and inhibit the activity of TGF-β[26]. Lack of vitamin A occurs during lipocyte activation both in cell culture and animal models, and this depletion may 'permit' the profibrogenic effect of TGF-β[26]. David *et al.* found that a supplement of retinoids can inhibit lipocyte proliferation and production of collagens *in vitro*[27]. These, and the clinical finding that vitamin A content depletion can be seen in most liver disorders, support the therapeutic application of retinoids as antifibrogenic agents[28]. However, overdose of vitamin A *per se* could result in liver fibrosis, and the toxicity of xenobiotics such as alcohol and drugs can be potentiated by concomitant administration of vitamin A, probably through the inducible metabolic pathway of microsomal cytochrome P450 IIE1[29–31]. These paradox phenomena obscure the routine use of retinoids in chronic liver diseases. Much work needs to be done to clarify the causal relationship between vitamin A depletion and lipocyte activation, and the therapeutic role of retinoids in fibrosis and cirrhosis with different aetiologies.

Lufironil

Lufironil [HOE 077, pyridine-2,4-dicarboxylic-di(2-methoxyethyl)amide] is a proinhibitor of prolyl 4-hydroxylase, which is a key enzyme catalysing the hydroxylation of peptide-bound proline residues in the newly synthesized procollagen α chain. Preclinical studies showed that lufironil could significantly attenuate liver collagen deposition in CCl_4- and bile duct ligation-induced rat fibrosis, but did not affect collagen contents in other organs[32,33]. This agent seems to be liver-selective and well tolerated during short-term administration. Its clinical efficacy for various liver fibrogenic disorders and long-term safety are to be clarified.

Lysyl oxidase inhibitor

Lysyl oxidase catalyses deamination of the ϵ-amino groups of part lysyl and hydroxylysyl residues in the newly secreted collagen chains forming aldehyde groups by which intra- and inter-collagen chains covalent cross-links are established[34]. This final post-translational modification makes collagen fibre more stable and resistant to collagenase. The previously reported β-aminopro-prionitrile can irreversibly inhibit the activity of lysyl oxidase, but its toxicity obscures its long-term application to humans[35]. It has been reported that *cis*-1,2-diaminocyclohexane and ethylenediamine are both effective inhibitors of lysyl oxidase, and a beneficial effect on experimental research is observed[36]. Further data on the therapeutic effect of this type of agent for liver fibrosis are awaited.

D-penicillamine

This is a copper chelator and can thus interfere with the lysyl oxidation of collagen which needs Cu^{2+} as cofactor. Owing to its overt side-effects and indefinite efficacy, D-penicillamine is rarely used in treating fibrogenic conditions, except in copper overload-related diseases such as Wilson's disease and Indian child cirrhosis[37].

Prostaglandin E₂

Basically prostaglandin E_2 (PGE_2) is regarded as a hepato-cytoprotective agent. By suppressing inflammation, and perhaps the acute-phase reaction, PGE_2 inhibits the release of various cytokines which may be profibrogenic[38].

Another action is to increase the intracellular cAMP levels, thereby enhancing collagen degradation within the cell. It has been reported that 16,16-dimethyl prostaglandin E_2 can decrease liver fibrosis in choline-deficient diet-fed rats[39]. There are no reports on its clinical efficacy for liver fibrosis.

Steroids

Besides their well-known anti-inflammatory and immunosuppressive action, steroids have direct effects on the expression of some ECM molecules. For example, *in vivo* dexamethasone can down-regulate the expression of type I collagen by rat hepatocytes and mesenchymal cells[40]. This type of drug has been tested on various chronic liver diseases, but no definitive antifibrotic effect is proven. Considering this, and the serious systemic side-effects in chronic use, steroids are rarely used for antifibrotic purposes, except for autoimmune hepatitis, in which clinical, biochemical, and even histological improvements can be achieved[41].

Zinc

Gimenez *et al.* reported that oral supplements of zinc, in the form of zinc sulphate solution, significantly decrease the collagen content in CCl_4 inhalation-induced liver fibrosis in the rat[42]. They also observed that zinc supplements increase the suppressed total collagenase activity of liver tissue in early stages of liver fibrosis, and inhibit elevated prolyl hydroxylase activity in late stages of liver cirrhosis. This could be simply explained by the fact that zinc will replace the iron, which is a cofactor of prolyl 4-hydroxylase, and collagenases *per se* are zinc-dependent metalloproteinases. Other mechanisms remain to be elucidated.

Pentoxifylline

Pentoxifylline is a methylxanthine used in peripheral vascular disorders because it can improve red blood cell deformability and blood flow. Peterson found that *in-vitro* pentoxifylline significantly reduced PDGF-stimulated proliferation of fibroblasts, and that *in vivo* it could decrease the collagen content in liver tissue in yellow phosphorus-induced liver fibrosis in pigs[43]. Whether this drug can halt liver fibrogenesis in other cell culture or animal models remains to be examined.

TGF-β and PDGF blocking agents

As mentioned above, TGF-β and PDGF are recognized as the most important profibrogenic cytokines. Therefore, it is an attractive approach to block the effect of the cytokines either by specific neutralizing antibodies or specific receptor antagonists. This strategy has already been explored in fibrogenesis of other sites such as large vessels, lungs and kidneys[44,45]. One preliminary study, in which application of TGF-β neutralizing antibodies inhibits collagen expression in rat fibrosis induced by bile duct ligation[46], showed promising results. Another extensively studied technique for blunting the activity of profibrogenetic cytokines is to block intracellular signal transduction by inhibitors of receptor-specific tyrosine kinase[47].

Antisense DNA

Advances in molecular cloning techniques have produced more data on the nuclear sequences and their regulation elements of the profibrogenic cytokines. Using antisense DNA to inhibit mRNA expression is technically achievable. Wu *et al.* reported that in cultured 3T3 cells expressing asialoglycoprotein receptors, expression of type I collagen mRNA could be significantly decreased by application of antisense oligonucleotides bound to asialo-orosomucoid-prolylysine[48]. This work is exciting, but there is still a long way to go before *in-vivo* use becomes practical.

TREATMENT OF LIVER FIBROSIS WITH TRADITIONAL CHINESE MEDICINE

In recent years considerable attention has been turned to the use of natural medicine in treating many intractable diseases, including chronic liver disease. Among them, traditional Chinese medicine (TCM) is important. TCM has had an even longer history than the Great Wall, the emblem of the ancient culture of China. The earliest record found so far was written on a silk work excavated from a Han tomb, together with a female corpse at Mawangdui in Hunan province. This record on silk is believed by archaeologists to have been in existence before the sixth century BC[49]. Two hundred years later the first description of liver disease appeared in the 'Plain Question' in 'Huangdi Internal classic of Medicine' which may date back to 475–221 BC. Since then, traditional medicinal herbs have been extensively used for the treatment of liver disease for thousands of years in China. In the past four decades Chinese physicians have tried to preserve the continuity of this traditional experience. Many experimental research and clinical trials have been carried out to explore and evaluate the therapeutic efficacy of single herbs or compound recipes of herbs on chronic liver diseases (Tables 1 and 2). A comprehensive review has been published recently[50].

Following the TCM theory, all the therapeutic recipes used for the treatment of liver diseases were prescribed on the basis of TCM syndrome diagnosis. The TCM diagnosis may differ greatly in different patients although they suffer from the same diseases. For each patient with hepatic disease the TCM diagnosis usually comprises two or more such syndromes. In clinical practice corresponding therapeutic principles should be adhered to, appropriate treatment and suitable herbs should be selected and used. For most patients with chronic hepatitis and cirrhosis, 'blood stasis' and 'liver stagnation' are common features in TCM syndrome diagnosis. In treatment, therefore, the therapeutic principle 'Huoxue huayu' should be adhered to. This term, in brief, means 'blood-activating and stasis-eliminating'. More than 30 herbs may be chosen for this purpose, and each formulation formed by different physicians may differ in composition but remain common in principle: invigorating blood circulation and removing stagnation and stasis.

Practising the same therapeutic principle, we also formulated a recipe, Composite *Salvia miltiorrhiza* (Compound 861, Cpd 861) which is compounded of 10 herbs[51]. Among the ten, *Salvia miltiorrhiza*, *Astragalus membranaceus* and *Spatholobus suberectus* are the major ones. This recipe was formed on the basis of daily experience in dealing with chronic liver diseases.

Table 1 Studies on antifibrotic herbs

	Model	*Attenuate*	*Reverse*	*Author*
Cucurbitacin B	Rat (CCl$_4$)	+		Han D. W., *et al.* 1979
Swertia, Lig Ustrum (oleanolic acid)	Rat (CCl$_4$)	+	–	Han D. W., *et al.* 1979
Glycyrrhizin	Rat (CCl$_4$)	+	–	Zhao M. Q., *et al.* 1983
Salvia miltiorrhiza	Rat (CCl$_4$)	+	–	Ma X. H., *et al.* 1988
Semen persicae	Rabbit (*Schistosoma*)	+	+	Liu P., *et al.* 1990
Cordyceps sinensis	Rat (immune injury)	+	+	Zhu J. X., *et al.* 1992
Astragalus	Rat (immune injury)	+	+	Ma H., *et al.* 1994

Table 2 Effect of herbal Cpd on liver fibrosis

	Model	*Attenuate*	*Reverse*	*Author*
Qiang Gan Ruan Jian decoction	Rat (CCl$_4$)	+	+	Han J. H., *et al.* 1979
Xiaoyao granule	Rat (CCl$_4$ + diet)	+		Ma X. H., *et al.* 1991
Kidney- and Yin-replenishing recipe	Rat (DMN)	+		Fan Z. B., *et al.* 1989
Cpd *Salvia miltiorrhizae* (Cpd 861)	Rat (immune injury)	+	+	Wang B. E., *et al.* 1990, 1993
Extract *Semen persicae* + *Cordyceps sinensis*	Rabbit (*Schistosoma*)	+	+	Liu, P., *et al* 1988
319 Capsule	Rat (CCl$_4$ + diet)	+	+	Liu C., *et al.* 1990

In view of its effectiveness in clinical practice, series of experimental research and clinical trials have been carried out with modern scientific modalities to evaluate the efficacy of this recipe in treating liver fibrosis.

Effect of Cpd 861 on experimental fibrosis

To evaluate the therapeutic effect of Cpd 861 on experimental liver fibrosis, its effect on fibrogenesis and degradation of ECM was investigated.

Material and method

Preparation of rat models of hepatic fibrosis.   An immune complex-induced model of liver fibrosis was produced using the method originally proposed by Paronetto and Popper[52], with modifications as reported by us previously[53]. Male Wistar rats, weighing 200–250 g, were sensitized with human albumin by sub-cutaneous injections at different sites, 4 mg each occasion, for four injections, at intervals of 14 days, 10 days and 10 days. Ten days after the fourth injection the rats were injected through the tail vein with an intravenous booster dose of albumin twice weekly for 8 weeks, with an initial dose of 2.5 mg, increasing to 4 mg.

Rats were divided into subgroups: (1) normal control group (N), (2) albumin-induced model group (M), (3) herbal prevention group (P), (4) herbal treatment or reversion group (R), and (5) herbal control group, if necessary.

Preparation of Cpd 861[51].   An extract of 10 herbs, with *Salvia miltiorrhiza*, *Astragalus membranaceus* and *Spatholobus suberectus* as chief components, was made by boiling, extraction and precipitation of the impurity with ethanol. This decoction was given to the animals by gastric gavage. The dosage was 1 ml per 100 g body weight, which is equivalent to seven times the orally adminis-tered dose by body weight for human patients.

Morphological methods.   Conventional histopathological study of the animal liver was done with haematoxylin–eosin stain and Masson trichrome stain. Ultrastructural observation was done on a JEM1200EX electron microscope.

Immunohistochemistry stain for collagen I, III and V was performed with related polyclonal antibodies by the ABC method[54]. Distribution of each col-lagen was examined with colour medical image analysis, and the area ratio of each collagen was calculated by comparing the area of collagen to the total area of liver tissue.

The microscopic grading criteria for fibrotic change in rat liver were as follows[57].

Grade 0: normal pattern.
Grade I: slight extending out of collagen fibre from the portal or central area.
Grade II: collagen fibres extending out, but not yet surrounding the whole lobule.
Grade III: extending collagen fibres connecting with each other and encircling whole lobules.

Grade IV: pseudolobule formation by thin septal fibrous band. Separated lobules were of even shape and large size.

Grade V: pseudolobule formation of uneven shapes and unequal sizes, separated by thick and thin fibrous septum.

Grade VI: nodule formation with encapsulation by thick bands.

Determination of total collagen content. Quantitative measurement of 4-hydroxyproline was done using the method described by Jamoll *et al.*[55] and modified by Zheng *et al.*[56]. Total collagen content was calculated by converting the amount of 4-hydroxyproline to collagen protein.

Lipocyte isolation and culture. Lipocyte isolation and culture was performed according to the method described by Friedman and Roll[58], and modified in our laboratory[59]. The second passage of lipocyte was used for the *in-vitro* experiment.

mRNA for I, III, and IV collagen quantitation[60]. cDNA probes for type I, III, and IV collagen and TGF-β, as well as β-actin, were prepared by random primer incorporation of digoxigenin-labelled deoxyuridine triphosphate with a commercial kit. Total RNA was isolated using a one-step method; 100 mg of liver was homogenized in 1 ml of solution D containing 4 mol/L guanidium isothiocyanate, 0.5% sarcosyl, 0.1 mol/L mercaptoethanol and 25 mmol/L sodium citrate. Then the homogenate was extracted with phenol-chloroform and the RNA in aqueous phase was precipitated with ethanol. Steady-state mRNA levels were assayed by dot–blot hybridization with digoxigenin-labelled probes for type I, III, IV collagen and for TGF-β. A β-actin probe was used as internal control.

Determination of collagenase activity in liver tissue and serum. Collagenase activity in liver tissue was measured using the method of Emonard and Grimaud[61] and Kato *et al.*[62]. Serum collagenase activity was detected with the method described by Rajabi *et al.*[63] and Murawaki *et al.*[64], with some modification.

Activity of collagenases was expressed directly with a value of d.p.m. measured by liquid scintillometry, since the quantity of liver tissue, incubation time and incubation temperature had been strictly defined and no conversion was necessary.

Design. The entire course of the experiment is divided into three stages:

1. Sensitization (with human albumin): 45 days. By the end of this stage, serum antibody to albumin is formed in 90% of the animals. On liver biopsy no fibrosis is formed histologically. No treatment is given during this period.
2. Intravenous booster of albumin period: 8 weeks. By the end of this period, liver biopsy showed that 75–80% of the animals had developed fibrosis, characterized by fine collagen bands encircling and/or extending into lobules.

3. After cessation of albumin administration fibrosis lasts more than 6 months. A model lasting longer than 270 days without reversion of fibrosis has been observed.

Prevention administration of Cpd 861 (P). Administration of Cpd 861 starts when sensitization is finished and the booster has just begun. Daily administration lasts until the end of the booster or longer, up to 3 months after cessation of albumin.

Reversion treatment of fibrosis (R) with Cpd 861. Administration started as soon as fibrosis had formed after cessation of albumin booster, to detect whether fibrosis could be reversed by Cpd 861.

Statistical analysis. For results of experiments, measurement data and enumeration data were analysed with chi-square test and Student's *t*-test, respectively. Ranked and matched data were processed with the Wilcoxon rank-sum test.

Results and discussion

Animal model. Two models have been used: a CCl_4-induced and an albumin immune complex-induced model. In the albumin-treated animals there was a significant increase of total collagen content indicated by a 5-fold rise in hydroxyproline content in liver as compared to control (Table 3). Regression of collagen deposition occurred in both models, but was slower in the albumin-induced model; this explains the longer period of albumin-induced fibrosis.

Quantification of specific mRNA species was determined by Northern blot hybridization analysis of total RNA. The albumin-treated model showed a less pronounced increase in type I procollagen mRNA, but a relatively greater increase in type III and IV procollagen mRNA. There was some increase in transforming growth factor β_1 in both models, but this was more marked in the CCl_4-induced model. A comparison of the two model systems suggests that a variety of mechanisms may be involved in the process of hepatic fibrogenesis. It appeared that an evident inflammatory response and elevated TGF-β level are associated with a marked increase in synthesis of type I collagen in the hepatotoxin model while other, as yet undefined, mediators may be responsible for the marked increase in type III and IV collagen found in the immune complex model[65].

Table 3 Hydroxyproline content in liver of control rats and rats administered human albumin (mg/g wet weight)

	Control	*Albumin-treated*
Weeks of treatment following sensitization		
2	0.89 ± 0.13*	2.09 ± 0.53
4	1.18 ± 0.20	3.33 ± 0.34
8	1.19 ± 0.27	5.28 ± 0.82
Months after last albumin treatment		
3	1.15 ± 0.31	5.17 ± 0.35
6	1.30 ± 0.26	4.73 ± 0.45

* Mean ± SD.

Antifibrotic effect of Cpd 861 on the rat model[57].   Histopathological analysis of the liver samples, taken at the end of experiment by haematoxylin–eosin stain and Masson trichrome stain, showed that fibrosis is much less severe in the prevention group and in the reversion group, as shown in Table 4. In the reversion group the herbal compound was given after cessation of the albumin booster, by which time fibrosis had already been formed, as shown by liver biopsy. The attenuation of fibrosis in the reversion group means that fibrolysis did occur, and this was induced by the herbs. Results of colchicine treatment, as a control, demonstrated that the antifibrotic effect was similar with both agents. Nevertheless, electron microscopic examination showed a different response of ultrastructural change in both groups. Compared to colchicine treatment, restoration of injured mitochondria and reappearance of hepatocyte microvilli seemed more marked in the herbal treatment group. This result is in accordance with that of the study on *Salvia miltiorrhiza* alone, published by us and others[66].

Table 4   Therapeutic effect of Cpd 861 on albumin-induced liver fibrosis

	0	*I*	*II*	*III*	*IV*	*V*	*VI*	*Total*
				Grading of fibrosis				
Normal control	20	0	0	0	0	0	0	20
Model	0	0	0	0	2	4	10	16
Colchicine	0	3	2	1	2	3	1	12
Cpd 861								
Prevention	0	2	1	2	1	1	0	7
Reversion	0	3	1	2	2	3	0	11

Colchicine vs model, $p<0.05$; Cpd 861 (prevention, reversion) vs model, $p<0.05$

Total collagen content.   Total collagen content of the liver tissue is regarded as a marker directly showing the severity of fibrosis. Biochemical determination of hydroxyproline concentration in liver was done after herbal treatment for comparison with normal control and model control. Total collagen, converted from hydroxyproline concentration in normals, is about 1 mg/g of liver wet weight. After albumin booster the content increased by 5-fold. After Cpd 861 treatment, total collagen content of the liver was decreased to around 4 mg/g by 2 months of treatment, and around 2.5 mg/g by 4 months of treatment ($p<0.05$) (Table 5). The reduction of liver collagen content was obviously due to herbal treatment.

Table 5   Total collagen content in liver before and after Cpd 861 (mg/g wet weight)

	Pre-treatment	*Post-treatment*	
		2 months	*4 months*
Normal control	0.971 ± 0.051	0.999 ± 0.044	1.043 ± 0.056
Model	5.699 ± 0.282	5.595 ± 0.275	5.523 ± 0.276
Cpd 861	5.615 ± 0.236	$4.212 \pm 0.266^{*}$	$2.451 \pm 0.215^{*\dagger}$

[*] vs Pre-treatment, $p<0.01$;   [†] 4 months vs 2 months, $p<0.01$

Table 6   Effect of Cpd 861 on area ratio of collagens (4 months treatment)

	Collagen I	Collagen III	Collagen IV	Total collagen
Normal control	0.62 ± 0.06	0.72 ± 0.09	0.68 ± 0.05	0.74 ± 0.08
Model	8.48 ± 0.92	8.53 ± 0.95	8.35 ± 0.61	9.75 ± 1.27
Cpd 861 treatment	4.98 ± 0.84[*]	4.52 ± 0.77[*]	4.88 ± 0.82[*]	5.01 ± 0.77[*]

[*] vs Model, $p<0.01$.

Quantitative measurement of collagen type I, III and IV in liver tissue.   The content of collagen I, III, V in the liver was measured by means of immuno-histochemistry stain with polyclonal antibodies. The amounts of total collagen demonstrated by Masson stain, and collagen I, III, V by immunohistochemical stain were analysed using a colour medical image analysis technique. The area ratio of each collagen was calculated by comparing the measured area of each collagen to the total tissue area. Area ratio represents the relative amount of single collagen, and comparison of the amount detected before and after herbal treatment indicates the therapeutic effect of Cpd 861 on different collagens. As shown in Table 6, collagen I, III and V were markedly increased in quantity in models, and were markedly decreased 4 months after Cpd 861 treatment (P). The result was in good accordance with total collagen content, and strongly suggested that Cpd 861 could effectively inhibit fibrogenesis in rats.

Inhibition of mRNA levels for procollagen I, III, IV and TGF-β in liver tissue[67]. As shown in Figs 1 and 2, density measurement of dot–blot hybridization indicated that the steady-state levels of mRNA for I, III and IV collagens was significantly decreased in the prevention group and the reversion group, as compared to the model group. As β-actin mRNA levels were not significantly changed, the result could be explained by the fact that the collagen genes were

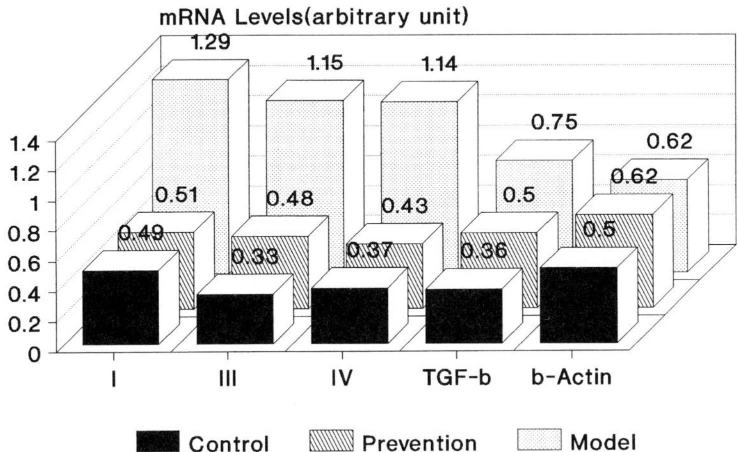

Fig. 1   Effect of Cpd 861 on collagen mRNA level after 5 months prevention

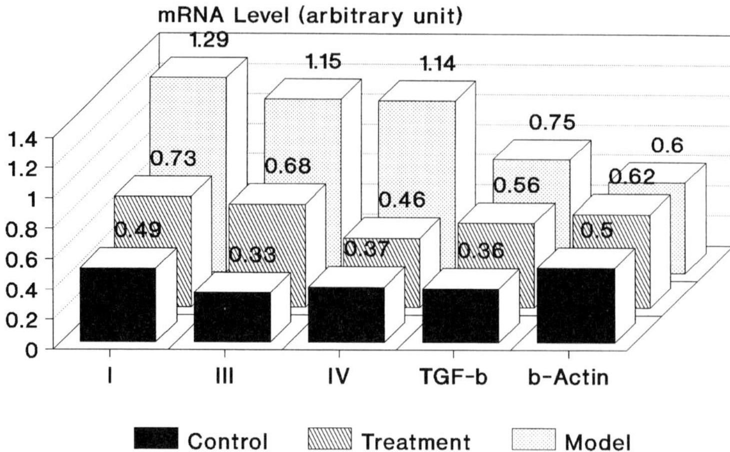

Fig. 2   Effect of Cpd 861 on collagen mRNA level after 2.5 months treatment

effectively inhibited by the herbal compound. The consistent increase in collagen mRNA in the model, and the substantial decrease after treatment, again illustrates the inhibitory effect on fibrogenesis. TGF-β mRNA levels were also found to be increased in models as compared to the normal control. This is in accordance with established knowledge that TGF-β, as a mediator, plays an important role in fibrogenesis. Inhibition of TGF-β mRNA level after herbal treatment may possibly explain part of the mechanism for the antifibrotic effect of the herbs.

Effect of Cpd 861 on collagen I, III and IV mRNA level in cultured rat lipocytes[68]. The *in-vitro* effect of the herbal compound on cultured lipocytes was examined by exposure of the second passage of the lipocyte culture to the liquid extract of compound *Salvia miltiorrhiza*. The results showed that collagen type IV mRNA levels, both in the herbal treatment group and the colchicine group, were remarkably decreased compared with the untreated control. Similar results were seen with I and III collagen mRNA. These results suggested that the antifibrotic effect of Cpd 861 may be partly due to modulation of collagen gene expression in lipocytes by the herbs, and gave support to the assumption that herbs suppress fibrogenesis by inhibiting gene expression in non-parenchymal cells.

Serum and liver tissue collagenase activity[69]. To elucidate whether the herbal compound has any effect on collagen degradation, active collagenase (A) activity and latent collagenase activity in liver tissue (L), serum collagenase (S) was detected during the course of herbal treatment. Results are shown in Tables 7 and 8. A, L and S were not altered significantly during the whole course of the experiment in normal controls or in the control group receiving herb Cpd 861 with no albumin administration.

Consecutive estimation of collagenase activity in the whole process of fibrosis in the rat model revealed that, during the sensitization stage, hepatic collage-

Table 7 Collagenase activity during the course of model formation (d.p.m.)

	Months	*A*	*L*	*A/L*	*S*
Presensitization	0	605.5 ± 42.3	1792.3 ± 124.9	0.339 ± 0.023	1229.8 ± 168.2
End of sensitization	1.5	597.5 ± 44.3	2032.2 ± 69.7	0.294 ± 0.023	1228.8 ± 161.9
Booster i.v.	2.5	1197.5 ± 152.5	3117.8 ± 453.7	0.335 ± 0.023	2306.5 ± 190.5
Cessation of booster	3.5	1027.5 ± 79.4	2971.5 ± 79.0	0.346 ± 0.028	1897.7 ± 247.8
	5.0	945 ± 72.7	2842.7 ± 443.5	0.336 ± 0.030	1980.1 ± 116.4
	6.5	805.3 ± 78.6	2428.5 ± 158.2	0.334 ± 0.047	1624.7 ± 114.9

A: Activated collagenase activity in liver tissue.
L: Latent collagenase activity in liver tissue.
S: Serum collagenase activity.

nase apparently showed no change, but was significantly increased after boosting with albumin. Thereafter increased enzyme activity was sustained at a higher level, although it tended to decline somewhat. In comparison to the model, on treatment with Cpd 861, hepatic collagenase activity was increased to 15% in the prevention group and 190% in the reversion treatment group ($p<0.01$) (Table 8 and Fig. 3). Serum collagenase activity showed a similar tendency. On the contrary, hepatic collagen content, detected concurrently with collagenase activity, showed marked attenuation on treatment with Cpd 861. Thus, the more pronounced activation of collagenase, and the resultant resolution of the fibrous tissue, seems to indicate that Cpd 861 is capable of stimulating degradation of ECM as part of its role in treating liver fibrosis, in addition to the inhibitory effect on fibrogenesis. The mechanism of the increase of collagenase activity in the process of fibrogenesis is not yet clear. It may be assumed that the albumin immune complex deposited in the liver can lead to injury to liver cells, and to subsequent release of various cytokines, such as TNF, IL-1, PDGF and TGF-β, which in turn incite activation of the lipocytes and then release of collagenase. Possible explanations for the decrease in enzyme activity might be: (1) decrease of collagenase gene expression, (2) inhibition of procollagenase activation, or (3) increase of specific inhibitors against activated collagenase. The mechanism for herbal Cpd 861 to increase collagenase activity is not yet

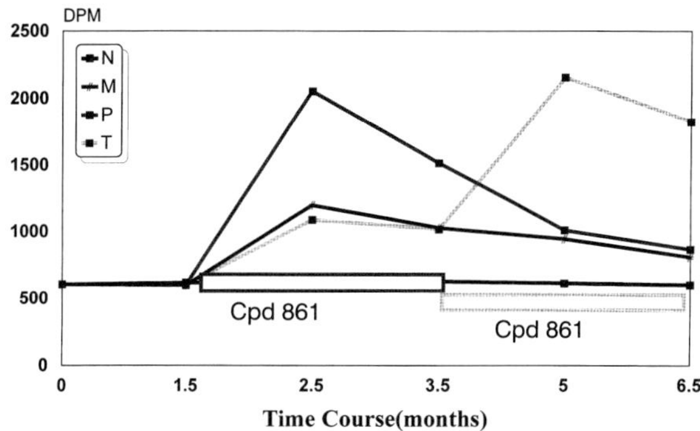

Fig. 3 Liver tissue collagenase activity

Table 8 Latent collagenase activity in liver tissue before and after Cpd 861 (d.p.m.)

	Cpd 861	NC	HC	M	P	R
Presensitization		1792.3 ± 124.9	1792.3 ± 124.9	1792.3 ± 124.9	1792.3 ± 124.9	1792.3 ± 124.9
Post-sensitization	P	1715.7 ± 223	1715.7 ± 223	2032.3 ± 69.7	1853.7 ± 97.4	1809.2 ± 154.9
Booster (middle)	P	1776.8 ± 128.2	1684 ± 136.8	3117.8 ± 453.7	4892 ± 175.8	3351.3 ± 353.2
Post-booster	R	1837.8 ± 107.8	1700.8 ± 133.9	2971.5 ± 79.0	3634.8 ± 175.5	2920.3 ± 57.0
Mid-treatment	R	847.2 ± 95.5	1718 ± 135.1	2842.7 ± 443.5	3208.3 ± 237.7	5935 ± 342.6
End-treatment	R	1857.7 ± 94.4	1773 ± 119.5	2428.5 ± 158.2	2882.8 ± 215.3	4275 ± 239.9

NC, Normal control; HC, Herbal control; M, Model; P, Prevention treatment; R, Reversion treatment.

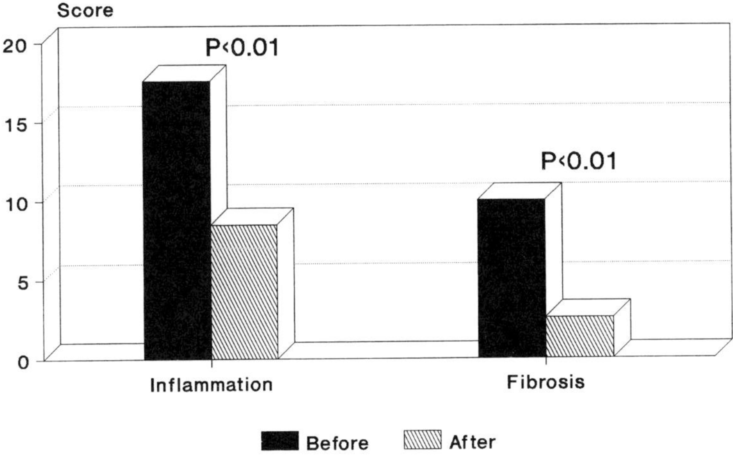

Fig. 4 Effect of Cpd 861 on human liver histology (12 cases)

clear. As shown above, Cpd 861 can inhibit biosynthesis of TGF-β, which is known to inhibit the expression of collagenase and to promote gene expression of the tissue inhibitor of metalloproteinase. Thus, as a result, inhibition of the expression of TGF-β by Cpd 861 will lead to an increase in collagenase activity.

Preliminary clinical application of Cpd 861 in treating chronic liver disease[57,70]

Based on the results of experimental studies, compound *Salvia miltiorrhiza* has been used in patients with chronic hepatitis to assess its clinical efficacy.

From 1993 to 1995, 60 cases of chronic hepatitis were put on open trial with Cpd 861. Among 60 cases, 46 were male and 14 female, age range 50–68 years. All had a history of chronic hepatitis B of more than 2 years (average duration of illness 13 years). All patients maintained daily intake of the drug orally for more than 2 years. At the 2-year follow-up, improvement of symptoms occurred in 50 cases (83%), including: disappearance of hypochondriac discomfort or pain in 67%, appetite improved in 60%, fatigue lessened in 60%, ALT returned to normal without relapse in 70%. On ultrasonography, the width of the portal vein was enlarged in 21 patients before treatment; among these 61.9% showed a decrease in diameter, no change in 19% and an increase in 9%. Among 27 cases with enlarged spleen, in 40.7% the spleen was decreased in size. Serum PIIIP and laminin were decreased to normal in 2 years (Table 9). Improvement in symptoms, decrease of ALT, normalization of serum PIIIP and laminin, as well as reduction of portal vein diameter and size of spleen, suggested that the therapeutic efficacy was promising.

In 12 patients with B-type chronic hepatitis, liver biopsy was performed before and after 6 months treatment with Cpd 861. The results showed significant attenuation of either inflammation or fibrosis (Table 10, Figure 4).

Table 9 Effect of Cpd 861 on serum PIIIP and laminin levels

	n	*PIIIP (U/ml)*	n	*Ln (U/ml)*
Pretreatment	60	0.956 ± 0.423	50	1.457 ± 0.420
Post-treatment 0.5 year	45	0.818 ± 0.320	35	1.243 ± 0.363
Post-treatment 2 years	50	$0.717 \pm 0.339^*$	36	$1.182 \pm 0.333^*$

* $p<0.01$.

Table 10 Liver histopathology of 12 patients pre- and post-treatment with Cpd 861

	Grading		*Staging*	
No.	*Pre-treatment*	*Post-treatment*	*Pre-treatment*	*Post-treatment*
1	G1$^-$	G2	S1$^-$	S1
2	G2	G1	S1	S0
3	G3	G2$^-$	S2	S2$^-$
4	G3	G1	S2$^-$	S0
5	G3	G1	S2	S1
6	G3$^-$	G2	S2$^-$	S1
7	G2	G1	S1	S0
8	G2	G1	S1	S0
9	G1	G1	S1	S1
10	G2$^-$	G1	S2$^-$	S1
11	G4	G2	S3	S1
12	G2$^+$	G1	S1$^+$	S0

The inflammatory activity score was reduced from 17.58 ± 7.63 to 8.50 ± 3.75 (Wilcoxon test, $p<0.01$), while the score for fibrosis (Masson stain and Sirius red stain) decreased from 10.00 ± 8.64 to 2.58 ± 2.47 (Wilcoxon test, $p<0.01$). On α-smooth muscle actin stain there were plenty of α-actin positive cells existing in the fibrous band, and the amount was markedly reduced after herbal treatment. This suggests that Cpd 861 could suppress fibrogenesis in humans as it did in the rat, and inhibition of the lipocyte proliferation probably plays an important role.

SUMMARY

In rats, compound *Salvia miltiorrhiza* can inhibit experimental liver fibrosis induced by the albumin immune complex. The antifibrotic action of the compound is due to its effect of suppressing fibrogenesis, and at the same time stimulating collagen degradation, as evidenced by decreased biosynthesis of total collagen and type I, III and V collagen in the liver, lowered expression of mRNA for procollagen I, III and IV in liver tissue, and decreased level of I, III and IV procollagen mRNA in cultured lipocyte and increased liver collagenase activity. The mechanism involved is as yet unknown, but inhibition of cytokine TGF-β may possibly play a role, as suppression of TGF-β increases collagenase activity and decreases the activity of the tissue inhibitor of metalloproteinase. Clinical use of this compound in treating chronic liver fibrosis is highly likely to occur.

Acknowledgment

We thank Drs H Ma, SS Yin and H You for their expert assistance in preparing this manuscript.

References

1. Greenwel P, Geerts A, Ogata I, Solis-Herruzo J-S, Rojkind M. Liver fibrosis. In: Arias IM, Boyer JL, Fausto N, *et al.* editors. The liver: biology and pathobiology, 3rd edn. New York: Raven Press; 1994:1367 81.
2. Gressner AM. Liver fibrosis: perspectives in pathobiological research and clinical outlook. Eur J Clin Chem Clin Biochem. 1991;29:293–311.
3. Pinzani M. Hepatic stellate (ITO) cells: expanding roles for a liver-specific pericyte. J Hepatol. 1995;22:700–6.
4. Nguyen MT, Herrine SK, Zern MA. Cytokines involvement in the liver. Curr Opin Gastroenterol. 1994;10:277–84.
5. Arthur MJP. Collagenases and liver fibrosis. J Hepatol. 1995;22(Suppl.2):43.
6. Diegelmann RF, Peterkofsky B. Inhibition of collagen secretion from bone and cultured fibroblasts by microtubular disruptive drugs. Proc Natl Acad Sci USA. 1972;69:892–6.
7. Harris ED Jr, Krane SM. Effects of colchicine on collagenase in cultures of rheumatoid synovium. Arthritis Rheum. 1971;14:669.
8. Tanner MS, Jackson D, Mowat AP. Hepatic collagen synthesis in a rat model of cirrhosis and its modification by colchicine. J Pathol. 1981;135:179–87.
9. Poo JL, Feldmann G, Moreau A, Gaudin C, Lebrec D. Early colchicine administration reduces hepatic fibrosis and portal hypertension in rats with bile duct ligation. J Hepatol. 1993;19:90–4.
10. Kershenobich D, Vargas F, Garcia-Tsao G, Tamayo RP, Gent M, Rojkind M. Colchicine in the treatment of cirrhosis of the liver. N Engl J Med. 1988;318:1709–13.
11. Bodenheimer H, Schaffner F, Pezzullo J. Evaluation of colchicine therapy in primary biliary cirrhosis. Gastroenterology. 1988;95:124–9.
12. Vuoristo M, Farkkila M, Karvonen A-L *et al.* A placebo-controlled trial of primary biliary cirrhosis treatment with colchicine and ursodeoxycholic acid. Gastroenterology. 1995;108:1470–8.
13. Wang YJ, Lee SD, Hsieh MC *et al.* A double-blind randomized controlled trial of colchicine in patients with hepatitis B virus-related postnecrotic cirrhosis. J Hepatol. 1994;21:872–7.
14. Lieber CS, Decarli LM, Mak KM, Kim C-I, Leo MA. Attenuations of alcohol-induced hepatic fibrosis by polyunsaturated lecithin. Hepatology. 1990 12:1390–8.
15. Lieber CS, Robins SJ, Li JJ *et al.* Phosphatidylcholine protects against fibrosis and cirrhosis in the baboon. Gastroenterology. 1994;106:152–9.
16. Li JJ, Kim C-I, Leo MA, Mak KM, Rojkind M, Lieber CS. Polyunsaturated lecithin prevents acetaldehyde-mediated hepatic collagen accumulation by stimulating collagenase activity in cultured lipocytes. Hepatology. 1992;15:373:81.
17. Rockey DC, Maher JJ, Jarnagin WR, Gabbiani G, Friedman SL. Inhibition of rat hepatic lipocyte activation in culture by interferon γ. Hepatology. 1992;16:776–84.
18. Mallat A, Preaux AM, Blazejewski S, Rosenbaum J, Dhumeaux D, Mavier P. Interferon α and γ inhibit proliferation and collagen synthesis of human Ito cells in culture. Hepatology. 1995;21:1003–10.
19. Elias I, Alpini G, Gubba S *et al.* Antiproliferative effects of γ-interferon in carbon tetrachloride (CCl_4)-induced cirrhosis. Hepatology. 1995;22:277A.
20. Sakaida I, Matsumura Y, Yasunaga M, Okita K. Interferon gamma treatment inhibits collagen deposition in pig serum-induced rat liver fibrosis *in vivo*. Hepatology. 1995;22:483A.
21. Czaja MJ, Weiner FR, Takahashi S *et al.* γ-Interferon treatment inhibits collagen deposition in murine schistosomiasis. Hepatology. 1989;10:795–800.
22. Shi Z, Stewart TA, Rockey DC. Liver injury and fibrosis in interferon γ gene knock-out mice. Hepatology. 1995;22:276A.
23. Castilla A, Prieto J, Fausto N. Transforming growth factors $\beta 1$ and α in chronic liver disease. Effects of interferon alpha therapy. N Engl J Med. 191;324:933–40.
24. Capra F, Casaril M, Gabrielli GB *et al.* α-Interferon in the treatment of chronic viral hepatitis: effects on fibrogenesis serum markers. J Hepatol. 1993;18:112–18.

25. Manabe N, Chevallier M, Chossegros P *et al.* Interferon-α2b therapy reduces liver fibrosis in chronic non-A, non-B hepatitis: a quantitative histological evaluation. Hepatology. 1993;18:1344–9.
26. Rojkind M, Greenwel P. The extracellular matrix of the liver. In: Arias IM *et al.* eds. The liver: biology and pathobiology, 3rd edn. New York: Raven Press; 1994:843–68.
27. David BH, Kramer RT, Davidson NO. Retinoic acid modulates rat Ito cell proliferation, collagen and transforming growth factor β production. J Clin Invest. 1990;86:2062–70.
28. Hendriks HFJ, Bosma A, Bruwer A. Fat-storing cells: hypo- and hypervitaminosis A and the relationship with liver fibrosis. Semin Liver Dis. 1993;13:72–80.
29. Leo MA, Lieber CS. Hepatic fibrosis after long-term administration of ethanol and moderate vitamin A supplementation in the rat. Hepatology. 1983;3:1–11.
30. Geubel AP, De Galocsy C, Alves N, Rahier J, Dive C. Liver damage caused by therapeutic vitamin A administration: estimate of dose related toxicity in 41 cases. Gastroenterology. 1991;100:1701–9.
31. Lieber CS. Alcohol and the liver: 1994 update. Gastroenterology. 1994;106:1085–1105.
32. Bickel M, Baader E, Brocks DG *et al.* Beneficial effects of inhibitors of prolyl 4-hydroxylase in CCl_4 induced fibrosis of the liver in rats. J Hepatol. 1991;13(Suppl. 3):S26–34.
33. Boker K, Schwarting G, Kauke G, Gunzler V, Schmidts E. Fibrosis of the liver in rats induced by bile duct ligation. J Hepatol. 1991;13(Suppl.3):S35–40.
34. Chojkier M, Brenner DA. Therapeutic strategies for hepatic fibrosis. Hepatology. 1988;8:176–82.
35. Franklin TJ. Current approaches to the therapy of fibrotic diseases. Biochem Pharmacol. 1995;49:267–73.
36. Tang SS, Simpson DE, Kagan HM. β-Quinone-directed irreversible inhibitors of lysyl oxidase. J Biol Chem. 1984;263:12963–9.
37. Pradhan AM, Bhave SA, Joshi VV, Bavdekar AR, Pandit AN, Tanner MS. Reversal of Indian childhood cirrhosis by D-penicillamine therapy. J Pediatr Gastroenterol Nutr. 1995;10:28–35.
38. Brenner DA, Alcorn JM. Therapy for hepatic fibrosis. Semin Liver Dis. 1990;10:75–83.
39. Ruwart MJ, Rush BD, Snyder KF *et al.* 16,16-Dimethyl prostaglandin E_2 delays collagen formation in nutritional injury in rat liver. Hepatology. 1988;8:61–4.
40. Jefferson DM, Reid LM, Giambrone M-A, Schafritz DA, Zern M. Effects of dexamethasone on albumin and collagen gene expression in primary cultures of adult rat hepatocytes. Hepatology. 1985;5:14–20.
41. Kirk AP, Jain S, Pocok S, Thomas HC, Sherlock S. Late results of the Royal Free Hospital prospective controlled trial of prednisolone therapy in hepatitis B surface antigen negative chronic active hepatitis. Gut. 1980;21:78–83.
42. Gimenez A, Pares A, Alie S *et al.* Fibrogenic and collagenolytic activity in carbon-tetrachloride-injured rats: beneficial effects of zinc administration. J Hepatol. 1994;21:292–8.
43. Peteerson TC. Pentoxifylline prevents fibrosis in an animal model and inhibits platelet-derived growth factor-driven proliferation of fibroblasts. Hepatology. 1993;17:486–93.
44. Ferns GAA, Raines EW, Sprugel KH, Motani AS, Redy MA, Ross R. Inhibition of neointimal smooth muscle accumulation after angioplasty by an antibody to PDGF. Science. 1991;253:1129–32.
45. Border WA, Nobel NA, Yamamoto T *et al.* Natural inhibitor of transforming growth factor-β protects against scarring in experimental kidney disease. Nature. 1992;360:361–4.
46. Strobel D, Wittekind C, Ruoslahti E, Hahn EG. *In vivo* application of a neutralizing TGF-β antibody in experimental liver fibrosis. J Hepatol. 1993;18(Suppl. 1):S63.
47. Levitzki A. Tyrphostins: tyrosine kinase blockers as novel antiproliferative agents and dissectors of signal transduction. FASEB J. 1992;6:3275–82.
48. Wu CH, Walton CM, Wu GY *et al.* Targeted inhibition of type I procollagen synthesis by anti-sense DNA oligonucleotides. Int Hepatol Commun. 1995;3(Suppl):S22.
49. Liu YC. The essential book of traditional Chinese medicine, Vol. I: Theory. New York: Columbia University Press; 1988.
50. Han DW. Hepatic pathophysiology, 1st edn. Taiyuan: Shanxi United University Press; 1992.
51. Wang BE, Sun M, Bai N *et al.* Therapeutic effect of composite huoxuehuayu herbs in treating experimental liver fibrosis. Trad Med Herbs. 1990;21:23–5.
52. Paronetto F, Popper H. Aggravation of hepatic lesions in mice by *in vivo* localization of immune complex (Auer Hepatitis). Am J Pathol. 1965;47:549.

53. Wang BE, Wang ZF, Yin WT *et al*. Experimental immune complex induced modal of liver fibrosis. Chin J Med. 1989;69:503–5.
54. Liu YF. Immunohistochemical stain. Beijing: People's Medical Publishing House; 1990:62–9.
55. Jamall IS, Finelli VN, Que Mee SS *et al*. A simple method to determine nanogram levels of 4-hydroxyproline in biological tissues. Anal Biochem. 1981;112:70–5.
56. Zheng SX, Cai WY, Qiu MC. *et al*. Modified method for determination of hydroxyproline in blood and urine. Chin J Clin Lab. 1983;6:133–6.
57. Wang BE, Wang HJ, Zhu JX, *et al*. Experimental and clinical study of the therapeutic effect of composite *Salviae miltiorrhizae* on liver fibrosis. Chin J Hepatol. 1993;1:69–72.
58. Friedman SL, Roll FJ. Isolation and culture of hepatic lipocyte, Kupffer cells, and sinusoidal endothelial cell by density gradient centrifugation with stractan. Anal Biochem. 1987;161:207–8.
59. Chen YJ, Wang BE, Ma XM *et al*. Isolation and culture of rat fat-storing cells. Chin J Hepatol. 1993;1:17–20.
60. Sambrook J, Fritsch EF, Maniatis T. Molecular cloning: a laboratory manual, 2nd edn. Cold Spring Harbor: Cold Spring Harbor Laboratory Press; 1989;7:53–5.
61. Emonard H, Grimaud JA. Active and latent collagenase activity during reversal of hepatic fibrosis in murine schistosomiasis. Hepatology. 1989;10:77–83.
62. Kato S, Murawaki Y, Hirayama C *et al*. Effects of ethanol feeding on hepatic collagen synthesis and degradation in rats. Res Commun Chem Pathol Pharmacol. 1985;47:163–80.
63. Rajabi M, Deon DD, Woessner TF. High levels of serum collagenase in premature labor: a potential biochemical marker. Obstet Gynecol. 1987;69:179–86.
64. Murawaki Y, Yamamoto H, Koda M *et al*. Serum collagenase activity reflects the amount of liver collagenase in chronic carbon tetrachloride-treated rats. Res Commun Chem Pathol Pharmacol. 1994;84:63–72.
65. Sun M, Wang BE, Annoni G, Esposti SD, Biempica L, Zern MA. Two rat models of hepatic fibrosis: a morphologic and molecular comparison. Lab Invest. 1990;63:467–75.
66. Liu EY, Wang BE, Zhu JX. Therapeutic efficacy of *Salvia miltiorrhiza* on liver fibrosis. Chin J Hepatol. 1993;1:93–96.
67. Jia JD, Wang BE, Dong Z *et al*. The effect of Cpd 861 on liver tissue collagen mRNA levels in experimental liver fibrosis in rat. Chin J Hepatol. 1996 (In press).
68. Jia JD, Wang BE, Ma XM. The effect of herbal Cpd 861 on type IV collagen mRNA levels in cultured rat lipocytes. Chin J Hepatol. 1996 (In press).
69. Wang AM (supervisor: Prof Wang Bao-en). Study on the effects of herbal Cpd 861 upon collagenase activities in experimental liver fibrosis (dissertation). Beijing: Capital University of Medical Sciences; 1995.
70. Wang HJ, Wang BE. Long-term follow-up result of compound Dan Shen granule (861 Chong Fu Ji) in treating hepatofibrosis. Chin J Integr Trad West Med Liver Dis. 1995;5:4–5.

Section V
Hepatocellular carcinoma

20
Surgical resection of hepatocellular carcinoma in 1380 patients

Z.-Y. TANG, Y.-Q. YU, X.-D. ZHOU, Z.-C. MA, Z. Q. WU and
X. P. JIANG

INTRODUCTION

Hepatocellular carcinoma (HCC), prevalent in southeast Asia and sub-Saharan Africa, has led to 250 000 annual deaths in the world, and is increasing in prevalence in some countries such as Japan, France and Italy[1,2]. In China, since the 1990s, HCC has surpassed gastric cancer to become the leading cancer killer in rural areas, and is ranked second in the cities[3]. Annual deaths from HCC in China have exceeded 130 000, which comprises around 45% of HCC deaths in the world[2].

The earliest liver cancer resection was done in the late nineteenth century; unfortunately, there was no substantial progress in the ensuing years. In the 1950s, based on the understanding of intrahepatic distribution of vessels and ducts, as well as biochemical change after major hepatic resection, lobectomy has been acknowledged as the only hope for a curative outcome[4,5]. In the 1960s, with progress in immunology, liver transplantation was advocated[6]. Since the 1970s, as a result of mass screening, small HCC resection has opened up a new area in clinical aspects of liver cancer research; limited resection instead of lobectomy has been advocated in patients with cirrhosis[7–9]. In the 1980s, with progress in medical imaging, advances were made both in small and large HCC; re-resection for subclinical recurrence was one of the effective approaches to prolong survival further after resection[10]. All of these factors resulted in a gradual improvement in survival after HCC resection.

GENERAL DATA AND THE ROLE OF SMALL HCC RESECTION

During the period 1958–94, of the 2254 pathologically proven HCC patients treated in the authors' institute, 1380 received resection. In these 1380 patients, abnormal serum α-fetoprotein (AFP) was found in 72.1% (362/1279). Small HCC amounted to 39.8% (549/831). Solitary tumour accounted for 68.0%.

Well-encapsulated tumour was found in 61.1% of patients. Tumour embolus was found in 38.4% of surgical specimens. Coexisting liver cirrhosis appeared in 85.6% of patients; 68.7% of the cirrhosis was macronodular cirrhosis. Limited resection and left lateral segmentectomy was performed in 64.9% of the series. The operative mortality was 2.9% (having been 23.4% in 1958–70, 4.6% in 1971–82, and 1.5% in 1983–94). The 5-year survival was 46.7% (having been 12.9% in 1958–70, 29.4% in 1971–82, and 53.5% in 1983–94), and 10-year 34.4%, whereas it was only 11.1% and 6.5% respectively for 874 patients with non-resectional treatment. By 1994, 184 patients survived more than 5 years, and 52 more than 10 years.

The superiority of small HCC resection was clear; when compared to large HCC resection, the resectability was higher (93.2% vs 49.9%), curative resection higher (95.1% vs 76.7%), operative mortality lower (1.3% vs 4.0%), 5-year survival higher (62.9% vs 34.6%), and number of 5-year survivors greater (109 vs 75), indicating that small HCC resection played an important role in obtaining long-term survivors, which agreed with our previous reports[11–13]. Similar results also appeared in the literature: of the 96 patients with 5-year survival, 91 were from HCC resection[14]. Okamoto et al. reported 79 patients with 5-year survival from 539 HCC resections[15]. Large series of small HCC resection have been found in the literature. Makuuchi et al. reported 362 small HCC resections; operative mortality was 1.7%, 5-year survival 43.7%[16].

HCC resection with acceptable results has also been found in the recent literature[17–20]. Wu and Chen reported 1102 HCC resections (85.2% associated with cirrhosis): operative mortality was 1.8%, 5-year survival was 28.4% in the entire series[17]. Lai et al. recently reported 343 HCC resections (73% associated with cirrhosis): operative mortality decreased to 4.5%, and 5-year survival increased to 35%[18]. In another series in the United States with lower occurrence of cirrhosis (33%), the 5-year survival of 106 HCC resections increased to 41%[19].

Table 1 Surgical data of 1380 patients with resection

	Percentage
Resectability	61.2
Curative resection	84.0
Palliative resection	16.0
Type of resection	
Limited	52.5
Left lateral segmentectomy	12.4
Left hemihepatectomy	14.1
Left trisegmentectomy	1.4
Right posterior lobectomy	4.6
Right hemihepatectomy	4.2
Right trisegmentectomy	0.3
Middle lobectomy	2.0
Two sites or more	8.7
Operative mortality	2.9
Survival	
5-year (n)	46.7 (184)
10-year (n)	34.4 (52)

Similar results were also reported in France: the 5-year survival was 40% in 68 HCC (median diameter 8.8 cm) resections in non-cirrhotic liver, the operative mortality was 2.9%[20]. In the authors' institute, with increasing experience in the resection of segment VIII HCC, resectability has been further increased[21].

FACTORS INFLUENCING RESECTABILITY AND PROGNOSIS

As shown in Table 2, analysis of factors influencing resectability revealed that small HCCs ($\leq$5 cm), solitary tumours, left lobe cancers, and encapsulated tumour had higher resectability. As shown in Table 3, analysis of factors influencing prognosis indicated that the following had higher 5-year survival when compared with their counterparts: small HCC (62.9% vs 34.6%), solitary HCC (52.1% vs 35.8%), encapsulated tumour (56.0% vs 31.6%), absence of tumour embolus (63.9% vs 40.8%), limited or left lobe resection (48.7% vs 34.5%), postoperative AFP $\leq$20 μg/L in AFP-producing HCC (57.2% vs 36.2%); no significant difference was found concerning coexistent cirrhosis and Edmondson's differentiation.

RELATION OF SOME GENE EXPRESSION AND SURVIVAL

Over-expression of nm23-H1 was reported associated with a lower recurrence rate after HCC resection[22–24]. In the authors' institute, studies on antimetastatic gene revealed that expression of nm23-H1 protein was positively correlated to 5-year survival, being 81.4% (n=46) vs 27.2% (n=41) (p<0.01). Expression of tissue inhibitor of metalloproteinase-2 (TIMP2) protein was also associated with longer 5-year survival after resection, being 71.9% (n=43) vs 39.3% (n=44)

Table 2 Factors influencing resectability

Factors	*Resection rate*
Tumour size	
$\leq$5 cm	93.2% (549/589)
>5 cm	49.9% (831/1665)
Number of nodules	
1	76.2% (927/1216)
2	77.0% (211/274)
>2	46.5% (226/486)
Tumour site	
Left lobe	92.7% (395/426)
Right lobe	72.5% (713/984)
Hilum	47.1% (56/119)
Both lobes	45.7% (209/457)
Tumour capsule	
Good	91.4% (774/847)
Poor	54.4% (492/904)
Cirrhosis	
No	72.3% (196/271)
Micronodular	74.0% (372/503)
Macronodular	66.8% (790/1183)

Table 3   Factors influencing survival after resection

Factors	n	3-year (%)	5-year (%)
Tumour size			
≤5 cm	549	74.5	62.9
>5 cm	831	44.1	34.6
Number of nodules			
1	927	63.8	52.3
>1	437	43.1	35.8
Tumour capsule			
Good	774	68.9	56.0
Poor	492	37.4	31.6
Tumour embolus			
Absent	698	71.9	63.9
Present	436	51.3	40.8
Edmonson's grading			
1	54	67.9	47.9
2	919	60.1	49.6
3	139	57.5	48.6
Cirrhosis			
No	196	63.6	47.1
Micronodular	372	62.0	55.1
Macronodular	789	53.4	42.9
Resection			
Limit, left lobe	1108	59.1	48.7
Right lobectomy	125	45.5	34.5
Postoperative AFP			
≤20 μg/L	329	70.5	57.2
>20 μg/L	450	42.2	36.2

($p<0.01$). Furthermore, patients with recurrence after resection showed higher positivity of TGF-α and EGF-receptor expression in HCC tissue, being 52.2% (12/23) vs 42.6% (20/47) for TGF-α, and 65.2% (15/23) vs 38.3% (18/47) for EGF-receptor[25,26].

RECURRENCE AFTER CURATIVE RESECTION

Recurrence is a major problem after curative resection of HCC. In the authors' institute the 5-year recurrence rate was as high as 61.5%, being 43.5% for small HCC resection. Using integration of hepatitis B virus DNA, loss of heterozygosity (LOH) pattern on chromosome 16, and p53 loss of heterozygosity, both unicentric and multicentric origin have been demonstrated in patients with recurrence[27–30]. For treatment of recurrence, re-resection for subclinical recurrence or solitary lung metastasis was advocated in 1984[10]. It remained the choice of treatment modality for recurrence in the ensuing years[31]. In the authors' institute, of the 97 patients with re-resection, the 5-year survival was 51.2% calculated from the first resection, and 38.7% from the re-resection[13]. Wu *et al.* reported 72 patients with re-resection: the 5-year survival was 49.5% after the first resection and 36.1% after the re-resection[32]; a similar result was also reported by Suenaga *et al.* (*n*=18), being 45% and 37% respectively[33].

In this series the 5-year survival after resection has increased from 12.9% (*n*=64) in 1958–70, 29.4% (*n*=174) in 1971–82, to 53.5% (*n*=1142) in 1983–94, which agreed with the increase in small HCC in the series, as well as the increase in the number of re-resections for recurrence (0, 27, and 114 patients, respectively).

In the authors' institute it has been found that HCC invasiveness-related onco-genes and growth factors included: P16 and P53 mutation, H-ras, c-erbB-2, nm23-H1, TGF-α, EGF-receptor, TIMP2, etc., and the positivities of these factors did not correlate well with tumour size. The biological approach will therefore probably be important in forthcoming years to further improve prognosis after resection. In the authors' institute a human HCC metastatic model in nude mice has recently been established[34], and antisense H-ras, as well as bispecific antibody (anti-CD3/anti-HBx) plus LAK cells have been demonstrated to inhibit tumour growth in this model[35]. TNF-gene liposome intra-lesional administration has also been proved to have an inhibitory effect on the HCC model in nude mice[36]. Experimental studies on gene therapy using adeno-virus-mediated human P53 tumour suppressor gene transfer or fibroblast-mediated human interferon-α gene therapy have also been reported[37,38]. Differentiation inducers such as retinoic acid have been reported to change the structure of N-glycan on the surface of the human HCC cell[39]. However, because of the complexity of gene therapy, as well as other biotherapies, studies on better combination of old modalities may still prove to be a useful approach.

FUTURE PROSPECTS

It is suggested that, besides early detection, biological characteristics of HCC are the major target to be studied to further improve long-term survival after resection. Problems remaining to be solved in the field of HCC resection include: the issue of 'cost-effectiveness' for screening of small HCC; the biological characteristics, particularly intraportal venous invasion, even in very small HCC; the multicentric origin of HCC; the coexistent cirrhosis, etc. All these remain great challenges.

Acknowledgement

This work was supported in part by China Medical Board Grant no. 93–583, 'Primary liver cancer'.

References

1. Kuroishi T, Hayakawa N, Kurihara M, Aoki K. Cancer mortality in 33 countries of the world (1953–1987). In: Tominaga S, Aoki K, Fujimoto I, Kuraihara M, editors. Cancer mortality and morbidity statistics (Japan and the world – 1994). Tokyo: Japanese Scientific Society Press; 1994:167–230.
2. Parkin DM, Stjernsward J, Muir CS. Estimates of the worldwide frequency of twelve major cancers. Bull WHO. 1984;62:163–82.
3. Centre for Health Statistics Information, Ministry of Public Health, P.R. China (editors). Selected edition on health statistics of China (1991–1994). Beijing: Ministry of Public Health, P.R. China; 1991:78–9.

4. Healey JE, Schroy PC, Sorensen RJ. The intrahepatic distribution of the hepatic artery in man. J Int Coll Surg. 1953;20:133–48.
5. Lortat-Jacob JL, Robert HG. Hepatectomie droite reglec. Nouv Presse Med. 1952;60:549–51.
6. Starzl TE (editor). Experience in hepatic transplantation. Philadelphia: Saunders;1969.
7. Shanghai Coordinating Group for Research in Liver Cancer, China (Tang ZY, Yu EX, Wu CE, Gu XY). Diagnosis and treatment of primary hepatocellular carcinoma in early stage – report of 134 cases. Chin Med J. 1979;92:801–6.
8. Tang ZY, Yu YQ, Lin ZY *et al.* Small hepatocellular carcinoma – clinical analysis of 30 cases. Chin Med J. 1979;59:35–40.
9. Tang ZY (editor). Subclinical hepatocellular carcinoma. Berlin: Springer; 1985.
10. Tang ZY, Yu YQ, Zhou XD. An important approach to prolonging survival further after radical resection of AFP positive hepatocellular carcinoma. J Exp Clin Cancer Res. 1984;3:359–66.
11. Tang ZY, Yu YQ, Zhou XD *et al.* Surgery of small hepatocellular carcinoma – analysis of 144 cases. Cancer. 1989;64:536–41.
12. Tang ZY, Yu YQ, Zhou XD *et al.* Small hepatocellular carcinoma – three decades' experience. In Jiang SJ, Xiao SD, editors. Proceedings of 1992 Shanghai International Symposium on Gastroenterology. Shanghai: Shanghai Science & Technical Literature Publisher; 1992:52–9.
13. Tang ZY, Yu YQ, Zhou XD. Evolution of surgery in the treatment of hepatocellular carcinoma from the 1950s to the 1990s. Semin Surg Oncol. 1993;9:293–7.
14. Du JH, Wang XH, Li XC. Clinical investigation of late treatment results of primary hepatocellular carcinoma. J Hepatobiliary Panc Splenic Surg. 1995;1:178–80 [in Chinese].
15. Okamoto E, Yamanaka N, Oriyama T *et al.* Determinants of long-term survival following hepatectomy for hepatocellular carcinoma, with special reference to patients surviving more than 10 years. J Hep Bil Panc Surg. 1994;94:1:107–12.
16. Makuuchi M, Kosuge T, Takayama T *et al.* Surgery of small liver cancers. Semin Surg Oncol. 1993;9:298–304.
17. Wu MC, Chen H. Hepatectomy for primary liver cancer in 1102 cases. Asian J Surg. 1994;17:14–16.
18. Lai ECS, Fan ST, Lo CM *et al.* Hepatic resection for hepatocellular carcinoma. Ann Surg. 1995;221:291–8.
19. Vauthey JN, Klimstra D, Franceschi D *et al.* Factors affecting long-term outcome after hepatic resection for hepatocellular carcinoma. Am J Surg. 1995;169;28–35.
20. Bismuth H, Chiche L, Castaing D. Surgical treatment of hepatocellular carcinomas in noncirrhotic liver: experience with 68 liver resections. World J Surg. 1995;19:35–41.
21. Yu YQ, Tang ZY, Ma ZC *et al.* Resection of segment VIII of liver for treatment of primary liver cancer. Arch Surg. 1993;128:224–7.
22. Boix L, Bruix J, Campo E *et al.* nm23-H1 expression and disease recurrence after surgical resection of small hepatocellular carcinoma. Gastroenterology. 1994;107:486–91.
23. Yamaguchi A, Urano T, Goi T *et al.* Expression of human nm23-H1 and nm23-H2 proteins in hepatocellular carcinoma. Cancer. 1994;73:2280–4.
24. Iizuka N, Oka M, Shimizu R *et al.* Expression of nm23-H1 gene in hepatocellular carcinoma. Biotherapy. 1994;8:715–18.
25. Wang XM, Tang ZY, Xue Q *et al.* Transforming growth factor α induces proliferation and expression of epidermal growth factor receptor in hepatocellular carcinoma cells. J Exp Clin Cancer Res. 1995;14:179–84.
26. Wang XM, Tang ZY, Zou HQ *et al.* Clinical significance of the expression of epidermal growth factor receptor in hepatocellular carcinoma. J Current Oncol 1995;2:22–4 [In Chinese].
27. Esumi M, Aritaka T, Arii M *et al.* Clonal origin of human hepatoma determined by integration of hepatitis B virus DNA. Cancer Res. 1986;46:5767–71.
28. Liang XH, Loncarevic IF, Tang ZY *et al.* Resection of hepatocellular carcinoma: oligocentric origin of recurrent and multinodular tumors. J Gastroenterol Hepatol. 1991;6:77–86.
29. Tsuda H, Oda T, Sakamoto M, Hirohashi S. Different pattern of chromosomal allele loss in multiple hepatocellular carcinoma as evidence of their different origin. Cancer Res. 1992;52:1504–9.
30. Hsu HC, Peng SY, Lai PL *et al.* Allelotype and loss of heterozygosity of P53 in primary and recurrent hepatocellular carcinoma: a study of 105 patients. Cancer. 1994;73:42–7.
31. Zhou XD, Tang ZY, Yu YQ *et al.* Recurrence after resection of α fetoprotein positive hepatocellular carcinoma. J Cancer Res Clin Oncol. 1994;120:369–73.

32. Wu MC, Chen H, Yan YQ. Rehepatectomy of primary liver cancer. Semin Surg Oncol. 1993;9:323–6.
33. Suenaga M, Sugiura H, Kokuba Y *et al.* Repeated hepatic resection for recurrent hepatocellular carcinoma in eighteen cases. Surgery. 1994;115:452–7.
34. Sun FX, Tang ZY, Liu KD *et al.* Growth pattern and metastatic behavior of orthotopically metastatic model of human hepatocellular carcinoma in nude mice. [In Chinese] Natl Med J China. 1995;75:673–5.
35. Liao Y, Tang ZY, Liu KD *et al.* Therapeutic effect and mechanism of anti-HBx/anti-CD3 BsAb retargeting LAK cells for lysis of LTNM4 xenografts in nude mice. Acta Acad Med Shanghai. 1995;22(Suppl.):55–9 [In Chinese].
36. Feng XS, Tang ZY, Zheng ZC *et al.* Preliminary studies on the effects of tumor necrosis factor gene transfer on the growth of human hepatocellular carcinoma cells in nude mice. Chin J Oncol. 1995;17:167–9 [In Chinese].
37. Drazan KE, Shen XD, Csete ME *et al. In vivo* adenovirus-mediated human P53 tumor suppressor gene transfer and expression in rat liver after resection. Surgery. 1994;116:197–204.
38. Cao XT, Wang JL, Zhang WP *et al.* Treatment of human hepatocellular carcinoma by fibroblast-mediated human interferon α gene therapy in combination with adoptive chemoimmunotherapy. J Cancer Res Clin Oncol. 1995;121:457–62.
39. Yang XP, Dong SC, Ju TZ *et al.* Retinoic acid changes the structure of N-glycan on the surface of human hepatocellular carcinoma cell and its enzymatic mechanism. Acta Acad Med Shanghai. 1995;22:324–8 [In Chinese].

21
Multimodality treatment of hepatocellular carcinoma

T. ICHIDA

INTRODUCTION

Surgical hepatic resection, chemo-lipiodolization with or without transcatheter arterial embolization (TAE) therapy and percutaneous ethanol injection (PEI) therapy have been major treatments for hepatocellular carcinoma during this decade at our institute, although we do use multimodality treatments of hepatocellular carcinoma such as irradiation, hyperthermia, immunotherapy, conventional chemotherapy and orthotopic liver transplantation.

Hepatocellular carcinoma originates mainly from chronic liver diseases such as hepatitis B and hepatitis C, by continuous infection with hepatitis viruses. According to the periodical survey and follow-up study of primary liver cancer in Japan by the Liver Cancer Study Group of Japan, approximately 95% of primary liver cancer comprised hepatocellular carcinoma. Among them, 70% was positive anti-HCV and 18% was hepatitis B surface antigen positive. Once hepatocellular carcinoma develops in the hepatic lobules, new hepatocellular carcinoma nodules should appear in different areas at different times. This indicates that there is no final achievement of a complete cure of hepatocellular carcinoma which came from chronic viral liver diseases, especially in hepatitis C virus-positive cases. Therefore, initial treatment is important in avoiding local recurrence and disturbance of hepatic functional reserves. Futhermore complete remission of the initial tumour gave us a period for survey of appearance of new tumour nodules in the hepatic lobes.

For the initial selection of treatment for hepatocellular carcinoma, we have to consider both tumour behaviour and host circumstances. Important tumour factors are tumour size, tumour location, numbers, histological differentiation, capsule formation, vascularity, vascular invasiveness, intrahepatic and extrahepatic metastasis, and as to tumour-bearing host hepatic functional reserve, non-tumorous pathology, ageing, cardiorenal function, and association of viral hepatitis are also important factors.

Considering these tumour and host factors, this chapter discusses the indication of each therapy for hepatocellular carcinoma, and attempts to elucidate suitable selection criteria for the initial treatment of the disease using clinical outcomes of non-surgical treatment in our data, as well as data from a national survey by the Liver Cancer Study Group of Japan[1–7].

PERCUTANEOUS ETHANOL INJECTION THERAPY

Clinical outcome

According to the results obtained in our department, the 1-, 2- and 3-year survival rates in hepatocellular carcinoma with tumours less than 2 cm maximum diameter were 92%, 84% and 75%, respectively, while the 4–5-year survival rate dropped markedly to 53%. As for advanced cases with tumours of 2 cm or more maximum diameter, the 1–2-year survival rate was also as high as 85% and 72%, but the 3–5-year survival rate tended to decrease to 59%, 42% and 39%, respectively (Table 1). To summarize the results obtained from both our institute and others, the 3-year survival rate was always high, but the survival curve began to decline in the 4th year, and the 5-year survival rate dropped markedly. The reason for the decrease after 3 or 5 years is the high incidence of recurrence in this treatment group. The recurrence rate after PEI therapy at 5 years was 71%, while the local recurrence rate after this therapy at 5 years was 30% (Table 2). A high incidence of recurrence in different lobes indicates that new tumours might develop in spite of local therapeutic control, because of

Table 1 Survival rate of percutaneous ethanol injection for hepatocellular carcinoma (percentages)

	<2 cm[*] (n = 41)	>2 cm[*] (n = 33)	Total[*] (n = 74)	Overall[†] (n = 562)
1-year survival	92	85	89	87
2-year survival	84	72	81	64
3-year survival	75	59	69	53
4-year survival	54	42	52	
5-year survival	54	39	46	

[*] Niigata University Hospital
[†] National Survey

Table 2 Tumour recurrence rate after percutaneous ethanol injection therapy (percentages)

	Local recurrence			New lesion recurrence		
	<2 cm (n = 41)	>2 cm (n = 32)	Total (n = 73)	<2 cm (n = 41)	>2 cm (n = 32)	Total (n = 73)
1-year	3	23	10	13	30	20
2-year	20	29	24	47	50	49
3-year	30	37	33	58	63	60
4-year	30	37	33	61	63	63
5-year	30	37	33	61	63	63

Niigata University Hospital

multicentric carcinogenesis of hepatocellular carcinoma. It is not unusual that liver cirrhosis is in premalignant condition. New tumours develop in different parts of the hepatic lobes after PEI therapy, as well as hepatic resection[8–15]. Clinical effort is necessary to decrease the incidence of local recurrence. However, without PEI therapy the results were significantly worse[16–18] in cases with tumours less than 2 cm[16–18]. Thus PEI therapy seems to be clinically useful[19–30].

Indications

Fundamentally, technical criteria of PEI therapy are as follows: (1) patients should have a secure route for tumour puncture on ultrasonography; (2) patients with ascites should be controlled by medical treatment; (3) indices of haemorrhagic tendency such as over 30 000 platelets/mm^3 and a bleeding time of less than 7 minutes and (4) excluding patients hypersensitive to local anaesthetics and ethanol. There is no critical restriction of liver functional reserve and tumour-bearing host for this therapy as required from liver surgical resection.

PEI therapy alone is actively performed in the treatment of small liver cancer based on the clinical fact that many of the tumours of less than 2 cm maximum diameter are well-differentiated hepatocellular carcinomas, and patients with this type of cancer show good long-term survival.

On the other hand, for patients with large cancers, PEI therapy is indicated as a part of multidisciplinary therapy, including TAE therapy and hepatectomy. Criteria for indication of PEI therapy as a part of multidisciplinary therapy are as follows: (1) all lesions delineated on ultrasonography, (2) tumour nodules greater than 2 cm, (3) recurrent cases after hepatectomy[31] and (4) nodules incompletely treated with lipiodol–TAE therapy[32–36].

Complications

Several complications of ethanol injection therapy, including neoplastic seeding[37–40], abscess formation[41,42], bile duct damage[43], liver atrophy[44] and portal thrombosis[45], were reported. However, these reports were of rare complications.

We therefore tried to elucidate the incidence of complications of this therapy in a multicentre study based on answers to questionnaires. According to the report of a meeting of the Study Group of Hepatic Tumor Biopsy (held on 27 October 1995, at Niigata), including 47 Japanese institutes, we summarize the incidence of complications of this therapy in Table 3[46]. In 6000 registered cases of hepatocellular carcinoma treated by PEI therapy, 241 complications were reported. The ones occurring most frequently were hepatic infarction with 72 cases (1.20%) and hypotension with 69 cases (1.15%). There were 10 fatal cases (0.17%) after PEI therapy, and five of these were hepatic insufficiency due to decompensated liver cirrhosis. Details of each case were not clear; however, we should assume that hepatic insufficiency can occur even during PEI therapy, which is regarded as a non-invasive treatment for hepatocellular carcinoma.

Fatal cases included one case each of hepatic infarction, abscess and biloma. These complications might be foreseen before and during PEI therapy because they might occur depending on puncture depth, puncture times and puncture

Table 3 Incidence of complication of PEI therapy (total 6000 cases in 47 institutes in Japan according to the Study Group of Hepatic Tumor Bio. in Niigata, October 1995)

Complication	Incidence	Treatment	Outcome
Hepatic infarction	72 (1.20%)		One death
Hypotension	69 (1.15%)	Conservative	Fair
Intraperitoneal bleeding	21 (0.35%)	Operation/TAE	Fair
Metastasis on the puncture line	14 (0.23%)	Operation/PEIT	Fair
Hepatic insufficiency	14 (0.23%)		Five deaths
Biliary bleeding	13 (0.22%)	Conservative	Fair
Haemothorax	11 (0.18%)	Conservative	Fair
Abscess	8 (0.13%)	Drainage	One death
Arrhythmia	4 (0.07%)	Conservative	Fair
Pneumothorax	3 (0.05%)	Conservative	Fair
Haemolysis	2 (0.03%)		Two deaths
Cholecystolithiasis	2 (0.03%)	Conservative	Fair
Pancreatitis	1 (0.02%)	Conservative	Fair
Cholecystitis	1 (0.02%)	Drainage	Fair
Portal thrombosis	1 (0.02%)	Conservative	Fair
Biloma	1 (0.02%)	Drainage	One death
Total	241 (4.02%)		10 deaths (0.17%)

skill. Two fatal cases due to haemolysis were not predictable, indicating alcoholic direct lethal toxicity.

In total the mortality in 6000 cases treated with PEI therapy was 0.17% and the frequency of complications was 4.02% in this study. We therefore conclude that this therapy is very useful for the treatment of hepatocellular carcinoma.

Tumour recurrence

MRI imaging is most popular for the evaluation of therapeutic effects after PEI therapy[47–53]; however, dynamic CT scanning might be a more simple procedure for the precise assessment of tumour necrosis and tumour regression[54–57], rather than enhanced ultrasound findings[58] and MRI imaging. We applied dynamic CT scanning to the assessment of tumour necrosis, and complete necrosis with tumour regression could be observed in 92% of our cases at 6 months after therapy. Important characteristics of PEI therapy are avoidance of local recurrence and detection of new tumours in other areas of the liver. However, our study revealed local recurrence in 30% of cases and recurrence in the whole liver in more than 70% after 5 years (Table 2). We thus need to treat hepatocellular carcinoma in complete remission with PEI therapy, and long survival times might depend on how we detect a new tumour appearance and how we manage recurrent tumours.

A high incidence of local recurrence is due to insufficient injection of ethanol, both intra-tumour and in the outer surrounding area. In the surrounding area and capsule, injected alcohol moves easily throughout the blood stream and disappears; it does not remain in the target area. This is one reason for the high incidence of local recurrence in PEI therapy. To solve this problem, percutaneus microwave coagulation therapy might be useful[59–61]. There are many arguments regarding this therapy with regard to size of puncture needle, sufficient coagulation time, coagulation area and unknown side-effects. Further studies of this therapy are necessary.

Transcatheter arterial embolization therapy

Indications

Intrahepatic haemodynamics in hepatocellular carcinoma[62] shows the state of portal invasion, which is a biological characteristic of hepatocellular carcinoma, and is an important indicator for the application of TAE therapy and decision-making in an area of embolization. When embolization is applied to bilateral lobes in the presence of tumour thrombi in a main portal trunk, or right or left portal vein, ischaemia is thought to be induced not only in the tumour region, but also in the non-tumour region, leading to hepatic insufficiency. This is because the blood supply to the corresponding lobes is completely arrested by obstruction of arterial blood flow in combination with the decrease in portal blood flow. Thus, we consider that TAE therapy is contraindicated for hepatocellular carcinoma with portal invasion by tumour thrombi. Criteria for indication of TAE therapy at our department are shown in Table 4.

Clinical outcome

Since patients subjected to TAE therapy show no certain tendencies of tumour size of hepatocellular carcinoma, or macroscopic advancement corresponding to the degree of progression, and the morphological background of the non-tumour region, it is difficult to compare therapeutic results collected from different institutes as to treatment of hepatocellular carcinoma with similar severity[63–94]. However, it has been generally accepted (based on nationwide research) that 1-year, 2-year, 3-year and 5-year survival rates after TAE therapy are 55.4%, 31.5%, 19.5% and 8.0%, respectively. These figures are from annual surveys and follow-up studies of primary liver cancer in Japan, issued by the Liver

Table 4   Criteria for indication of transcatheter arterial embolization for hepatocellular carcinoma

Host factor
1. As for patients with ascites, it should be controlled by medical treatment
2. Contraindicated for patients with formation of an apparent arterial–venous shunt
3. Contraindication for patients with severe jaundice (3.0 mg/dl or more total bilirubin)
4. Contraindication for patients with a marked decrease in a blood-clotting protein (50% or less on thrombin test and hepaplastin test)
5. Contraindicated for patients having a transaminase of 300 IU/L or more
6. Contraindicated for patients having less than 0.06 by Indocyanine Green test for K indexes

Tumour factor
1. Portal tumour thrombosis classified as VP0 to VP2 is eligible, but contraindicated for portal trunk obstruction
2. Contraindicated for patients with hepatocellular carcinoma occupying 60% or more of the liver, except segmental TAE therapy
3. Principal indications of hepatocellular carcinoma are stage II, III and IVa
4. Diffuse type of hepatocellular carcinoma should be avoided because of arterial–portal shunt
5. Contra-indicated with no apparent tumour staining in angiography (DSA)

Cancer Study Group of Japan (n=7633). TAE therapy is thought to have been properly selected when it produced about 3 years prolongation of life, because this therapy is characterized as a conservative therapy, rather than a radical therapy, when used for the treatment of hepatocellular carcinoma.

Colour Doppler sonography[95,96] might be useful to check blood supply after TAE therapy, as well as CT and MRI studies[97], and damage in non-tumorous areas should be confirmed by histological survey[98–100], as well as damage to the biliary arterial system such as bile duct necrosis and biloma[101]. The therapeutic effects of TAE therapy should be confirmed taking account of loss of arterial blood supply after embolization by imaging. In spite of cases with incomplete embolization[102,103] and those giving unsatisfactory clinical results in preoperative procedures[104–108], recent survival rates after TAE therapy have been elevated by concomitant use of arterial infusion of lipiodol containing an anti-cancer agent, and by application of segmental TAE (Table 5).

Table 5 Clinical result of lipiodol–transcatheter arterial embolization therapy for hepatocellular carcinoma (percentages)

Survival	Stage I (n = 5)	Stage II (n = 17)	Stage III (n = 18)	Stage IV (n =30)	Total (n = 70)
1-year	100	77	92	64	77
2-year	100	75	71	25	52
3-year	–	66	54	6	40
4-year	–	57	35	5	29
5-year	–	53	31	5	25

Niigata University Hospital

Segmental lipiodol–TAE therapy

Segmental lipiodol–TAE therapy was conducted in cases of hepatocellular carcinoma at stage I, II and a part of III, with complete necrosis of tumours within a small restricted area. If the tumour is located within one segment of the hepatic lobe, a lipiodol-containing anti-cancer agent should first be injected into the regional artery of the segment using a superselective angiographic technique, and then embolize with gel form particles[109–111]. Although one or two segments

Table 6 Segmental lipiodol–TAE therapy versus overall lipiodol–TAE (percentages)

	Segmental lipiodol–TAE (n = 30)		Lipiodol–TAE (n = 64)	
	Survival	Non-recurrence survival	Survival	Non-recurrence survival
1-year survival	100	76	76	35
2-year survival	96	55	51	20
3-year survival	70	43	38	20
4-year survival	70	–	30	–
5-year survival	–	–	21	–

Niigata University Hospital

of hepatic lobes were embolized, leading to partial ischaemic infarction, this ischaemic damage could be minimized, and does not have a dramatic influence on whole hepatic functional reserve. Furthermore, this segmental lipiodol–TAE therapy achieved a low incidence of local recurrence of hepatocellular carcinoma (Table 6). Single or repeated segmental lipiodol–TAE therapy should be performed even for advanced hepatocellular carcinoma with local recurrence under complete local control.

Chemo-lipiodolization

Indications

Lipiodol, an oily contrast medium, was originally developed as a contrast medium for lymphatic vessels. Since it has affinity to the liver tissue when used as a contrast medium in angiography, this medium was once used as a sensitizer for CT scanning. It was later found that lipiodol remained in the liver for a relatively long period of time, but was more predominantly and rapidly deposited in the tumour tissue of hepatocellular carcinomas. This suggests that micro-bubbles of lipiodol are simply trapped in tumour capillaries and sinusoids, and at the same time they also adhere to tumour vascular walls. Utilizing these characteristics a suspension or emulsion of lipiodol, supplemented with an anti-cancer agent, is arterially infused to a tumour nutritional vessel. Targeting therapy has been tentatively performed to obtain intra-tumour accumulation, and to sustain release of an anti-cancer agent[112–119].

For 5 years we have also used an emulsion of lipiodol (CELE: CDDP–epirubicin–lipiodol emulsion), containing 80 mg of CDDP, 60 mg of epirubicin, and lipiodol, mixed with phosphatidylcholine and Iopamidol (iopamiron 300), a non-ionic contrast medium[114,115].

We perform arterial infusion of CELE in all patients eligible for administration prior to TAE therapy. Contraindications of this arterial infusion involve mainly anti-cancer agents; this therapy should not be given to patients with moderate renal and/or cardiac diseases. The therapy is also contraindicated for patients with a history of delayed shock due to the non-ionic contrast medium, although such cases are rarely observed. Indications and contraindications for this therapy are decided according to the patient's general condition, but are not restricted by local conditions. Thus this therapy takes no account of the state of patency of the portal trunk or the location of the tumour. However, the influence of lipiodolization on cirrhotic liver, such as temporary disturbance of blood supply[120], should be considered, and adverse effects[121] taken into account.

Clinical results

Many patients undergoing single infusion of CELE into the hepatic artery for the treatment of hepatocellular carcinoma classified as stage IV are ineligible for TAE therapy. Occlusion of a portal trunk is observed in more than half of these patients. Clinical results of the arterial infusion of CELE showed that 1-, 2- and 3-year survival rates were 66%, 31% and 12%, respectively in 36 patients with advanced hepatocellular carcinoma at our institute. The Liver Cancer Study Group of Japan published clinical outcomes of chemolipiodolization infusion with multiple anti-cancer agents in 6809 patients with hepatocellular carcinoma, and the 1-, 2- and 3-year survival rates were 17.0%, 5.7% and 2.7%, respectively.

Hepatic resection

Indications of hepatic resection depended on hepatic functional reserve and localization in hepatic lobes without extrahepatic metastasis[122–135]. Overall outcomes of hepatic resection reported by the Liver Cancer Study Group of Japan revealed that 1-, 2-, 3- and 5-year survival rates were 80.3%, 68.0%, 57.3% and 40.8%, respectively in 9099 patients with hepatocellular carcinoma during the past decade. In the past hepatic resection was the only method for the treatment of hepatocellular carcinoma in a cancer-free state. However, at present we have numerous means of treatment with sufficient results in the cancer-free state besides hepatic resection. Therefore, considering time-lapse multicentric carcinogenesis of hepatocellular carcinoma, we have doubts as to the use of invasive therapy such as hepatic resection, especially in liver cirrhosis[136–140]. We need to pay attention to excessive damage to patients during the initial treatment; then it would be better to attempt complete remission of treated nodules for at least 1 year. Minimal functional damage and complete remission of treated tumour is important.

If hepatocellular carcinoma is detected without any chronic liver disease, any influence of viral hepatitis or any disturbance of hepatic functional reserve, we recommend hepatic resection.

Clinical outcome of treatment in stage I hepatocellular carcinoma

To compare therapeutic procedures regarding survival rate, we discuss stage I hepatocellular carcinoma, which shows a relatively long survival rate after treatment. We summarize the clinical outcomes of stage I hepatocellular carcinoma treated with PEI therapy and lipiodol–TAE therapy in our institute, and those of hepatic resection[141,142] in a national survey, in Table 7. The survival rates in cases with hepatic resection and PEI therapy were similar. This result indicates that minimally invasive treatment of hepatocellular carcinoma is required at the initial indication of hepatocellular carcinoma with chronic liver diseases, because of time-lapse multicentric carcinogenesis in chronic liver diseases. The

Table 7 Therapeutic outcome of stage I hepatocellular carcinoma (percentages)

	Hepatic resection	*Lipiodol–TAE*	*Percutaneous ethanol injections*	
	*(n = 1562)**	*(n = 5)†*	*(n = 41)†*	*(n = 301)**
1-year survival	90	100	91	95
3-year survival	73	100	79	55
5-year survival	55	—	53	—

* Liver Cancer Study Group of Japan (1982–1991), 1994
† Niigata University Hospital

author emphasizes that no excessive damage by hepatic resection is favourable for the treatment of hepatocellular carcinoma in the early stages.

Selection criteria in the treatment of hepatocellular carcinoma

We have discussed clinical results in the treatment of hepatocellular carcinoma with several medical procedures, as mentioned above. Based on these clinical outcomes, and the indication of each major therapy, we propose selection criteria for the initial treatment of hepatocellular carcinoma as shown in Table 8. We are sure that the indication of each therapy is useful in the treatment of hepatocellular carcinoma to achieve longer survival times.

Table 8 Selection criteria of treatment for hepatocellular carcinoma

Stage	Factor	With liver cirrhosis	Without liver cirrhosis
I	Well differentiated	PEI	PEI
	Moderate–poor	PEI	PEI or hepatic resection
II	Well (<3 cm)	PEI	PEI
	>3 cm	Hepatic resection or lipiodol–TAE	Hepatic resection
	Multiple	Lipiodol–TAE and/or PEI	Hepatic resection or lipiodol–TAE or PEI
III	Solid	Hepatic resection or lipiodol–TAE	Hepatic resection or lipiodol–TAE
	Multiple	Lipiodol–TAE and PEI	Lipiodol–TAE and PEI
IVa		Lipiodol–TAE and PEI	Lipiodol–TAE and PEI
IVb		Chemo-lipiodolization/ chemotherapy	Chemo-lipiodolization/ chemotherapy

PEI, percutaneous ethanol injection therapy; TAE, transcatheter arterial embolization therapy

Chemotherapy (Table 9)

Until now many kinds of anti-cancer agent have been used for hepatocellular carcinoma orally, intravenously and arterially. Oral administration of 5-fluorouracil (5-FU), tegafur (FT207), uracil–tegafur (UFT) and carmofur was

Table 9 Anti-cancer agents for hepatocellular carcinoma

General:
  Alkylating agents: nothing
  Antimetabolites: froxuridine (FUDR), fluorouracil (5-FU), tegafur (FT207), tegafur uracil (UFT), carmofur
  Antitumour antibiotics: adriamycin, epirubicin, mitomycin C, neocarcinostatin, mitoxantrone
  Plant products: VP-16 (etoposide)
  Miscellaneous: CDDP

Intravenously:

	adriamycin	epirubicin	5-FU	CDDP	mitomycin C	mitoxantrone	VP-16
Efficacy rate	5–27%	17%	2%	5%	15%	20%	16%

Intra-arterially:
  neocarcinostatin, adriamycin, epirubicin, mitomycin C, 5-FU, CDDP, VP-16

not evaluated as being effective for hepatocellular carcinoma[143]. Tests of intravenous administration of 5-FU, mitomycin C, adriamycin[144], epirubicin[145], cis-diamminodichloroplatinum[146], mitoxantrone[147] and VP-16 were conducted worldwide, and adriamycin, epirubicin and mitoxantrone were evaluated as effective drugs for hepatocellular carcinoma with a 15–27% efficacy rate. Intra-arterial regional infusion therapy is very popular for the treatment of hepatocellular carcinoma because of the advantage of the arterial blood supply to this tumour[148–150]. Theoretically, initially an anti-cancer agent of a high concentration level passes through the liver tissues in active form, then these drugs are metabolized to the inactive form through the liver and excreted into the lung and kidney. This indicates that intra-arterial administration via the hepatic artery can achieve high concentrations of the active form of drugs in tumour tissues, and can decrease the side-effects of these drugs in the inactive form via the liver tissues. Adriamycin[151], epirubicin and CDDP[152] are reported to be the most effective drugs in the treatment of hepatocellular carcinoma using a transcatheter arterial infusion technique with a 24–40% efficacy rate.

SUMMARY

For the treatment of hepatocellular carcinoma it is first important to prevent chronic viral-infected liver diseases from progressing to hepatocellular carcinoma using interferon, anti-inflammatory drugs, herbal medicine, retinoids or an antiviral agent. Secondly, we have to detect hepatocellular carcinoma at the earliest stage with a single nodule without any vascular invasiveness and well-differentiated histology, and to treat it initially with a regional therapy with minimum invasiveness, such as PEI therapy, PMCT and segmental lipiodol–TAE therapy. Third, progressive hepatocellular carcinoma should be treated using a multimodality regimen[153–155].

References

1. Ishikawa K. Follow-up study of patients with primary liver cancer: Report 3. Acta Hepatol Jpn. 1976;17:460–5 [in Japanese, Abstract in English].
2. Liver Cancer Study Group of Japan. Primary liver cancer. Cancer. 1980;45:2663–9.
3. Liver Cancer Study Group of Japan. Primary liver cancer in Japan. Cancer. 1984;54:1747–55.
4. Liver Cancer Study Group of Japan. Primary liver cancer in Japan. Sixth report. Cancer. 1987;60:1400–11.
5. Liver Cancer Study Group of Japan. Primary liver cancer in Japan, Clinicopathological features and results of surgical treatment. Ann Surg. 1990;211:277–87.
6. Liver Cancer Study Group of Japan. Predictive factors for long term prognosis after partial hepatectomy for patients with hepatocellular carcinoma in Japan. Cancer. 1994;74:2772–7.
7. Liver Cancer Study Group of Japan. Survey and follow-up study of primary liver cancer in Japan – Report 11. Acta Hepatol Jpn. 1995;36:208–18 [in Japanese, Abstract in English].
8. Nagao T, Inoue S, Yoshini F et al. Post-operative recurrence of hepatocellular carcinoma. Ann Surg. 1990;211:28–33.
9. Jwo SC, Chiu JH, Chau GY, Loong CC, Lui WY. Risk factors linked to tumor recurrence of human hepatocellular carcinoma after hepatic resection. Hepatology. 1992;16:1367–71.
10. Nagasue N, Uchida M, Makino Y et al. Incidence and factors associated with intrahepatic recurrence following resection of hepatocellular carcinoma. Gastroenterology. 1993;105:488–94.

11. Ouchi K, Matsubara S, Fukuhara K, Tominaga T, Matsuno S. Recurrence of hepatocellular carcinoma in the liver remnant after hepatic resection. Am J Surg. 1993;166:270–3.
12. Nakajima Y, Ohmura T, Kimura J *et al.* Role of surgical treatment for recurrent hepatocellular carcinoma after hepatic resection. World J Surg. 1993;17:792–5.
13. Chen MF, Hwang TL, Jeng LB, Wang CS, Jan YY, Chen SC. Postoperative recurrence of hepatocellular carcinoma. Two hundred five consecutive patients who underwent hepatic resection in 15 years. Arch Surg. 1994;129:738–42.
14. Okada S, Shimada K, Yamamoto J *et al.* Predictive factors for postoperative recurrence of hepatocellular carcinoma. Gastroenterology. 1994;106:1618–24.
15. Takenaka K, Adachi E, Nishizaki T *et al.* Possible multicentric occurrence of hepatocellular carcinoma: a clinicopathological study. Hepatology. 1994;19:889–94.
16. Okuda K, Ohnishi T, Obata H *et al.* Natural history of hepatocellular carcinoma and prognosis in relation to treatment. Cancer. 56:918–928, 1985.
17. Ebara M, Ohto M, Shinagawa T *et al.* Natural history of minute hepatocellular carcinoma smaller than three centimeters complicating cirrhosis. Gastroenterology. 1986;90:289–98.
18. Livraghi T, Bolondi L, Buscarini L *et al.* No treatment, resection and ethanol injection in hepatocellular carcinoma: a retrospective analysis of survival in 391 patients with cirrhosis. Italian Cooperative HCC Study Group. J Hepatol. 1995;22:522–6.
19. Sugiura N, Tanaka K, Ohto M *et al.* Treatment of small hepatocellular carcinoma with percutaneous ethanol injection under US guidance. Acta Hepatol Jpn. 1983;24:920 [in Japanese].
20. Livraghi T, Festi D, Monti F *et al.* US-guided percutaneous alcohol injection of small hepatic and abdominal tumors. Radiology. 1986;161:309–12.
21. Sheu JC, Sung JL, Huang GT *et al.* Intratumor injection of absolute ethanol under ultrasound guidance for the treatment of small hepatocellular carcinoma. Hepato-Gastroenterology. 1987;34:255–61.
22. Shiina S, Yasuda H, Muto H *et al.* Percutaneous ethanol injection in the treatment of liver neoplasms. Am J Roentgenol. 1987;149:949–52.
23. Seki T, Nonaka T, Kubota Y *et al.* Ultrasonically guided percutaneous ethanol injection therapy for hepatocellular carcinoma. Am J Gastroenterol. 1989;84:1400–7.
24. Ebara M, Ohto M, Sugihara N *et al.* Percutaneus ethanol injection for the treatment of small hepatocellular carcinoma: study of 95 patients. J Gastroenterol Hepatol. 1990;5:616–26.
25. Vilana R, Bruix J, Bru C, Ayuso C, Sole M, Rodes J. Tumor size determines the efficacy of percutaneous ethanol injection for the treatment of small hepatocellular carcinoma. Hepatology. 1992;16:353–7.
26. Livraghi T, Bolondi L, Lazzaroni S *et al.* Percutaneous ethanol injection in the treatment of hepatocellular carcinoma in cirrhosis: a study on 207 patients. Cancer. 1992;69:925–9.
27. Shiina S, Tagawa K, Niwa Y *et al.* Percutaneous ethanol injection therapy for hepatocellular carcinoma: results in 146 patients. Am J Roentgenol. 1993;160:1023–8.
28. Kotoh K, Sakai H, Sakamoto S *et al.* The effect of percutaneous ethanol injection therapy on small solitary hepatocellular carcinoma is comparable to that of hepatectomy. Am J Gastroenterol. 1994;89:194–8.
29. Honda N, Guo Q, Uchida H, Ohishi H, Hiasa Y. Percutaneous hot saline injection therapy for hepatic tumors: an alternative to percutaneous ethanol injection therapy. Radiology. 1994;190:53–7.
30. Livraghi T, Giorgio A, Marin G *et al.* Hepatocellular carcinoma and cirrhosis in 746 patients: long-term results of percutaneous ethanol injection. Radiology. 1995;197:101–8.
31. Tanikawa K, Majima Y. Percutaneous ethanol injection therapy for recurrent hepatocellular carcinoma. Hepato-Gastroenterology. 1993;40:324–7.
32. Tanaka K, Okazaki H, Nakamura S *et al.* Hepatocellular carcinoma treated with a combination therapy of transcatheter arterial embolization and percutaneous ethanol injection. Radiology. 1991;179:713–17.
33. Tanaka K, Nakamura S, Numata K *et al.* Hepatocellular carcinoma: treatment with percutaneous ethanol injection and transcatheter arterial embolization. Radiology. 1992;185:457–60.
34. Lencioni R, Vignali C, Caramella D, Cioni R, Mazzeo S, Bartolozzi C. Transcatheter arterial embolization followed by percutaneous ethanol injection in the treatment of hepatocellular carcinoma. Cardiovasc Intervent Radiol. 1994;17:70–5.
35. Koda M, Okamoto K, Miyoshi Y *et al.* Combination therapy with transcatheter arterial embolization and percutaneous ethanol injection for advanced hepatocellular carcinoma. Hepato-Gastroenterology. 1994;41:25–9.

36. Kato T, Saito Y, Niwa M, Ishiguro J, Ogoshi K. Combination therapy of transcatheter chemoembolization and percutaneous ethanol injection therapy for unresectable hepatocellular carcinoma. Cancer Chemother Pharmacol. 1994;33:S115–18.
37. Cedrone A, Rapaccini GL, Pompili M *et al.* Neoplastic seeding complicating percutaneous ethanol injection for treatment of hepatocellular carcinoma. Radiology. 1992;183:787–8.
38. Goletti O, De Negri F, Pucciarelli M *et al.* Subcutaneous seeding after percutaneous ethanol injection of liver metastasis. Radiology. 1992;183:785–6.
39. Cedrone A, Rapaccini GL, Pompili M, Grattagliano A, Aliotta A, Trombino C. Neoplastic seeding complicating percutaneous ethanol injection for treatment of hepatocellular carcinoma. Radiology. 1992;183:787–8.
40. Shimada M, Maeda T, Saito A, Morotomi I, Kano T. Needle track seeding after percutaneous ethanol injection therapy for small hepatocellular carcinoma. J Surg Oncol. 1995;58:247–81.
41. Solinas A, Erbella GS, Distrutti E *et al.* Abscess formation in hepatocellular carcinoma: complications of percutaneous ultrasound-guided ethanol injection. J Clin Ultrasound. 1993;21:531–3.
42. Okada S, Aoki K, Okazaki N *et al.* Liver abscess after percutaneous ethanol injection (PEI) therapy for hepatocellular carcinoma. A case report. Hepato-Gastroenterology. 1993;40:496–8.
43. Koda M, Okamoto K, Miyoshi Y *et al.* Hepatic vascular and bile duct injury after ethanol injection therapy for hepatocellular carcinoma. Gastrointest Radiol. 1992;17:167–9.
44. Motoo Y, Okai T, Matsui O *et al.* Liver atrophy after transcatheter embolization and percutaneous ethanol injection therapy for a minute hepatocellular carcinoma. Gastrointest Radiol. 1991;16:164–6.
45. Lencioni R, Caramella D, Sanguinetti F, Battolla L, Falaschi F, Bartolozzi C. Portal vein thrombosis after percutaneous ethanol injection for hepatocellular carcinoma: value of color Doppler sonography in distinguishing chemical and tumor thrombi. Am J Roentogenol. 1995;164:1125–30.
46. Ichida T, Tanaka M, Tanikawa K *et al.* Low incidence of fatal complication after PEI therapy – multicenter analysis of 6.000 cases of PEI therapy in Japan. (in preparation)
47. Kubota Y, Nakano T, Seki T *et al.* Validity of MRI imaging for monitoring effects of percutaneous ethanol injection for HCC. Hepato-Gastroenterology. 1989;36:262–5.
48. Sironi S, Livraghi T, DelMaschio A. Small hepatocellular carcinoma treated with percutaneous ethanol injection: MR imaging findings. Radiology. 1991;180:333–6.
49. Sironi S, Livraghi T, Angeli E *et al.* Small hepatocellular carcinoma: MR follow-up of treatment with percutaneous ethanol injection. Radiology. 1993;187:119–23.
50. Sironi S, De Cobelli F, Livraghi T *et al.* Small hepatocellular carcinoma treated with percutaneous ethanol injection: unenhanced and gadolinium-enhanced MR imaging follow-up. Radiology. 1994;192:407–12.
51. Bartolozzi C, Lencioni R, Caramella D, Mazzeo S, Ciancia EM. Treatment of hepatocellular carcinoma with percutaneous ethanol injection: evaluation with contrast-enhanced MR imaging. Am J Roentgenol. 1994;162:827–31.
52. Usui H, Itai Y. Percutaneous ethanol injection therapy for hepatocellular carcinoma:validity of MR imaging in the evaluation of treatment effect. Radiation Med. 1995;13:103–8.
53. Ito K, Honjo K, Fujita T, Awaya H, Matsumoto T, Matsunaga N. Enhanced MR imaging of the liver after ethanol treatment of hepatocellular carcinoma: evaluation of areas of hyperperfusion adjacent to the tumor. Am J Roentgenol. 1995;164:1413–17.
54. Lencioni R, Caramella D, Bartolozzi C. Response of hepatocellular carcinoma to percutaneous ethanol injection: CT and MR evaluation. J Comput Assist Tomogr. 1993;17:723–9.
55. Joseph FB, Baumgarten DA, Bernardino ME. Hepatocellular carcinoma: CT appearance after percutaneous ethanol ablation therapy. Work in progress. Radiology. 1993;186:553–6.
56. Lencioni R, Caramella D, Vignali C, Russo R, Paolicchi A, Bartolozzi C. Lipiodol–CT in the detection of tumor persistence in hepatocellular carcinoma treated with percutaneous ethanol injection. Acta Radiol. 1994;35:323–8.
57. Ebara M, Kita K, Sugiura N *et al.* Therapeutic effect of percutaneous ethanol injection on small hepatocellular carcinoma: evaluation with CT. Radiology. 1995;195:371–7.
58. Imari Y, Sakamoto S, Shiomichi S *et al.* Hepatocellular carcinoma not detected with plain US: treatment with percutaneous ethanol injection under guidance with enhanced US. Radiology. 1992;185:497–500.
59. Seki T, Wakabayashi M, Nakagawa T *et al.* Ultrasonically guided percutaneous microwave coagulation therapy for small hepatocellular carcinoma. Cancer. 1994;74:817–25.

60. Watanabe Y, Sato M, Abe Y *et al.* Laparoscopic microwave coagulo-necrotic therapy for hepatocellular carcinoma: a feasible study of an alternative option for poor-risk patients. J Laparoend Surg. 1995;5:169–75.
61. Murakami R, Yoshimatsu S, Yamashita Y, Matsukawa T, Takahashi M, Sagara K. Treatment of hepatocellular carcinoma: value of percutaneous microwave coagulation. Am J Roentgenol. 1995;164:1159–64.
62. Breedis C, Young G. The blood supply of neoplasms in the liver. Am J Pathol. 1954;30:969–77.
63. Benmark S, Rosengren K. Angiographic study of the collateral circulation to the liver after ligation of the hepatic artery in man. Am J Surg. 1970;119:620–4.
64. Almersjo O, Bengmark S, Rudenstam CM *et al.* Evaluation of hepatic dearterialization in primary and secondary cancer of the liver. Am J Surg. 1972;124:5–9.
65. Balasegaram M. Complete hepatic dearterialization for primary carcinoma of the liver. Am J Surg. 1972;124:340–5.
66. Larmi TKI, Karkola P, Klintrup HE *et al.* Treatment of patients with hepatic tumors and jaundice by ligation of the hepatic artery. Arch Surg. 1974;108:178–83.
67. Chung VC, Wallace S. Hepatic arterial embolization in the treatment of hepatic neoplasms. Radiology. 1981;140:51–8.
68. Ichida T, Kojima T, Nakano M *et al.* Clinico-pathological study of transcatheter arterial embolization therapy for hepatocellular carcinoma: first report. Acta Hepatol Jpn. 1981;22:1264–75 [in Japanese, Abstract in English].
69. Yamada R, Sato M, Kawabata M *et al.* Hepatic artery embolization in 120 patients with unresectable hepatoma. Radiology. 1983;148:397–401.
70. Chung VP, Soo CS, Carrasco CH *et al.* Superselective catheterization technique in hepatic angiography. Am J Roentgenol. 1983;141:803–11.
71. Ohnishi K, Tsuchiya S, Nakayama T *et al.* Arterial chemoembolization of hepatocellular carcinoma with mitomycin C microcapsules. Radiology. 1984;152:51–5.
72. Soga K, Nomoto M, Ichida T *et al.* Clinical evaluation of transcatheter arterial embolization and one-shot chemotherapy in hepatocellular carcinoma. Hepato-Gastroenterology. 1988;35:116–20.
73. Takayasu K, Murakami Y, Moriyama N *et al.* Clinical and radiological assessments of the results of hepatectomy for small hepatocellular carcinoma and therapeutic arterial embolization for postoperative recurrence. Cancer. 1989;64:1848–52.
74. Kasugai H, Kojima J, Tatsuta M *et al.* Treatment of hepatocellular carcinoma by transcatheter arterial embolization combined with intra-arterial infusion of a mixture of cisplatin and ethiodized oil. Gastroenterology. 1989;97:965–71.
75. Yamada R, Kishi K, Sonomura T *et al.* Transcatheter arterial embolization in unresectable hepatocellular carcinoma. Cardiovasc Intervent Radiol. 1990;13:135–9.
76. Venook AP, Stagg RJ, Lewis BJ *et al.* Chemoembolization for hepatocellular carcinoma. J Clin Oncol. 1990;8:1108–14.
77. Pelletier G, Roche A, Ink O. A randomized trial of hepatic arterial chemoembolization in patients with unresectable hepatocellular carcinoma. J Hepatol. 1990;11:181–4.
78. Ikeda K, Kumada H, Saitoh S *et al.* Effect of repeated transcatheter arterial embolization on the survival time in patients with hepatocellular carcinoma – analysis by the Cox proportional hazard model. Cancer. 1991;68:2150–4.
79. Raoul JL, Heresbach D, Bretagne JF *et al.* Chemoembolization of hepatocellular carcinomas. A study of the biodistribution and pharmacokinetics of doxorubicin. Cancer. 1992;70:585–90.
80. Nakao N, Kamino K, Miura K, Takayasu Y, Ohnishi M, Miura T. Transcatheter arterial embolization in hepatocellular carcinoma: a long-term follow-up. Radiat Med. 1992;10:13–18.
81. Shinjo H, Okazaki M, Higashihara H, Koganemaru F, Okumura M. Hepatocellular carcinoma: a multivariate analysis of prognostic features in patients treated with hepatic arterial embolization. Am J Gastroenterol. 1992;87:1154–9.
82. Bismuth H, Morino M, Sherlock D *et al.* Primary treatment of hepatocellular carcinoma by arterial chemoembolization. Am J Surg. 1992;163:387–94.
83. Hsieh M, Chang W, Wang L *et al.* Treatment of hepatocellular carcinoma by transcatheter arterial chemoembolization and analysis of prognostic factors. Cancer Chemother Pharmacol. 1992;31:S82–5.

84. Yoshimi F, Nagao T, Inoue S *et al.* Comparison of hepatectomy and transcatheter arterial chemoembolization for the treatment of hepatocellular carcinoma: necessity for prospective randomized trial. Hepatology. 1992;16:702–6.

85. Savastano S, Feltrin GP, Neri D *et al.* Palliative treatment of hepatocellular carcinoma with transcatheter arterial embolization. Acta Radiol. 1993;34:26–9.

86. Ngan H, Lai CL, Fan ST, Lai EC, Yuen WK, Tso WK. Treatment of inoperable hepatocellular carcinoma by transcatheter arterial chemoembolization using an emulsion of cisplatin in iodized oil and gelfoam. Clin Radiol. 1993;47:315–20.

87. Uchida H, Matsuo N, Sakaguchi H, Nagano N, Nishimine K, Ohishi H. Segmental embolotherapy for hepatic cancer: keys to success. Cardiovasc Intervent Radiol. 1993;16:67–71.

88. Shiono T, Yoshikawa K, Hisamatsu K, Takenaka E. Efficacy of emulsion containing Gd-DTPA and lipiodol in hepatic transcatheter arterial embolization. Radiat Med. 1993;11:187–90.

89. Clouse ME, Stokes KR, Kruskal JB, Perry LJ, Stuart KE, Nasser IA. Chemoembolization for hepatocellular carcinoma: epinephrine followed by a doxorubicin-ethiodized oil emulsion and gelatin sponge powder. J Vasc Intervent Radiol. 1993;4:717–25.

90. Struk D, Rankin RN, Karlik SJ. Stability studies on chemoembolization mixtures. Dialysis studies of doxorubicin and lipiodol with Avitene, Gelfoam, and Angiostat. Invest Radiol. 1993;28:1024–7.

91. Stuart K, Stokes K, Jenkins R, Trey C, Clouse M. Treatment of hepatocellular carcinoma using doxorubicin/ethiodized oil/gelatin powder chemoembolization. Cancer. 1993;72:3202–9.

92. Chang JM, Tzeng WS, Pan HB, Yang CF, Lai KH. Transcatheter arterial embolization with or without cisplatin treatment of hepatocellular carcinoma. A randomized controlled study. Cancer. 1994;74:2449–53.

93. Taniguchi K, Nakata K, Kato Y *et al.* Treatment of hepatocellular carcinoma with transcatheter arterial embolization. Analysis of prognostic factors. Cancer. 1994;73:1341–5.

94. Ikeda K, Saitoh S, Koida I *et al.* A prospective randomized evaluation of a compound of tegafur and uracil as an adjuvant chemotherapy of hepatocellular carcinoma treated with transcatheter arterial chemoembolization. Am J Clin Oncol. 1995;18:204–10.

95. Tanaka K, Inoue S, Numata K *et al.* Color Doppler sonography of hepatocellular carcinoma before and after treatment by transcatheter arterial embolization. Am J Roentgenol. 1992;158:541–6.

96. Lin ZY, Chang WY, Wang LY *et al.* Duplex pulsed Doppler sonography of hepatocellular carcinoma treated with transcatheter arterial embolization. J Ultrasound Med. 1991;10:619–23.

97. Bartolozzi C, Lencioni R, Caramella D, Falaschi F, Cioni R, DiCoscio G. Hepatocellular carcinoma: CT and MR features after transcatheter arterial embolization and percutaneous ethanol injection. Radiology. 1994;191:123–8.

98. Choi BI, Kim HC, Jan JK *et al.* Therapeutic effect of transcatheter oily chemoembolization therapy for encapsulated nodular hepatocellular carcinoma: CT and pathologic findings. Radiology. 1992;182:709–13.

99. Khan KN, Nakata K, Kusumoto Y *et al.* Evaluation of nontumorous tissue damage by transcatheter arterial embolization for hepatocellular carcinoma. Cancer Res. 1991;51:5667–71.

100. Tai DI, Chen HY, Wang PW *et al.* Hepatobiliary imaging of functional and morphological changes following hepatic arterial embolization in hepatocellular carcinoma. J Nucl Med. 1995;36:1590–4.

101. Kobayashi S, Nakanuma Y, Terada T, Matsui O. Postmortem survey of bile duct necrosis and biloma in hepatocellular carcinoma after transcatheter arterial chemoembolization therapy: relevance to microvascular damage of peribiliary capillary plexus. Am J Gastroenterol. 1993;88:1410–15.

102. Gunji T, Kawauchi N, Ohnishi S *et al.* Treatment of hepatocellular carcinoma associated with advanced cirrhosis by transcatheter arterial chemoembolization using autologous blood clot: a preliminary report. Hepatology. 1992:15;252–7.

103. Nishioka Y, Kyotani S, Okamura M *et al.* A study of embolizing materials for chemoembolization therapy of hepatocellular carcinoma: embolic effect of cisplatin albumin microspheres using chitin and chitosan in dogs, and changes of cisplatin content in blood and tissue. Chem Pharm Bull. 1992;40:267–8.

104. Hwang T, Chen M, Lee T *et al.* Resection of hepatocellular carcinoma after transcatheter arterial embolization. Arch Surg. 1987;122:756–9.

105. Yu Y, Xu D, Zhou X *et al.* Experience with liver resection after hepatic arterial chemoembolization for hepatocellular carcinoma. Cancer. 1993;71:62–5.
106. Nagasue N, Galizia G, Kohno H *et al.* Adverse effects of preoperative hepatic artery chemoembolization for resectable hepatocellular carcinoma: a retrospective comparison of 138 liver resections. Surgery. 1993;217:149–54.
107. Teng GJ, He SC, Guo JH, Cai XL, Gao GR. Preoperative transcatheter hepatic arterial embolization for hepatic malignancy. Invest Radiol. 1993;28:235–41.
108. Adachi E, Matsumata T, Nishizaki T, Hashimoto H, Tsuneyoshi M, Sugimachi K. Effects of preoperative transcatheter hepatic arterial chemoembolization for hepatocellular carcinoma. The relationship between postoperative course and tumor necrosis. Cancer. 1993;72:3593–8.
109. Matsuo N, Uchida H, Nishimine K *et al.* Segmental transcatheter hepatic artery chemoembolization with iodized oil for hepatocellular carcinoma: antitumor effect and influence on normal tissue. J Vasc Intervent Radiol. 1993;4:543–9.
110. Park JH, Han JK, Chung JW, Choi BI, Han MC, Kim YI. Superselective transcatheter arterial embolization with ethanol and iodized oil for hepatocellular carcinoma. J Vasc Intervent Radiol. 1993;4:333–9.
111. Matsui O, Kadoya M, Yoshikawa J *et al.* Small hepatocellular carcinoma: treatment with subsegmental transcatheter arterial embolization [see comments]. [Review] Radiology. 1993;188:79–83.
112. Konno T, Maeda H, Iwai K *et al.* Effect of arterial administration of high molecular weight anti-cancer agent SMANCS with lipid lymphographic agent on hepatoma: a preliminary report. Eur J Cancer Clin Oncol. 1983;19:1053.
113. Isomoto I, Aikawa H, Mori H *et al.* Intraarterial injection therapy of newly developed cis-platin–phosphatidyl choline–lipiodol suspension for hepatocellular carcinoma. Radiat Med. 1992;10:19–25.
114. Ichida T, Katoh M, Hayakawa M *et al.* Treatment of hepatocellular carcinoma with CDDP–epirubicin–lipiodol suspension: a pilot clinico-pharmacological study. Cancer Chemother Pharmacol. 1992;31:s51–4.
115. Ichida T, Katoh M, Hayakawa M *et al.* Therapeutic effect of a CDDP–epirubicin–lipiodol emulsion on advanced hepatocellular carcinoma. Cancer Chemother Pharmacol. 1994;33:s74–8.
116. Nakao N, Uchida H, Kamino K *et al.* Determination of the optimum dose level of lipiodol in transcatheter arterial embolization of primary hepatocellular carcinoma based on retrospective multivariate analysis. Cardiovasc Intervent Radiol. 1994;17:76–80.
117. Urata K, Mitsumata K, Kamakura T, Hasuo K, Sugimachi K. Lipiodolization for unresectable hepatocellular carcinoma: an analysis of 205 patients using univariate and multivariate analysis. J Surg Oncol. 1994;56:8.
118. Stefanini GF, Amorati P, Biselli M *et al.* Efficacy of transarterial targeted treatments on survival of patients with hepatocellular carcinoma: an Italian experience. Cancer. 1995;75:2427–34.
119. Groupe D'Etude et de Traitement du Carcinome Hepatocellulaire. A comparison of lipiodol chemoembolization and conservative treatment for unresectable hepatocellular carcinoma. N Engl J Med. 1995;332:1256–61.
120. Nishizaki T, Takenaka K, Yoshida K, Ikeda T, Sugimachi K. Influence of lipiodolization on a cirrhotic liver. J Surg Oncol. 1995;58:263–8.
121. Kosakai I, Ichida T, Yamaguchi O, Asakura H. Delayed anoxic pseudolobular necrosis (terminal hepatic necrosis) after chemo-lipiodolization for hepatocellular carcinoma. Am J Gastroenterol. 1996;91:1263–5.
122. Nagasue N, Yukaya H, Ogawa Y *et al.* Clinical experience with 118 hepatic resections for hepatocellular carcinoma. Surgery. 1986;99:694–701.
123. Nagao T, Goto S, Kawano N *et al.* Hepatic resection for hepatocellular carcinoma: clinical features and long-term prognosis. Ann Surg. 1987;205:33–40.
124. Sesto ME. Vogt DP, Hermann RE. Hepatic resection in 128 patients: a 24-year experience. Surgery. 1987;102:846–51.
125. Iwatsuki S, Starzl TE. Personal experience with 411 hepatic resections. Ann Surg. 1988;208:421–34.
126. Chen M, Hwang T, Jeng LB *et al.* Hepatic resection in 120 patients with hepatocellular carcinoma. Arch Surg. 1989;124:1025–8.

127. Tsuzuki T, Sugioka A, Ueda M *et al.* Hepatic resection for hepatocellular carcinoma. Surgery. 1990;107:511–20.
128. Ozawa K, Takayasu T, Kumada K *et al.* Experience with 225 hepatic resections for hepatocellular carcinoma over a 4-year period. Am J Surg. 1991;161:677–82.
129. Arii S, Tobe T. Results of surgical treatment: follow up study by Liver Cancer Study Group of Japan. In: Tobe T, Kameda H, Okudaira M *et al.*, editors. Primary liver cancer in Japan. Tokyo: Springer-Verlag; 1992:243–55.
130. Zhou XD, Yu YQ, Tang ZY *et al.* Surgical treatment of hepatocellular carcinoma. Hepato-Gastroenterology. 1993;40:333–6.
131. Kosuge T, Makuuchi M, Takayama T, Yamamoto J, Shimada K, Yamasaki S. Long-term results after resection of hepatocellular carcinoma; experience of 480 cases. Hepatogastroenterology. 1993;40:328–32.
132. Nagasue N, Kohno H, Chang YC *et al.* Liver resection for hepatocellular carcinoma. Results of 229 consecutive patients during 11 years. Ann Surg. 1993;217:375–84.
133. Lygidakis NJ, Pothoulakis J, Konstantinidou AE, Spanos H. Hepatocellular carcinoma: surgical resection versus surgical resection combined with pre-and post-operative locoregional immunotherapy-chemotherapy. A prospective randomized study. Anticancer Res. 1995;15:543–50.
134. Lai EC, Fan ST, Lo CM, Chu KM, Liu CL, Wong J. Hepatic resection for hepatocellular carcinoma. An audit of 343 patients. Ann Surg. 1995;221:291–8.
135. Kawasaki S, Makuuchi M, Miyagawa S *et al.* Results of hepatic resection for hepatocellular carcinoma. World J Surg. 1995;19:31–4.
136. Kinami Y, Takashima S, Miyazaki I. Hepatic resection for hepatocellular carcinoma associated with cirrhosis. World J Surg. 1986;10:294–301.
137. Bismuth H, Houssin D, Ornowski J, Meriggi F. Liver resections in cirrhotic patients: a western experience. World J Surg. 1986;10:311–17.
138. Gozzetti G, Mazziotti A, Cavallari A *et al.* Clinical experience with hepatic resections for hepatocellular carcinoma in patients with cirrhosis. Surg Gynecol Obstet. 1988;166:503–10.
139. Franco D, Capussotti L, Smadja C *et al.* Resection of hepatocellular carcinoma. Results in 72 European patients with cirrhosis. Gastroenterology. 1990;98:733–78.
140. Sasaki Y, Imaoka S, Masutani S *et al.* Influence of coexisting cirrhosis on ling-term prognosis after surgery in patients with hepatocellular carcinoma. Surgery. 1992;112:515–21.
141. Nagao T, Nagashima I, Inoue S, Omori Y, Kawano N, Morioka Y. Hepatic resection for minute hepatocellular carcinoma. Surg Today. 1992;22:110–14.
142. Chen MF, Hwang TL, Jeng LB. Hepatic resection for 28 patients with small hepatocellular carcinoma. Int Surg. 1992;77:72–6.
143. Ihde DC, Matthews MJ, Makuch RW *et al.* Prognostic factors in patients with hepatocellular carcinoma receiving systemic chemotherapy: identification of two groups of patients with prospects for prolonged survival. Am J Med. 1985;78:399–406.
144. Olweny CLM, Toya T, Katongole-Mbiddle E *et al.* Treatment of hepatocellular carcinoma with adriamycin: preliminary communication. Cancer. 1975;39:1250–7.
145. Cersosismo RJ, Hong WK. Epirubicin; a review of the pharmacology, clinical activity and adverse effects of an adriamycin analog. J Clin Oncol. 1986;4:425–39.
146. Melia W, Westably D, Williams R. Diamminodichloride platinum (cis-platinum) in the treatment of hepatocellular carcinoma. Clin Oncol. 1981;7:275–80.
147. Falkson G, Coetzer BJ, Terblanche APS *et al.* Phase II trial of mitoxantrone in patients with primary liver cancer. Cancer Treat Rep. 1984;68:1311–12.
148. Ramming KP. The effectiveness of hepatic artery infusion in treatment of primary hepatobiliary tumors. Semin Oncol. 1983;10:199–205.
149. Nakamura K, Takashima S, Takada K *et al.* Clinical evaluation of intermittent arterial infusion chemotherapy with an implanted reservoir for hepatocellular carcinoma. Cancer Chemother Pharmacol. 1992;31(Suppl. 1):S93–8.
150. Minoyama A, Yoshikawa M, Ebara M, Saisho H, Sugiura N, Ohto M. Study of repeated arterial infusion chemotherapy with a subcutaneously implanted reservoir for advanced hepatocellular carcinoma. J Gastroenterol. 1995;30:356–66.
151. Bern MM, McDermott W, Cody B *et al.* Intraarterial hepatic infusion and intravenous Adriamycin for treatment of hepatocellular carcinoma. A clinical pharmacology report. Cancer. 1978;42:399–405.

152. Kajanti M, Rissanen P, Virkkunen P *et al.* regional intraarterial infusion of cisplatin in primary hepatocellular carcinoma. A phase II study. Cancer. 1986;58:2386–8.
153. Yamasaki S, Hasegawa H, Makuuchi M, Takayama T, Kosuge T, Shimada K. Choice of treatments for small hepatocellular carcinoma: hepatectomy, embolization or ethanol injection. J Gastroenterol Hepatol. 1991;6:408–13.
154. Tanikawa K. Multidisciplinary treatment of hepatocellular carcinoma: follow up study by Liver Cancer Study Group of Japan. In Tobe T, Kameda H, Okudaira M *et al.*, editors. Primary liver cancer in Japan. Tokyo: Springer-Verlag; 1992:139–51.
155. Farmer DG, Rosove MH, Shaked A, Busuttil RW. Current treatment modalities for hepatocellular carcinoma. Ann Surg. 1994;219:236–47.

Section VI
Gallstone disease

22
Pathogenesis of cholesterol and pigment gallstones

M. C. CAREY

INTRODUCTION

Gallstones are a common phase separation disease[1,2] that results from the condensation and precipitation of cholesterol crystals or amorphous calcium bilirubinates in the gallbladder and biliary tree[3,4]. The principal pathophysiological defect in each case is supersaturation of bile with the precipitating solute[3,4].

CHOLESTEROL GALLSTONES

All cholesterol stones are composed principally of cholesterol monohydrate crystals[3]. They form in the gallbladder in sterile supersaturated bile that results from hepatic hypersecretion of cholesterol. The aetiology of cholesterol hypersecretion is not known. It is clearly related to an intracellular homeostatic defect that directs more endogenous and exogenous unesterified hepatic cholesterol into bile[5]. Biliary phospholipids, mostly lecithin, are known to originate from the endoplasmic reticulum and from there transfer to the canalicular membrane, most probably via a specific phosphatidylcholine transfer protein[6]. They are then translocated across the membrane under the influence of an ATP-driven P-glycoprotein (mdr2/MDR3 gene product)[7], and then vesiculate from specific lipid domains on the exoplasmic leaflet of the canalicular membrane[8]. The vesiculation and detachment of unilamellar vesicles into the canalicular lumen is thought to be bile salt-dependent[3]. Nonetheless, the processes whereby unesterified cholesterol molecules are conveyed from the canalicular membrane into bile, presumably into these canalicular vesicles, is not known[9]. Bile salt molecules traffic out of the liver independently[10], and as they are progressively concentrated in the canalicular space and ductules, they induce a phase change in unilamellar vesicles from a lamellar phase to rods (hexagonal phase) and from rods to micelles[11]. In cholesterol stone disease, defective motility of the gallbladder, mucin hypersecretion and gelation, as well as rapid nucleation, may be related to mucosal and muscle injury from gallbladder absorption of biliary cholesterol molecules[3]. Gallbladder dysmotility leads to more frequent cycling and reduction in size of the bile salt pool, and as a result of excessive exposure to the anaerobic flora there is increased bile salt hydrophobicity which amplifies the lithogenic state in many ways[3]. Recent studies on the heritability of cholesterol gallstones induced by a lithogenic diet in the inbred mouse suggest that the presence of *Lith* genes affect the rate and severity of cholelithogenesis[12].

PIGMENT GALLSTONES

Pigment gallstones of the 'black' variety are composed principally of poly-merized calcium hydrogen bilirubinate[4,13], $[Ca(HUCB)_2]_n$. These form in the gallbladder in sterile bile that is supersaturated with the calcium salt of the mono-acid form of unconjugated bilirubin. Supersaturation with this highly insoluble salt occurs in bile when the ion-product of the salt exceeds the solubil-ity product[4]. Usually this results from endogenous β-glucuronidase activity or spontaneous alkaline hydrolysis of an excess of conjugated bilirubins following their hypersecretion into bile[13]. Two common conditions lead to hepatic hyper-secretion of conjugated bilirubins: (a) intravascular haemolysis which may be congenital or acquired, and either chronic or intermittent[4,13], and (b) entero-hepatic cycling of bilirubin, acquired as a consequence of bilirubin reabsorption often associated with bile salt malabsorption from the small to the large intes-tine[14], e.g. ileal Crohn's disease, resection or bypass, cystic fibrosis and starch-rich diets. Pigment gallstones of the 'brown' variety occur secondary to chronic anaerobic infection of the biliary tree. Frequently the initiating event in develop-ing countries is parasitic infestation. Brown stones can form anywhere in the biliary system, including the gallbladder and the intrahepatic ducts[4,13,15]. They are composed principally of unpolymerized calcium bilirubinates and calcium soaps[4]. These stones are characterized by their faeculent odour, greasy putty-like consistency, and irregular round or cylindrical shape. They contain numerous rod-shaped anaerobic bacteria throughout, and bacterial 'skeletons' are visual-ized within their structure by electron microscopy[15]. Because biliary lecithin and bile salt conjugates are hydrolysed in addition to bilirubin conjugates, 'brown' pigment stones also contain substantial quantities of unesterified cholesterol[4]. Whether pronucleation defects exist outside of bile in formation of 'black' pigment stones has not been clarified, but 'dysmotility' from mechanical obstruction and chronic anaerobic bacterial infection appears crucial in the formation of 'brown' pigment gallstones[4].

Acknowledgements

The author's work is supported by National Institutes of Health (USPHS) grants DK36588 and DK36856, and his laboratory is managed and administered by Mss Monika R. Leonard and Susan R. Edins.

References

1. Berndt H, Nurnberg D, Pannwitz H. Prevalence of cholelithiasis. Results of an epidemiologic study using sonography in East Germany, Z Gastroenterol. 1989;27:662–6.

2. Acalovskschi M, Pascu M, Iobagin S *et al.* Increasing gallstone prevalence and cholecystectomy rate in a large Romanian town. A necropsy study. Dig Dis Sci. 1995;40:2582–6.
3. Carey, MC. Formation and growth of cholesterol gallstones: the new synthesis. In: Fromm H, Leuschner U, editors. Bile acids–cholestasis–gallstones (Falk Symposium No. 84). Dordrecht: Kluwer; 1996;147–75.
4. Cahalane MJ, Neubrand MW, Carey MC. Physical–chemical pathogenesis of pigment gallstones, Semin Liver Dis. 1988;8:317–28.
5. Ito J, Kawata S, Imar Y, Kakimoto H, Trzaskos JM, Matsuzawa Y. Hepatic cholesterol metabolism in patients with cholesterol gallstones: enhanced intracellular transport of cholesterol. Gastroenterology. 1996;110:1617–27.
6. Cohen DE, Leonard MR, Carey MC. *In-vitro* evidence that phospholipid secretion into bile may be coordinated intracellularly by the combined actions of bile salts and the specific phosphatidylcholine transfer protein of liver. Biochemistry. 1994;33:9975–80.
7. Smit, JJM, Schinkel AM, Oude Elferink RPJ *et al.* Homozygous disruption of the murine mdr2 P-glycoprotein gene leads to a complete absence of phospholipid from bile and to liver disease. Cell. 1993;75:451–62.
8. Crawford JM, Möckel G-M, Crawford AR *et al.* Imaging biliary lipid secretion in the rat: ultrastructural evidence for vesiculation of the hepatocyte canalicular membrane, J Lipid Res. 1995;36:2147–63.
9. Robins SJ, Fasulo JM, Pritzker CR, Patton GM. Hepatic transport and secretion of unesterified cholesterol in the rat is traced by the plant sterol sitostanol. J Lipid Res. 1996;37:15–21.
10. Meier PJ. Hepatocellular transport systems: from carrier identification in membrane vesicles to cloned proteins. J Hepatol. 1996;24(Suppl. 1):29–35.
11. Cohen DE, Kaler EW, Carey MC. Cholesterol carriers in human bile: are lamellae involved? Hepatology. 1993;18:1522–32.
12. Khanuja B, Cheah Y-C, Hunt M *et al. Lith 1*, a major gene affecting cholesterol gallstone formation among inbred strains of mice. Proc Natl Acad Sci USA. 1995;92:7729–33.
13. Leuschner U, Güldütuna S, Hellstern A. Pathogenesis of pigment stones and medical treatment, J Gastroenterol Hepatol. 1994;9:87–98.
14. Brink MA, Méndez-Sánchez N, Carey MC. Bilirubin cycles enterohepatically after ileal resection in the rat, Gastroenterology. 1996;110:1945–57.
15. Cetta F. The role of bacteria in pigment gallstone disease. Ann Surg. 1991;213:315–26.

23
Non-surgical management of gallstone disease

G. PAUMGARTNER

INTRODUCTION

During recent decades considerable advances in the surgical and non-surgical treatment of gallstone disease have been made, and the physician is increasingly faced with the questions: (1) Which patients with gallstone disease require therapeutic intervention? and (2) Which therapeutic interventions are applicable in individual patients?

The decision for or against a specific therapeutic intervention must take into account the balance between the risks of the disease and the risks of the treatment, between the patient's complaints and the discomfort from therapy, and between the expected benefits and costs of therapy. For this evaluation the stage of the gallstone disease must be defined[1]. There are three stages of cholelithiasis, namely (1) the asymptomatic stage, (2) the symptomatic stage without complications, and (3) the symptomatic stage with complications, such as acute cholecystitis, choledocholithiasis, biliary pancreatitis and gallbladder cancer. The various stages of gallstone disease differ with regard to the natural history of the disease, and therefore require different therapeutic approaches.

EXPECTANT MANAGEMENT

Expectant management is indicated in the large number of patients with asymptomatic gallbladder stones, which are usually detected during routine ultrasound examinations[2,3]. This recommendation is based on the observation that the natural history of asymptomatic gallstones is generally benign[2]. Several large studies with a follow-up of 10–20 years, which have been reviewed by Ransohoff and Gracie[2], show that asymptomatic gallstone disease is a rather benign disease. In the study of Gracie and Ransohoff[4], the average risk of developing biliary pain was about 2% per year during the first 5 years of follow-up and then decreased to about 0.5% during the third 5 years. A biliary complication occurred only in three of 123 asymptomatic persons, and in all three an episode of pain preceded the complication and thus provided a 'warning' symptom. This study, however, has the shortcoming that mainly male subjects were included.

Recently, the results of a large population study by the GREPCO group in Italy[5] became available. This prospective study in a free-living population used ultrasonography for the detection of gallstones. It showed that the cumulative probability of developing symptoms was 26% after 10 years. The cumulative probability of developing complications after 10 years was only 3%. The annual incidence of complications (0.3%) in this study was somewhat higher than in the study of Gracie and Ransohoff[4], but lower than that reported by Friedman *et al.* (1%)[6]. The study of the GREPCO group[5] reported no deaths due to gallstone disease except for one asymptomatic patient who died of gallbladder carcinoma.

Taking into account the total number of approximately 6500 person-years of follow-up included in published cohort studies, the calculated incidence of gallbladder carcinoma in asymptomatic subjects can be estimated to be about 0.015% per year[5]. Ransohoff and Gracie[2] estimated that the incidence of gallbladder cancer in an asymptomatic gallstone subject aged 50 years or older is about 0.02% per year. Incidence rates in certain ethnic groups (Pima Indians and other New World Indians) and in subgroups of gallstone patients (porcelain gallbladder, stones with a diameter larger than 3 cm), however, may be higher[1].

Decision analysis tells us that with the low risks of asymptomatic gallstone disease even a perfect prophylactic therapy with no morbidity and no mortality would result in only a very small gain in life expectancy in asymptomatic subjects with gallstones, namely in the order of about 1–2 weeks[2]. It may therefore be concluded that asymptomatic gallstones, in general, should be managed expectantly. Exceptions are gallstones in patients with porcelain gallbladder, American Indians and possibly patients with very large gallstones because of an increased risk of gallbladder cancer[1,3].

THERAPEUTIC INTERVENTION

Patients with a history of biliary colic (symptomatic gallbladder stones) are at a substantially higher risk of recurrent biliary pain and complications than patients with asymptomatic stones. The majority of symptomatic patients develop pain again, and the risk of biliary complications is 1–2% per year. Several studies show that, within 5–30 years of follow-up, 66% had recurrent biliary pain or complications and 28% developed complications[7]. A study in Sirmione has recently confirmed that persistence or recurrence of pain in previously symptomatic subjects is frequent and occurs in about 50% of the patients[7]. The risk of complications is higher in patients who have frequent and severe symptoms[8]. About 30% of patients who have had only one attack of biliary pain do not have further episodes of pain[2]. A therapeutic intervention should therefore be recommended for most patients with symptomatic gallstones. However, if the patient with a first attack of biliary pain wants to try a period of watchful waiting to see if pain recurs, this is acceptable[2]. The complicated forms of cholecystolithiasis usually require prompt surgical therapy. Table 1 lists the various treatment options for symptomatic gallstones according to their invasiveness, with oral

Table 1 Treatment options for symptomatic gallstones according to increasing invasiveness

1. Oral bile acid dissolution therapy
2. Extracorporeal shockwave lithotripsy
3. Topical dissolution therapy
4. Laparoscopic cholecystectomy
5. Open cholecystectomy

bile acid dissolution therapy being the least, open cholecystectomy being the most invasive procedure.

Laparoscopic or open cholecystectomy must be regarded as the standard treatment for patients with symptomatic gallstones[1,3]. Laparoscopic cholecystectomy has the advantage that stone clearance can be achieved independently of the type, number and size of the stones, and independently of gallbladder function, but it has the disadvantages of an invasive procedure with general anaesthesia, the risk of bile duct injury[9] and a small mortality rate[10]. Many patients are reluctant to undergo surgery or general anaesthesia despite the low risks of morbidity and mortality, and they opt for the least invasive treatment that can be justified on medical grounds. In a small number of patients, non-surgical therapy may be suitable when there is a high operative risk.

In a subset of patients without complications of their gallstone disease, non-surgical treatments, such as oral bile acid dissolution therapy or extracorporeal shockwave lithotripsy, are possible. They have the advantage of being non-invasive procedures with low morbidity and no or negligible mortality. There are a number of common requirements of non-surgical gallstone treatment; they include certain stone characteristics such as the presence of cholesterol stones without calcifications, a maximal size and number of stones, as well as normal gallbladder function[11,12]. In the following, only the two non-invasive forms of non-surgical gallstone therapy, oral bile acid dissolution therapy and extracorporeal shock-wave lithotripsy, will be discussed. With the introduction of laparoscopic cholecystectomy, topical dissolution therapy, which, in contrast to oral dissolution therapy and shockwave lithotripsy is invasive, has practically been abandoned, and will therefore not be discussed.

Oral bile acid dissolution therapy

Therapy with bile acids is aimed at reversing the condition that is the prerequisite for the formation of cholesterol gallstones, namely supersaturation of bile with cholesterol[13]. Removal of cholesterol from the stone can occur by micellar solubilization and/or formation of a liquid crystalline phase. Both mechanisms may be operative simultaneously.

Bile acid dissolution therapy can be performed with ursodeoxycholic acid alone at a dose of 8–12 mg/kg body weight per day[11]. A combination of reduced doses of ursodeoxycholic acid and chenodeoxycholic acid may also be employed[14,15]. This is based on the assumption that the side-effects of a full dose of chenodeoxycholic acid can be avoided, and that the desired effects of both bile acids on bile desaturation and gallstone dissolution are additive. Because of different mechanisms of action of chenodeoxycholic acid and ursodeoxycholic acid, the concept has been raised that the combination of these two bile acids may be even more effective for gallstone dissolution than monotherapy with ursodeoxycholic acid. For the dissolution of stone fragments after shockwave lithotripsy, combination therapy (7 mg/kg per day of each bile acid) and monotherapy with ursodeoxycholic acid (11 mg/kg per day) were equally effective[16]. Since the combination caused diarrhoea more often, monotherapy with ursodeoxycholic acid appears to be the preferable treatment.

A recent meta-analysis[17] has included all randomized trials of gallstone dissolution by ursodeoxycholic acid in patients with radiolucent gallstones in a visualizing gallbladder. Ursodeoxycholic acid completely dissolved the stones in 37% of all patients. In patients with gallstones up to 10 mm in diameter the dissolution rate was 49%. Stones larger than 10 mm dissolved in only 29%[17]. The best results – complete dissolution in more than 70% of the patients – have been observed in patients with floating stones smaller than 5 mm in diameter. The time required for complete stone dissolution shows wide variation. In the majority of patients who respond, the gallstone diameter decreases linearly with treatment time. The rate of decrease varies considerably between patients, the median rate[18] being 0.7 mm/month. On the basis of these findings we employ the selection criteria for oral bile acid dissolution therapy shown in Table 2.

Table 2 Selection criteria for oral bile acid dissolution therapy

---

1. *Gallbladder*
   Opacification on oral cholecystogram
2. *Stones*
   Radiolucency on X-ray
   Computerized tomography: stones isodense or hypodense to bile
   Stone diameter: ≤5 mm (optimal), 6–10 mm (acceptable)

Extracorporeal shockwave lithotripsy

The efficacy of oral bile acid dissolution therapy is not limited only by gallstone size but also by the fact that some stones apparently do not respond even if they are mainly composed of cholesterol. This may be related to surface properties of the stones. Thus, there is a good rationale for first fragmenting the stone and then dissolving the remaining fragments. In order to reach this goal, extracorporeal shockwave lithotripsy of gallstones has been introduced by Sauerbruch *et al.*[19].

Shockwaves are high-pressure waves that obey the laws of acoustics, but they differ from sound waves and conventional ultrasound waves by being highly distorted from the normal representation of sinusoidally varying acoustic pressure waves. They are characterized by a positive-pressure pulse of short duration with an extremely short rise time. The positive pressure pulse is followed by a negative-pressure pulse of much lower amplitude but longer duration[20]. Because most human tissues have an acoustic impedance approximately equal to that of water, shockwaves can be transmitted into the body with little attenuation. In order to create a limited area of high pressure at the location of the stone, while keeping the pressure in the surrounding tissue relatively low, the shockwaves are focused. This makes it possible to keep tissue damage outside the focal area to a minimum[20]. Lithotripters of different manufacturers vary with respect to the mechanisms used for shockwave generation, focusing and targeting[20]. Shockwaves can be generated by the use of an underwater spark-gap (electrohydraulic principle), piezoelectric crystals or an electromagnetic membrane. In spark-gap lithotripters shockwaves are focused by an ellipsoidal metal reflector. In order to focus piezoelectrically generated shockwaves the piezoelectric crystals are mounted on a spherical dish. Electromagnetically generated shockwaves are usually focused by acoustic lenses, but a metal reflector also can be used.

Most groups have combined extracorporeal shockwave lithotripsy with adjuvant bile acid dissolution therapy. However, complete clearance of the stones can also be achieved by biliary lithotripsy without adjuvant bile acid therapy when the fragments are very small (<2 mm or fragments below the resolution of the ultrasound) and the gallbladder contracts well[21–24].

In a study of extracorporeal shockwave lithotripsy combined with adjuvant bile acid therapy, we included patients with symptomatic, uncomplicated cholecystolithiasis, one to three radiolucent stones with diameters 5–30 mm, no calcifications or at most a thin radiopaque rim (<3 mm) in a gallbladder that opacified on an oral cholecystogram[12,25]. For evaluation of efficacy the patients were then classified according to the number, diameter, and radiolucency of the stones. Figure 1 shows the results of the combination of lithotripsy plus adjuvant bile acid therapy, expressed as the percentage of patients free of stones 6 months, 12 months, and 18 months after lithotripsy[11]. It can be seen that the

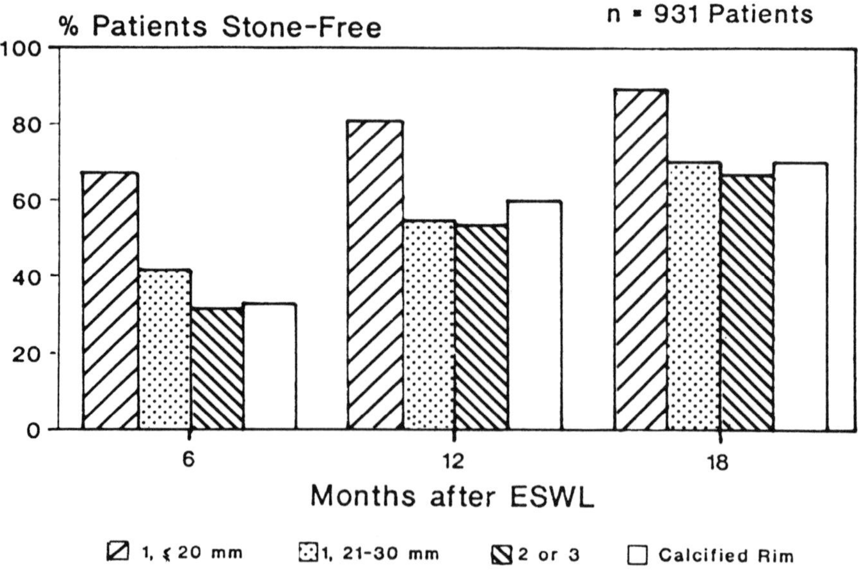

Fig. 1 Percentage of patients free of stones at various time points after extracorporeal shockwave lithotripsy and adjuvant bile acid therapy calculated by actuarial analysis. ▨ , Patients with a single stone ≤20 mm in diameter; ▨ , patients with a single stone 21–30 mm in diameter; ▨ , patients with two or three stones with a cumulative diameter ≤30 mm; ▢ , patients with a single stone exhibiting a thin (<3 cm) calcified rim. Reproduced from Paumgartner et al.[11]

efficacy of this treatment depended on the number and size of the stones, as well as on the presence or absence of a calcified rim. The best results were obtained in the group of patients with a single radiolucent stone up to 20 mm in diameter. In this group nearly 70% of patients became stone-free at 6 months, 80% at 12 months, and nearly 90% at 18 months.

Quantitative assessment of gallbladder motor function was not used to select patients for shockwave lithotripsy in most studies. Recent findings[26] confirm previous reports[23,27] that gallbladder emptying is a major determinant of stone clearance. Sixty-six per cent of the patients with an ejection fraction of more than 60% cleared all their fragments from the gallbladder as early as 3 months after a lithotripsy[26]. By contrast, of those with an ejection fraction smaller than 60%, only 29% cleared their fragments within the same time period. Therefore, it is advisable to determine gallbladder emptying induced by a test meal, and to select only patients for extracorporeal shockwave lithotripsy who exhibit gallbladder emptying of more than 60% of the fasting volume.

On the basis of our findings we recommend the selection criteria for extracorporeal shockwave lithotripsy shown in Table 3.

Table 3   Selection criteria for extracorporeal shockwave lithotripsy

1. *Gallbladder*
   Opacification on oral cholecystogram or sonographic evidence for patency of cystic duct
   (gallbladder contraction following a test meal)
   Gallbladder emptying >60% of fasting volume
2. *Stones*
   Radiolucency on X-ray
   Stone number: 1
   Stone diameter: 5–20 mm

In a recently performed, randomized multicentre study we have found that, in patients with good gallbladder emptying and a high degree of stone fragmentation, adjuvant bile acid therapy does not further improve early stone clearance[24]. Therefore, we are now testing the strategy of sequential lithotripsy dissolution therapy. This strategy consists of so-called 'pulverization' of the stone (single radiolucent stone with a diameter less than 20 mm) by repeated high-energy lithotripsy as a first step, followed by bile acid dissolution therapy as a second step 3 months later, only if stone fragments persist.

Side-effects and complications directly related to extracorporeal shockwave lithotripsy have been minimal[12]. Transient gross haematuria occurred in 4% and liver haematoma in one out of 1500 patients. Fragment-related adverse effects were biliary colic in 34%; mild biliary pancreatitis in 2%, cholestasis in 1% and cholecystitis in 1%. Endoscopic sphincterotomy had to be performed in 1%, surgery because of acute cholecystitis in 0.2% and elective cholecystectomy in about 3% of the patients[12].

RECURRENCE

Patients who have successfully undergone a gallbladder-preserving treatment for gallstones are at risk of stone recurrence. The cumulative recurrence at 4 years after successful bile acid dissolution therapy is only about 10% in patients who initially had a single stone, but about 45% in patients who initially had multiple stones[28]. In our group of patients treated with shockwave lithotripsy and bile acids, 90% of the patients have had single stones. Reccurence rate in this group of patients was 20% after 4 years[29]. Besides initial stone number, incomplete gallbladder emptying[30,31] and increased conversion of cholic acid to deoxychoic acid[30] are risk factors for gallstone recurrence.

References

1. Paumgartner G. Nonoperative management of gallstone disease. In Sleisenger KH, Fordtran JS, editors. Gastrointestinal disease: pathophysiology/diagnosis/managment. Philadelpha: WB Saunders; 1994:1844–57.
2. Ransohoff DF, Gracie WA. Treatment of gallstones. Ann Intern Med. 1993;11:606–19.
3. Paumgartner G, Carr-Locke DL, Dubois F, Roda E, Thistle JL. Strategies in the treatment of gallstone disease. Gastroenterol Int. 1993;6:65–75.
4. Gracie WA, Ransohoff DF. The natural history of silent gallstones: the innocent gallstone is not a myth. N Engl J Med. 1982;307:798–803.
5. Attili AF, De Santis A, Capri R, Recipe AM, Maselli S and the GREPCO Group. The natural history of gallstones: the GREPCO experience. Hepatology. 1995;21:656–60.
6. Friedman GD, Ravioli CA, Fireman B. Prognosis of gallstones with mild or no symptoms: 25 years of follow-up in health maintenance organization. J Chron Dis. 1989;42:127.
7. Sama C, Morselli Labate AM, Taroni F, Barbara L. Epidemiology and natural history of gallstone disease. Semin Liver Dis. 1990;10:149–58.
8. Lund J. Surgical indications in cholelithiasis: prophylactic cholecystectomy elucidated on the basis of long-term follow up on 526 nonoperated cases. Ann Surg. 1960;151:153–62.
9. Strasberg SM, Hertl M, Soper NJ. An analysis of the problem of biliary injury during laparoscopic cholecystectomy. J Am Coll Surg. 1995;180:101–25.
10. The Southern Surgeons Club. A prospective analysis of 1518 laparoscopic cholecystectomies. N Engl J Med. 1991;324:1072–8.
11. Paumgartner G, Pauletzki J, Sackmann M. Ursodeoxycholic acid treatment of cholesterol gallstone disease. Scand J Gastroenterol. 1994;29(Suppl.204):27–31.
12. Sackmann M, Pauletzki J, Sauerbruch T, Holl J, Schelling G, Paumgartner G. The Munich gallbladder lithotripsy study: results of the first 5 years with 711 patients. Ann Intern Med. 1991;114:290–6.
13. Paumgartner G, Sauerbruch T. Gallstones: Pathogenesis. Lancet. 1991;338:1117–24.
14. Roehrkasse R, Fromm H, Malavolti, M, Tunuguntla AK, Ceryak S. Gallstone dissolution treatment with a combination of chenodeoxycholic and ursodeoxycholic acids. Studies of safety, efficacy and effects on bile lithogenicity, bile acid pool, and serum lipids. Dig Dis Sci. 1986;31:1032–40.
15. Podda M, Zuin M, Battezzati PM, Ghezzi C, De Fazio C, Dioguardi ML. Efficacy and safety of a combination of chenodeoxycholic acid and ursodeoxycholic acid for gallstone dissolution: a comparison with ursodeoxycholic acid alone. Gastroenterology. 1989;96:222–9.
16. Sackmann M, Pauletzki J, Aydemir U *et al.* Efficacy and safety of ursodeoxycholic acid for dissolution of gallstone fragments: comparison with the combination of ursodeoxycholic acid and chenodeoxycholic acid. Hepatology. 1991;14:1136–41.
17. May GR, Sutherland LR, Shaffer EA. Efficacy of bile acid therapy for gallstone dissolution: a meta-analysis of randomized trials. Aliment Pharmacol Ther. 1993;7:139–48.
18. Senior JR, Johnson MF, DeTurck DM Bazzoli F, Roda E. *In vivo* kinetics of radiolucent gallstone dissolution by oral dihydroxy bile acids. Gastroenterology. 1990;99:243–51.
19. Sauerbruch T, Delius M, Paumgartner G *et al.* Fragmentation of gallstones by extracorporeal shock waves. N Engl J Med. 1986;314:818–22.

20. Paumgartner G. Shock-wave lithotripsy of gallstones. AJR. 1989;153:235–42.
21. Tsuchiya Y, Ishihara F, Kajiyama G *et al.* Repeated piezoelectric lithotripsy for gallstones with and without ursodeoxycholic acid dissolution: a multicenter study. J Gastroenterol. 1995;30:768–74.
22. Soehendra N, Nam V-C, Binmoeller KF, Koch H, Bohnacker S, Schreiber WH. Pulverisation of calcified and non-calcified gall bladder stones: extracorporeal shock wave lithotripsy used alone. Gut. 1994;35:417–22.
23. Donald JJ, Fache JS, Burhenne HJ. Biliary lithotripsy: correlation between gallbladder contractility before treatment and the success of treatment. AJR 1991;157:287–9.
24. Sauter G,. Kullak-Ublick GA, Schumacher R *et al.* Gallstone clearance after repeated high-energy shock-wave lithotripsy is not further improved by ursodiol. Gastroenterology. 1996;110 A475.
25. Sackmann M, Pauletzki J, Delius M *et al.* Noninvasive therapy of gallbladder calculi with a radiopaque rim. Gastroenterology. 1992;102:988–93.
26. Pauletzki J, Sailer C, Klueppelberg U *et al.* Gallbladder emptying determines early gallstone clearance after shock-wave lithotripsy. Gastroenterology, 1994;107:1496–502.
27. Sackmann M, Eder H, Spengler U, Pauletzki J, Holl J, Paumgartner G. Gallbladder emptying is an important factor in fragment disappearance after shock wave lithotripsy. J Hepatol. 1993;17:62–6.
28. Villanova N, Bazzoli F, Taroni F *et al.* Gallstone recurrence after successful oral bile acid treatment. Gastroenterology. 1989;97:726–31.
29. Sackmann M, Niller, H, Klueppelberg U *et al.* Gallstone recurrence after shock-wave therapy. Gastroenterology. 1994;106:225–30.
30. Berr F, Mayer M, Sackmann MF, Sauerbruch T, Holl J, Paumgartner G. Pathogenic factors in early recurrence of cholesterol gallstones. Gastroenterology. 1994;106:215–24.
31. Pauletzki J, Althaus R, Holl J, Sackmann M, Paumgartner G. Gallbladder emptying is a determinant of gallstone recurrence after lithotripsy. Gastroenterology. 1995;108:A432.

24
Surgical treatment of gallbladder stones

S. M. STRASBERG

INTRODUCTION

Laparoscopic cholecystectomy has become the standard treatment for gallbladder stones. Introduced in 1989 this treatment revolutionized cholecystolithotherapy. It was demanded by patients because it provided a rapid permanent cure of the disease, with little pain and inconvenience, at reasonable cost and with few side-effects. It has become widely disseminated around the world and there has been a yearly increase in the percentage of cholecystectomies performed by laparoscopy to the point that open cholecystectomy is a vanishing procedure. In this chapter the indications and contraindications to the procedure, and its negative outcomes, will be discussed.

INDICATIONS AND CONTRAINDICATIONS TO LAPAROSCOPIC CHOLECYSTECTOMY

Asymptomatic cholelithiasis

Cholelithiasis may be divided into three clinical stages: the asymptomatic stage, the symptomatic stage and the complicated stage. Many studies dating back to the beginning of this century have documented the natural history of asymptomatic cholecystitis. Taken together these studies permit the following conclusions. Asymptomatic cholelithiasis is an extremely common problem. Most persons with asymptomatic cholelithiasis will remain asymptomatic (75–80%). Patients who lose their asymptomatic status almost always develop pain for some time before they develop complications of the disease. In other words there is usually a regular progression through the clinical stages of the disease, and asymptomatic patients are rarely suddenly struck by a life-threatening complication. This is an important feature of the natural history, since there is no rationale for treatment of asymptomatic cholelithiasis on the basis of preventing complications. The policy of watchful waiting in asymptomatic cholelithiasis has been found to be safe in all of these studies, with no deaths and few complications attributable to this clinical strategy.

There are two caveats to this approach. The first is that cholecystectomy rarely *is* indicated in asymptomatic gallstone disease. An absolute indication is the precancerous state known as the porcelain gallbladder. It has been suggested that stones larger than 3 cm in diameter are associated with a higher risk of development of gallbladder cancer. It is also well known that certain populations, such as Bolivians and Chileans, have a much higher incidence of gallstone-associated gallbladder cancer. It is not possible to give authoritative recommendations either in patients with large stones or in specific populations; however, it is clear that outside these groups there is no basis for recommending cholecystectomy in asymptomatic patients in order to avoid the occurrence of gallbladder carcinoma. The incidence of the problem is so low that prophylactic cholecystectomy is not justified. Relative indications for cholecystectomy in asymptomatic patients, which include consideration of psychological needs, are cholelithiasis in children, a family history of gallbladder cancer, the concomitant presence of choledocholithiasis and sickle-cell anaemia in patients prone to sickling crises. The second caveat is based on the fact that patients with asymptomatic stones may have gastrointestinal symptoms and even abdominal pain, while patients with symptomatic stones may have atypical pain. Coming to the correct diagnosis may be difficult, and sometimes cholecystectomy must be recommended in patients with atypical pain not accounted for by other processes[1]. The common feature to all of the exceptions to the policy of no treatment for patients with asymptomatic stones is that these exceptions are rare.

The advent of a new procedure requires reconsideration of risks and indications. Laparoscopic cholecystectomy is a safer procedure on a per-patient basis. It is also more economical, especially when indirect or societal costs are considered. However, in order to be indicated in asymptomatic patients a procedure would have to approximate the safety and cost of vaccination for infectious disease. Therefore, the preceding statements regarding asymptomatic cholelithiasis are as true today as they were during the era of open cholecystectomy. However, whether these guidelines are being followed has been questioned, since several studies have documented a large increase (33–66%) in the number of cholecystectomies since the introduction of the laparoscopic technique [2–4]. As a result, although mortality as well as cost have fallen on a per-procedure basis, the total number of cholecystectomy-related deaths[4] and cost of treating gallstones by cholecystectomy[2,4] have not decreased.

The causes of the increase in the number of cholecystectomies have not been determined. One likely contributing factor is that symptomatic patients who would have refused open cholecystectomy are more likely to agree to the laparoscopic procedure. Another might be that patients are being referred for treatment at an earlier stage of disease. Increased numbers of procedures reflecting referral at an earlier stage of disease would be expected to cause a temporary increase in the cholecystectomy rates, with return to somewhat lower and more stable levels after several years. A third possible factor is that indications for surgery have been widened inappropriately, e.g. for treatment of asymptomatic patients or for treatment of patients with minimal or questionable symptoms of cholelithiasis.

We examined the disposition of 194 patients with cholelithiasis referred to our surgical unit just before the advent of laparoscopic cholecystectomy[1]. Of patients advised to have open cholecystectomy, 16% refused; in the laparoscopic era only one out of our first 500 patients refused. These data suggested that a substantial part of the increase in overall numbers of cholecystectomies reflects a much greater patient acceptance of this new procedure. In addition, 13% of the referred patients were advised against having cholecystectomy, because they were asymptomatic or because their symptoms were attributed to another cause. Although the increase in cholecystectomy rates has been known for about 2 years now, there have been no definitive studies that have actually determined the cause.

Symptomatic cholelithiasis

Laparoscopic cholecystectomy is unquestionably the major treatment for symptomatic cholelithiasis today. It has almost entirely displaced other therapies, and has attained the stature of the accepted first-line procedure for this disease. In this section we will focus on contraindications to laparoscopic cholecystectomy in symptomatic patients, and certain special conditions. Contraindications to laparoscopic cholecystectomy in complicated disease will be discussed separately.

Contraindications to laparoscopic cholecystectomy in the symptomatic patient

These may be divided into patient-based and surgeon-based contraindications, and the contraindications may be relative or absolute.

Patient-based contraindications.   The only absolute contraindications today are the inability to withstand a general anaesthetic, intractable bleeding disorder and end-stage liver disease. These are rare events in a patient requiring treatment for symptomatic cholelithiasis. However, a few patients have such severe cardiac or pulmonary disease that the procedure cannot be performed, especially when cardiac ejection fractions are less than 20%. Patients with pre-existing obstructive lung disease may retain CO_2 disproportionately during laparoscopic cholecystectomy under CO_2 pneumoperitoneum[5]. The presence of a ventriculoperitoneal shunt is not a contraindication[6]. Relative contraindications are pregnancy and milder stages of liver disease. Cirrhosis itself is only a relative contraindication.

Surgeon-based contraindications.   The difficulty of the procedure can be determined by the presence of certain preoperative factors. Previous attacks of cholecystitis comprise a risk factor for difficult cholecystectomy[7]. Maleness, advanced age, and many previous attacks of pain are additive risk factors for difficult cholecystectomy[7]. It has been shown that the probability of complications rises with inexperience and the difficulty of the procedure. Therefore, for inexperienced operators, these factors constitute a relative contraindication for the procedure.

Special situations in laparoscopic cholecystectomy

Pregnancy. Pregnant patients are preferably managed conservatively until delivery, but sometimes patients require operation for worsening biliary colic, acute cholecystitis unresponsive to medical management, and some cases of choledocholithiasis and gallstone pancreatitis[8]. Several recent reports indicate that laparoscopic cholecystectomy can be performed safely in pregnancy[8]. The safest time for laparoscopic cholecystectomy is the second trimester.

Cirrhosis. Cirrhosis is a relative contraindication to laparoscopic cholecystectomy[9,10] due to the danger of operating in the face of portal hypertension and coagulopathy. However, many early cirrhotics do not have these problems, and laparoscopic cholecystectomy may be performed safely in such patients[9,10].

Diabetics. Prophylactic cholecystectomy has been occasionally advocated in diabetics. However, there is no evidence to support this policy. There is good evidence to support a strategy of early cholecystectomy in the symptomatic patient. Diabetics tend to present with acute cholecystitis more frequently once they become symptomatic, and diabetics also withstand complications less well.

Laparoscopic cholecystectomy in children. Laparoscopic cholecystectomy in children is quite successful. Vinograd *et al.*[11] summarized their experience in 14 children. The gallbladder was successfully removed in 13 patients. The times to discharge and return to normal activities were brief. In another series of uncomplicated laparoscopic cholecystectomies in 12 children, Davidoff *et al.*[12] demonstrated decreased pain and ileus, improved cosmesis, shortened hospitalization, and faster return to activity as compared to open cholecystectomy. We have managed choledocholithiasis and biliary pancreatitis in children with laparoscopic techniques similar to those used in adults[13].

Complicated cholelithiasis

Acute cholecystitis

Randomized controlled trials performed in the open cholecystectomy era demonstrated benefits of early versus interval cholecystectomy for acute cholecystitis[14,15]. No trials exist for the laparoscopic procedure. When laparoscopic cholecystectomy was first introduced acute cholecystitis was considered to be a contraindication. Gradually it became clear that laparoscopic cholecystectomy can be performed safely during the phase of acute inflammation[16–18]. Patients enjoy the same postoperative benefits as in elective laparoscopic cholecystectomy. Laparoscopic cholecystectomy for acute inflammation is a longer procedure than open operation, but median postoperative stay is lower[16,17].

Conversion rates are higher when laparoscopic cholecystectomy is performed for acute cholecystitis[18], especially when empyema and gangrenous cholecystitis are present. However, the conversion rate for acute oedematous cholecystitis is the same as that for chronic cholecystitis with fibrosis. Rattner *et al.*[19] evaluated clinical factors associated with conversion. Patients requiring conversion to open cholecystectomy had longer durations of symptoms, higher white blood cell counts, higher alkaline phosphatase, and higher APACHE II scores.

Ultrasonographic findings, such as gallbladder distension, wall thickness and pericholecystic fluid, did not correlate with the success of laparoscopic cholecystectomy.

Several studies have commented on the relationship between biliary injury and performance of laparoscopic cholecystectomy during the acute phase of inflammation. Certainly there can be an increased degree of technical difficulty during acute inflammation. Laparoscopic cholecystectomy should not be attempted if the inflammation has been present for more than 72 hours, because of increased vascularity and tissue oedema. In these circumstances non-operative therapy should be initiated, and elective 'interval' laparoscopic cholecystectomy be performed 2–3 months later. Although conversion rates are somewhat higher[7], interval laparoscopic cholecystectomy can usually be successfully completed, and this procedure has all the usual advantages of a laparoscopic cholecystectomy over an open cholecystectomy. Surgeons should be experienced in performance of elective laparoscopic cholecystectomy before operating in the presence of acute inflammation, and should be ready to convert when unable to identify anatomical structures, or to control bleeding. Laparoscopic cholecystectomy is also contraindicated in the presence of gallbladder rupture with peritonitis, since the abdomen cannot be properly cleaned laparoscopically.

When patients fail conservative therapy we prefer to perform percutaneous cholecystostomy[20] followed by interval laparoscopic cholecystectomy, rather than open cholecystectomy in the acute phase. The former preserves the minimally invasive nature of the treatment.

Gallstone pancreatitis

Gallstones are a common cause of acute pancreatitis. In the era of open cholecystectomy studies showed that cholecystectomy should be performed during the initial admission for the attack of gallstone pancreatitis[21]. This strategy avoided bouts of pancreatitis in the interval between the initial attack and cholecystectomy, and diminished the total duration of hospitalization. With laparoscopic cholecystectomy the issues are the need for preoperative endoscopic retrograde cholangiopancreatography (ERCP) and, once again, the timing of the cholecystectomy. Preoperative ERCP was performed routinely in two series totalling 40 patients; common bile duct (CBD) stones were seen and removed in 29% and 43% of patients[22,23]. Laparoscopic cholecystectomy was subsequently performed in 100% and 88% of the patients. In one series the technical difficulty of laparoscopic cholecystectomy in the presence of acute gallstone pancreatitis was judged to be increased[22]. There was no relationship between the presence of CBD stones and severity of pancreatitis. In these series, median postoperative stay was 2 days and there were no procedure-related complications. In two other series of laparoscopic cholecystectomy procedures in the setting of acute biliary pancreatitis, preoperative ERCP was not performed[24,25]. Intraoperative cholangiograms were obtained in 76% and 83% of patients respectively, and CBD stones were discovered in 11% of patients in both series. We recently reviewed the outcomes of 57 patients with gallstone pancreatitis, 86% of whom underwent laparoscopic cholecystectomy[26]. Open cholecystectomy was performed in 14%

of patients due to presumed contraindications to the laparoscopic approach, including pancreatic necrosis requiring debridement. Preoperative ERCP was performed in 59% of patients and CBD stones were discovered and treated successfully by sphincterotomy in 30% of the entire group. Thus, ERCP was negative in half of those patients examined. Of the six patients with CBD stones demonstrated by laparoscopic intraoperative cholangiography, transcystic duct clearance was successful in five. Small stones were allowed to remain in place in the other patient who had undergone preoperative sphincterotomy and the stones subsequently passed spontaneously. In another series of 71 patients with gallstone pancreatitis[27], preoperative ERCP performed in 22 patients revealed CBD stones in seven, i.e. 32% of those studied and 10% of the whole group.

Based on historical data and these recent reports, the following recommendations for the current management of acute gallstone pancreatitis are suggested:

1. Urgent ERCP with sphincterotomy if necessary is indicated for those patients with severe ongoing pancreatitis, cholangitis, or CBD stones demonstrated by sonographic examination.
2. Laparoscopic cholecystectomy may be performed in most patients during the index admission without preoperative ERCP; intraoperative cholangiography should be performed routinely, with laparoscopic extraction of CBD stones if demonstrated. Postoperative ERCP should be used for residual stones where endoscopic expertise is high.
3. As effective debridement of necrotic pancreas is presently not feasible laparoscopically, clinical evidence of necrotizing pancreatitis should prompt a computerized tomography (CT) scan; if necrosis is identified, open operative debridement combined with cholecystectomy is the procedure of choice.

Acute cholangitis. There is no place for laparoscopic cholecystectomy in the treatment of this life-threatening condition. Laparoscopic cholecystectomy is performed as an interval procedure after recovery.

COMPLICATIONS OF LAPAROSCOPIC CHOLECYSTECTOMY

Biliary injuries

This is the most important problem in laparoscopic cholecystectomy. We recently reviewed this subject[28]. Biliary injury causes great morbidity and cost. Four reliable reports[3,29–31] suggest that the major bile duct injury rate is between 0.3% and 0.6%. If all biliary injuries are considered the injury rate ranges from 0.6% to 1.5%. This is 3–4 times higher than reported rates for open cholecystectomy.

Most reports include both major bile duct injuries and 'bilomas' or 'bile leaks'. The latter are more common during laparoscopic cholecystectomy than in open cholecystectomy. To deal with this development we proposed a classification more appropriate for the laparoscopic era[28] (Fig. 1). Type A injuries are injuries to minor ducts without loss of continuity of the biliary tree. Almost all such injuries are due to failure to properly occlude the cystic duct, or are due to an injury to a small bile duct in the liver bed. Type B and C injuries

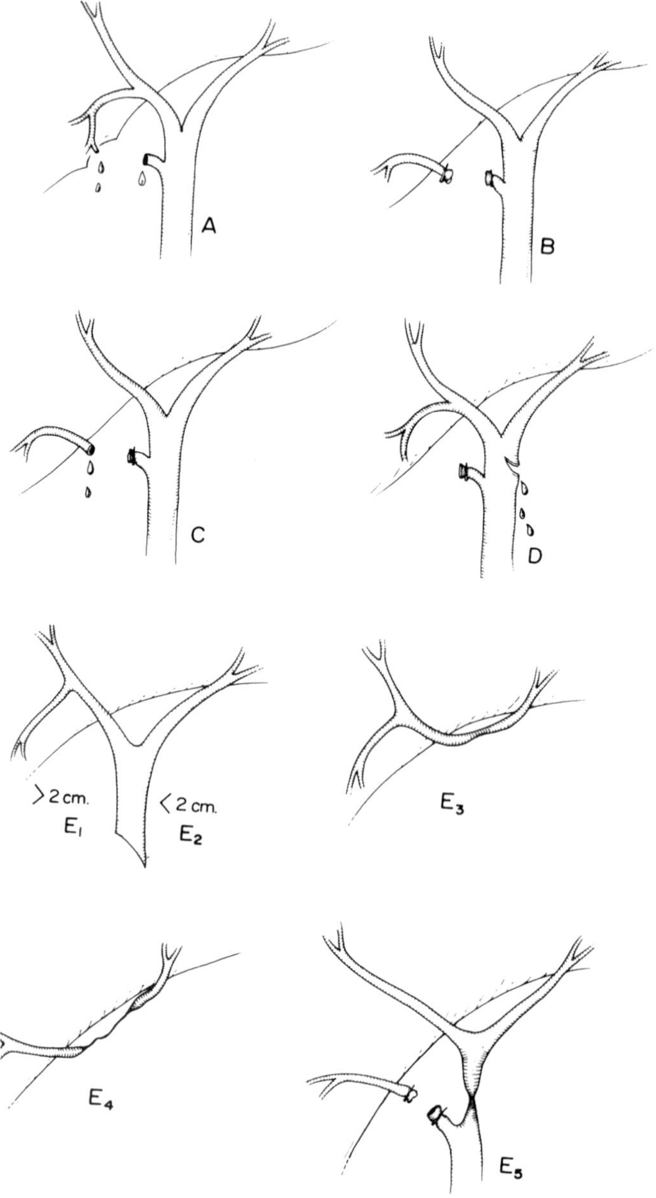

Fig. 1 A new classification of laparoscopic injuries to the biliary tract. The injuries type A to E are illustrated. Type E injuries are subdivided according to the Bismuth classification. Type A injuries originate from small bile ducts that are entered in the liver bed or from the cystic duct. Type B and C injuries almost always involve aberrant right hepatic ducts. Type A, C, D, and some E injuries may cause bilomas or fistulae. Type B and other type E injuries occlude the biliary tree and bilomas do not occur. The notations >2 cm and <2 cm in type E1 and type E2 indicate the length of common hepatic duct remaining. (By permission of the *Journal of the American College of Surgeons*)

are injuries to aberrant right hepatic bile ducts. Although aberrant right bile ducts are present in only 2% of patients, it seems such patients are very susceptible to injury during laparoscopic surgery. In type B injuries the ducts are occluded, while in type C transection is the problem; both have the common feature of discontinuity of the biliary tree, but have different clinical presentations. Type D injuries, like type A injuries, are lateral injuries, but are more serious because they involve the main ducts and can progress to type E injuries. Type E injuries are also injuries to the main bile ducts. There are five types and these are grouped according to the Bismuth classification of major ductal injuries produced at open cholecystectomy. Type A and E injuries predominate in reports from referral centres[28]. However, it is likely that type D and A injuries are really the most common, since most of these injuries can be treated locally without referral to a tertiary centre.

Risk factors include experience of the surgeon, local operative risk factors such as acute and chronic inflammation, and aberrant anatomy, especially of the right duct. Direct causes of injury are misidentification of ductal anatomy or technical errors. Misidentification of the common duct as the cystic duct leads to type D or E[28] injuries, and misidentification of an aberrant right duct as the cystic duct leads to type B or C injuries. Misidentification tends to occur in the presence of acute or chronic inflammation. The technical causes of biliary injury are injudicious use of cautery, improper closure of the cystic duct and too deep a plane of dissection on the liver bed. Prevention of injury requires that the operation be performed by trained surgeons who avoid difficult situations such as acute cholecystitis until experience is gained. The key to avoiding injury due to misidentification is conclusive identification of the cystic duct and artery, since these are the structures to be divided[28]. Routine operative cholangiography has not lessened injury in published series, although it may lessen the extent of injury, by providing early diagnosis[28]. The most serious technical problem is cautery injury. This may be avoided by either not using cautery in the portal dissection, or using it on low settings and only on small pieces of tissue that are lifted off underlying structures.

Biliary injuries are best managed by a team of biliary endoscopists, interventional radiologists and hepatobiliary–pancreatic surgeons. The clinical presentations of type A and type E injury tend to be distinct[28]. Type A injuries are usually recognized in the early postoperative period. Type E injuries are most often recognized during the first week after surgery also, but some are also recognized intraoperatively and a few (5%) present more than 1 month after surgery. Type A injuries usually present with pain and sepsis, due to an intraperitoneal collection of bile. In some cases the presentation is a bile fistula. Patients with type A injuries are almost never jaundiced. Conversely most patients with type E injuries appear with painless jaundice.

If a biliary injury is diagnosed intraoperatively conversion and immediate repair are almost always mandatory. For patients first presenting in the postoperative period, investigation depends on the mode of presentation, i.e. pain/sepsis, jaundice, or fistula. With pain/sepsis, ultrasound or CT is used to search for intraperitoneal fluid collections. Collections are drained percutaneously to determine if they contain bile and, if so, scintigraphy is done to determine if the leak is continuing. If there is a continuing bile, diagnostic ERCP is done. In almost all type A injuries, some type D injuries and a few type E injuries, treatment occurs during the same ERCP procedure. Type A injuries are treated by endoscopic sphincterotomy and an internal stent or a nasobiliary catheter. In patients presenting with jaundice ERCP is the first investigation. The distal duct will usually be found to be occluded or transected, and continuity to the proximal duct lost. In these cases percutaneous transhepatic cholangiography (PTC) is needed to outline the proximal ducts and to provide bile drainage. Stenting may be performed at this time by ERCP or PTC if the problem is a stenosis. In our experience stenting usually fails unless the stenotic segment is short (less than 1 cm), or partial. With an external bile fistula the first investigation should be a fistulagram. Subsequent management depends upon results.

Surgery is required in type A and D injuries that have failed closed treatment, type B injuries that need treatment, all type C injuries, and most type E injuries. Hepatico-jejunostomy is the treatment of choice for type B, C and E injuries[28]. Percutaneous stents are useful guides to the position of the ducts. The timing of surgery must take into account the degree of inflammation present, and often it is wise to delay surgery until acute inflammation has subsided. The principles of repair are to recognize all injured ducts and establish a wide mucosa-to-mucosa anastomosis without tension, with good blood supply. Most severe injuries are best treated at specialized hepatic–pancreatic–biliary (HPB) surgery units. There has been no long-term follow-up of laparoscopic biliary injuries. It is likely that the long-term recurrence will be in the order of 20%, most recurrences presenting in the first 3 years after repair.

Other complications of laparoscopic cholecystectomy

Cardiopulmonary complications are less common after laparoscopic surgery than after open surgery. This is probably due to reduction in postoperative upper abdominal pain and resulting improvement in pulmonary function[32]. The commonest complication is a wound infection, occurring in 1–2% of patients; this is a minor problem compared to infection of a laparotomy incision. There have been other major, but rare, complications such as bowel or vascular injuries[33], which may almost always be avoided by open pneumoperitoneum using the Hasson technique[34]. There are reports of hernias at the umbilical trocar site; these are avoidable by suture of this incision when the trocar is removed. Spillage of stones during laparoscopic cholecystectomy is not a rare event, occurring in about 10% of operations. Leaving stones in the peritoneal cavity may result in intra-abdominal abscess, subcutaneous abscess and later discharge of stones through the abdominal wall, or through the lung and trachea[35,36].

References

1. Strasberg SM, Clavien P-A. Cholecystolithiasis. Lithotherapy for the 1990s. Hepatology. 1992;16:820–39.
2. Lagoretta AP, Silber JH, Constantino GN, Kobylinski RW, Zatz SL. Increased cholecystectomy rate after the introduction of laparoscopic cholecystectomy. J Am Med Assoc. 1993;270:1429–32.
3. Orlando III R, Russell JC, Lynch J, Mattie A. Laparoscopic cholecystectomy, a statewide experience. Arch Surg. 1993;128:494–9.

4. Steiner CA, Bass EB, Talamini MA, Pitt HA, Steinberg EP. Surgical rates and operative mortality for open and laparoscopic cholecystectomy in Maryland. N Engl J Med. 1994;330:403–8.

5. Goodale RL, Beebe DS, McNevin MP *et al.* Hemodynamic, respiratory and metabolic effects of laparoscopic cholecystectomy. Am J Surg. 1993;166:533–7.

6. Collure DW, Bumpers HL, Luchette FA, Weaver WL, Hoover EL. Laparoscopic cholecystectomy in patients with ventriculoperitoneal (VP) shunts. Surg Endosc. 1995;9:409–10.

7. Sanabria JR, Gallanger S, Croxford R, Strasberg SM. Risk factors in laparoscopic cholecystectomy for conversion to open cholecystectomy. J Am Coll Surg. 1994;179:696–704

8. Strasberg SM Callery, MP Soper NJ. Hepatobiliary surgery during pregnancy. In: Reyes HB, Leuschner U, Arias IM, editors. Pregnancy, sex hormones and the liver. Dordrecht: Kluwer; 1996:282–94.

9. D'Albuquerque LA, de Miranda MP, Genzini T, Copstein JL, de Oliveira e Silva A. Laparoscopic cholecystectomy in cirrhotic patients. Surg Laparosc Endosc. 1995;5:272–6.

10. Lacy AM, Balaguer C, Andrade E *et al.* Laparoscopic cholecystectomy in cirrhotic patients. Indication or contradiction? Surg Endosc. 1995;9:407–8.

11. Vinograd I, Halevy A, Klin B *et al.* Laparoscopic cholecystectomy: treatment of choice for cholelithiasis in children. World J Surg. 1993;17:263–6.

12. Davidoff AM, Branum GD, Murray EA *et al.* The technique of laparoscopic cholecystectomy in children. Ann Surg. 1992;215:186–91.

13. Callery MP, Soper NJ. Laparoscopic management of complicated biliary tract disease in children. Surg Laparosc Endosc. (In press).

14. Jarvinin H, Hastbacka J. Early cholecystectomy for acute cholecystitis. A randomized controlled study. Ann Surg. 1980;191:501–5.

15. Lahtinen J, Alhava EM, Aukee S. Acute cholecystitis treated by early and delayed surgery. A controlled clinical trial. Scand J Gastroenterol. 1978;13:673–8.

16. Zucker KA, Flowers JL, Bailey RW, Graham SM, Bueli J, Imbembo AL. Laparoscopic management of acute cholecystitis. Am J Surg. 1993;165:508–14.

17. Cox MR, Wilson TG, Luck AJ, Jeans PL, Padbury RTA, Toouli J. Laparoscopic cholecystectomy for acute inflammation of the gallbladder. Ann Surg. 1993;218:630–4.

18. Wilson RG, Macintyre IM, Nixon SJ, Saunders JH, Varma JS, King PM. Laparoscopic cholecystectomy as a safe and effective treatment for severe acute cholecystitis. Br J Med. 1992;305:394–5.

19. Rattner DW, Ferguson C, Warshaw AL. Factors associated with successful laparoscopic cholecystectomy for acute cholecystitis. Ann Surg. 1993;217:233–6.

20. Picus D, Hicks ME, Darcy MD *et al.* Percutaneous cholecystolithotomy: analysis of results and complications in 58 consecutive patients. Radiology. 1992;183:779–84.

21. Kelly TR, Wagner DS. Gallstone pancreatitis: a prospective randomized trial of timing of surgery. Surgery. 1988;104:600–5.

22. Tate JJT, Lau WY, Li AKC. Laparoscopic cholecystectomy for biliary pancreatitis. Br J Surg. 1994;81:720–2.

23. Rhodes M, Armonstrong CP, Longstaff A, Cawthorn S. Laparoscopic cholecystectomy with endoscopic retrograde cholangiopancreatography for acute gallstone pancreatitis. Br J Surg. 1993;80:247.

24. Graham LD, Burrus RG, Burns RP, Chandler KE, Barker DE. Laparoscopic cholecystectomy in biliary pancreatitis. Am Surg. 1994;60:40–3.

25. Taylor EW, Dunham RH, Bloch JH. Laparoscopic management of gallstone pancreatitis. J Laparoendosc Surg. 1994;4:121–5.

26. Soper NJ, Brunt LM, Callery MP, Edmundowicz SA, Aliperti G. Role of laparoscopic cholecystectomy in the management of acute gallstone pancreatitis. Am J Surg. 1994;167:42–51.

27. de Virgilio C, Verbin C, Chang L, Linder S, Stabile BE, Klein S. Gallstone pancreatitis. The role of preoperative endoscopic retrograde cholangiopancreatography. Arch Surg. 1994;129:909–13.

28. Strasberg SM, Hertl M, Soper NJ. An analysis of the problem of biliary injury during laparoscopic cholecystectomy. J Am Coll Surg. 1995;180:101–25.

29. Bernard HR, Hartman TW. Complications after laparoscopic cholecystectomy. Am J Surg. 1993;165:533–5.

30. Wherry DC, Rog CG, Marohn MR, Rich NM. An external audit of laparoscopic cholecystectomy performed in medical treatment facilities of the Department of Defense. Ann Surg. 1994;220:626–34.

31. Adamsen S, Hansen OH, Jensen PF *et al.* Bile duct injury in laparoscopic cholecystectomy in Denmark. Gastroenterology. 1995;108:404.
32. Coelho JC, de Araujo RP, Marchesini JB, Coelho IC, de Araujo LR. Pulmonary function after cholecystectomy performed through Kocher's incision, a mini-incision and laparoscopy. World J Surg. 1993;17:544–6.
33. Alpegren KN, Scheeres DE. Aortic injury. A catastrophic complication of laparoscopic cholecystectomy. Surg Endosc. 1994;8:689–91.
34. Strasberg SM, Sanabria JR, Clavien P-A. Complications of laparoscopic cholecystectomy. Can J Surg. 1992;35:275–80.
35. Leslie KA, Rankin RN, Duff JH. Lost gallstones during laparoscopic cholecystectomy: are they really benign? Can J Surg. 1994;37:240–2.
36. Downie GH, Robbins MK, Sousa JJ, Paradowski LJ. Cholelithoptysis. A complication following laparoscopic cholecystectomy. Chest. 1993;103:616–17.

25
Therapy of choledocholithiasis – endoscopic techniques

S. BOHNACKER, K. F. BINMOELLER and N. SOEHENDRA

INTRODUCTION

Having been introduced by Demling, Classen[1] and Kawai et al.[2] in 1974, endoscopic papillotomy (EPT) is now established as treatment of choice for choledocholithiasis. Dilatation of the papilla, as suggested by Staritz et al.[3], is suitable only for smaller stones, and is therefore not widely accepted. In multicentre studies on long-term results of EPT[4], earlier concerns about the possible consequences of duodenobiliary reflux have proved to be clinically insignificant. EPT can be tailored according to the number and size of stones. Technically EPT is no more difficult than dilatation; in contrast, it facilitates the insertion of accessories and extraction of larger stones. Following EPT, smaller stones or fragments easily missed on fluoroscopy can pass spontaneously.

TECHNIQUE OF PAPILLOTOMY

Endoscopic incision of the papilla of Vater is usually performed using the Erlanger papillotome. This instrument consists of an approximately 20 mm cutting steel wire mounted on the tip of a 5–6 Fr catheter. After cannulation of the common bile duct the papillotome is retracted until approximately half of the cutting wire is visible in the porus of the papilla. Then the incision in an 11–12 o'clock direction is performed. Selective cannulation of the common bile duct is mandatory for this procedure, to avoid injury to the pancreatic duct.

Two modifications have been added to the original technique to allow for successful management of difficult cases:

1. *Wire-guided papillotomy*: cannulation of the common bile duct is often easier over a hydrophilic wire (Terumo, Tokyo, Japan or Tracer wire, Wilson-Cook Medical Inc., USA). A double-lumen papillotome can then be inserted over the wire.
2. *Precut*: this technique can be useful if selective cannulation of the common bile duct fails. The roof of the papilla is incised to visualize the orifices of

the common bile duct and pancreatic duct. This facilitates the selective cannulation of either duct. If the technique is mastered this method can be very helpful. However, if attempted inexpertly it may induce a higher complication rate[5].

The Billroth-II resected stomach remains a challenge to endoscopists owing to the altered anatomical situation. Particular experience and special devices are required for successful negotiation of the caudo-cranial working direction[6]. In patients with a very long afferent loop (e.g. after antecolic or Roux-en-Y anastomosis), the duodenal stump is often beyond reach. Such patients may be successfully treated using a combined percutaneous–transhepatic and endoscopic approach ('rendezvous' technique).

TECHNIQUE OF STONE EXTRACTION

Following successful papillotomy, stones should be removed in the same session to prevent impaction and cholangitis. Spontaneous passage can be expected only in the case of small stones. Stone extraction from the common bile duct is best performed with a Dormia basket; balloon catheters are suitable for smaller and soft stones. If complete clearance cannot be achieved in one session, a nasobiliary catheter or an endoprosthesis should be placed, to prevent complications from stone impaction. A nasobiliary catheter is more inconvenient for the patient, but offers the possibility of rinsing the bile duct and allows for repeat cholangiography to assess the status of ductal clearance.

Difficult stone extraction is usually due to larger size and/or number of stones. Impacted stones pose a special therapeutic problem. For these cases various lithotripsy techniques are currently available.

TECHNIQUE OF INTRADUCTAL LITHOTRIPSY

Fragmentation of stones prior to extraction is necessary if stones are impacted or too large (larger than 20 mm). For the transpapillary route, mechanical, electrohydraulic and laser lithotripsy, using the mother/babyscope system, are available.

Mechanical lithotripsy (ML)

This technique is the most simple one. The stone is entrapped into the basket and crushed against a metal probe[7]. However, this method can be applied only if the stone is not impacted and can be engaged completely into the basket. Mechanical lithotripsy can be performed either through the endoscope (TTS Lithotriptor from Olympus) or after withdrawal of the endoscope (Lithotriptor from Wilson-Cook). The Wilson-Cook lithotriptor is used mainly for emergency cases in which the stone captured in the basket becomes impacted in the distal CBD.

Electrohydraulic lithotripsy (EHL)

Shockwaves generated by the electrohydraulic lithotriptor (Lithotron EL 23, Fa. Walz Electronic Inc., Germany) are very effective for crushing large impacted bile duct stones. Exact targeting of the electrode on the stone is mandatory, as tissue injury is possible. In other words, EHL can be performed only under direct endoscopic vision. A motherscope is therefore required, through which a babyscope is introduced transpapillary into the bile duct (TJF M20 and CHF B20, Olympus Optical Co., Japan). The babyscope has a 1.7 mm working channel to accommodate the 4.5 Fr EHL probe. A nasobiliary catheter is placed to allow for continuous water irrigation, providing clear vision and liquid medium around the stone for effective conduction of shockwaves.

Laser-induced shockwave lithotripsy (LISL)

Shockwaves induced by pulsed laser (Nd: YAG laser and dye laser) are also effective for disintegrating bile duct stones[8] but their efficacy is less than that of EHL. The advantage of LISL compared to EHL is that the very thin laser probe can be passed through a thinner babyscope, which may be introduced through a standard duodenoscope, avoiding the need for the motherscope. However, for EHL, 3 Fr probes are now available, so that a thinner babyscope that fits to the regular therapeutic duodenoscope can be used.

The rhodamine-6G laser lithotriptor 'Lithognost' (Fa. Telemit Corp., Germany) shows promise. The machine provides stone tissue recognition sensors that allow lithotripsy to be performed without endoscopic monitoring. The high cost of this laser machine may be partly balanced by the fact that a mother–babyscope system is not necessary[9].

EXTRACORPOREAL SHOCKWAVE LITHOTRIPSY (ESWL)

ESWL is also effective for fragmentation of common bile duct (CBD) stones. For treatment of bile duct stones, especially those located in the distal CBD, a machine with fluoroscopic guidance may be required, since visualization of stones in this area by ultrasound is often difficult. Not all CBD stones can be fragmented by ESWL. According to a German multicentre study the success rate of ESWL amounted to 86% with a morbidity rate of 36% (mostly minor complications) and a mortality rate of 1.8%[10]. We use ESWL preferably for treatment of intrahepatic stones.

POSSIBILITIES AND LIMITATIONS OF ENDOSCOPIC CBD STONE EXTRACTION

The results of endoscopic treatment of choledocholithiasis are highly endoscopist-dependent. Success rates vary according to local situations. Papillotomy may be successful in almost all cases if all techniques are mastered. Procedure-related complications include acute pancreatitis, bleeding and perforation with an average rate of less than 5%. The mortality rate is less than 0.5%[11,12].

Patients with Billroth-II resected stomach or Roux-en-Y anastomosis may be difficult or even impossible to treat because of long afferent loops. The 'rendezvous' technique using a combined endoscopic and percutaneous–transhepatic approach is associated with a higher procedural risk, complication rates being approximately twice as high compared to endoscopic transpapillary treatment. The risks of this technique have therefore to be weighed carefully against those of surgery, and an individual decision should be made in each case, taking the experience and infrastructure availability into consideration.

So-called difficult bile duct stones are encountered in 13.7% of our patients with bile duct stones[13]. Most of these were stones measuring more than 20 mm. Following fragmentation using mechanical lithotripsy, 30.6% of these stones could be removed completely from the bile duct. In another 60.2% of cases the stones were impacted and had to be fragmented by EHL. Following successful lithotripsy using EHL, complete clearance of the bile duct could be achieved in all cases. There were no complications except for one biliary leakage, which could be managed conservatively. This complication occurred in a patient with Mirizzi's syndrome and obviously resulted from stone-induced pressure necrosis. There was no procedure-related mortality. In 781 cases with bile duct stones (mean age of patients 72 years), the overall success rate of endoscopic treatment was 99.5%. Of these patients, 10 (1.3%) had intrahepatic stones and underwent ESWL treatment. In three cases complete stone clearance could not be achieved because of ductal strictures. One patient of poor surgical risk died of suppurative cholangitis and septicaemia.

CBD stones can be removed endoscopically in almost 100% of cases when all available methods are applied. Even impacted cystic duct stones obstructing the common bile duct (Mirizzi's syndrome) can be removed by the endoscopic transpapillary approach using EHL[14]. Surgical exploration of the bile duct is rarely necessary. For those few patients in whom endoscopy fails, the percutaneous–transhepatic approach can be attempted. For inoperable patients with stone-induced obstructive jaundice, endoscopic stenting may be a sufficient palliative measure[15]. Our treatment algorithm for difficult bile duct stones is shown in Fig. 1.

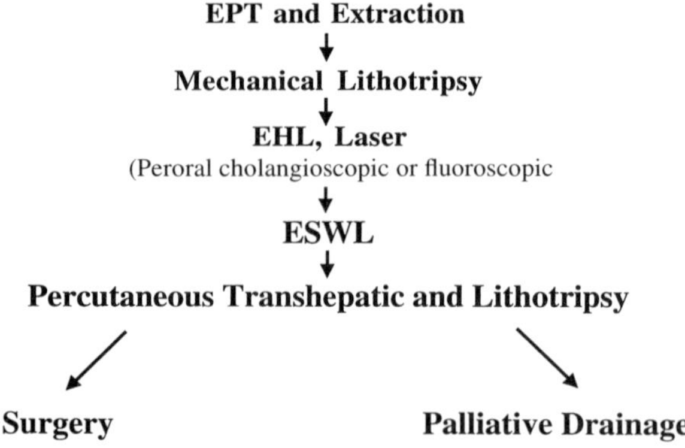

Fig. 1 Algorithm for the treatment of bile duct stones

LAPAROSCOPIC REMOVAL OF BILE DUCT STONES?

Further advances in laparoscopic surgery have raised the question of whether bile duct stones should be removed during laparoscopic cholecystectomy[16–18]. At the current stage of development we consider only the transcystic approach without choledochotomy to be a reasonable alternative to transpapillary endoscopic stone extraction. The results of the laparoscopic approach are difficult to interpret since patients are highly selected. The question that needs to be answered is: what proportion of patients with symptomatic CBD stones are reasonable candidates for laparoscopic–transcystic stone removal? We performed a 1-year study in which all patients referred to our unit for endoscopic treatment of choledocholithiasis were also evaluated for their suitability for laparoscopic–transcystic stone extraction. A patient found to meet one or more of the following criteria was determined to be 'unsuitable' for laparoscopic–transcystic stone extraction: (a) clinical jaundice, cholangitis, pancreatitis; (b) stone larger than 10 mm; (c) stone number greater than three; (d) stone(s) proximal to the cystic duct insertion; (e) stone impaction; (f) microlithiasis. According to these criteria the laparoscopic method was found to be unsuitable in 99% of all patients.

The Society of American Gastrointestinal Endoscopic Surgeons have recently conducted a survey on laparoscopic treatment of choledocholithiasis: 83% of their members voted for endoscopic stone removal prior to laparoscopic surgery and 80% for endoscopic treatment after surgery[19]. This can be explained by the high success rate and low procedural risk of endoscopic stone extraction, and technical inadequacies and limited experience with the laparoscopic method. Further developments in laparoscopic surgery will determine whether the laparoscopic approach will play a larger role relative to the endoscopic approach. At present we recommend the algorithm for the management of symptomatic cholelithiasis as shown in Fig. 2.

References

1. Classen M, Demling L. Endoskopische Sphinkterotomie der Papilla Vateri und Steinextraktion aus dem Ductus choledochus. Dtsch Med Wochenschr. 1974;99:496.
2. Kawai K, Akasaka Y, Murakami K. Endoscopic sphincterotomy of the ampulla of Vater. Gastrointest Endosc. 1974;20:148.
3. Staritz M, Ewe K, Meyer zum Büschenfelde KH. Endoscopic papillary balloon dilation (EPD) for the treatment of common bile duct stones and papillary stenosis. Endoscopy. 1983;15:197.
4. Seifert E. Long-term follow up after endoscopic sphincterotomy (EST). Endoscopy. 1988;20:232.
5. Shakoor T, Geenen JE. Pre-cut papillotomy. Gastrointest Endosc. 1992;38:623.
6. Soehendra N, Kempeneers I, Reynders-Frederix V. Ein neues Papillotom für den Billroth-II-Magen. Dtsch Med Wochenschr. 1980;105:362.
7. Demling L, Seuberth K, Riemann JF. A mechanical lithotripter. Endoscopy. 1982;14:100.
8. Ell C, Lux G, Hochberger J, Müller D, Demling L. Laser lithotripsy of common bile duct stones. Gut. 1988;29:746.
9. Ell C, Hochberger J, May A et al. Laser lithotripsy of difficult bile duct stones by means of rhodamine-6G laser and an integrated automatic stone-tissue detection system. Gastrointest Endosc. 1993;39:755.
10. Sauerbruch T, Stern M. The study group for shock-wave lithotripsy of bile duct stones. Fragmentation of bile duct stones by extracorporeal shock waves. Gastroenterology. 1989;96:146.

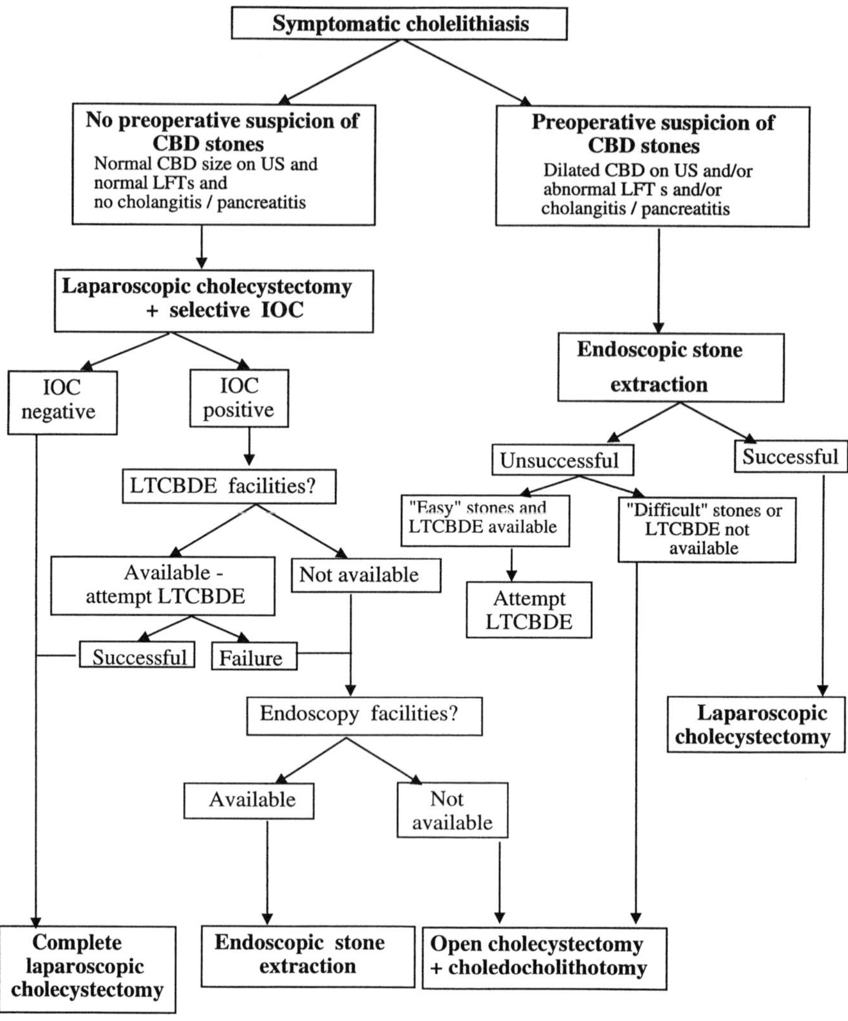

Fig. 2 Algorithm for the treatment of symptomatic cholelithiasis. CBD = common bile duct, LTCBDE = laparoscopic–transcystic common bile duct exploration, LFTs = liver function tests, US = ultrasound, IOC = intraoperative cholangiography

11. Cotton PB, Lehman G, Vennes J *et al.* Endoscopic sphincterotomy complications and their management: an attempt at consensus. Gastrointest Endosc. 1991;37:383.

12. Seifert E, Schulte F, Chalybäus C. Quo vadis endoskopische Sphinkterotomie? Z Gastroenterol. 1989;27:77.

13. Binmoeller KF, Brückner M, Thonke F, Soehendra N. Treatment of difficult bile duct stones using mechanical, electrohydraulic and extracorporeal shock wave lithotripsy. Endoscopy. 1993;25:201.

14. Binmoeller KF, Thonke F, Soehendra N. Endoscopic treatment of Mirizzi's syndrome. Gastrointest Endosc. 1993;39:532.

15. Cotton PB, Forbes A, Leung JWC, Dineen L. Endoscopic stenting for long-term treatment of large bile duct stones: 2- to 5-year follow-up. Gastrointest Endosc. 1987;33:411.
16. Petelin JB. Laparoscopic management of common bile duct pathology. Surg Endosc. 1993;7:117(A).
17. Phillips EH, Carroll BJ, Fallas MJ. Laparoscopic transcystic duct common duct exploration. Surg Endosc. 1993;7:116(A).
18. BGES (Belgian Group for Endoscopic Surgery), De Weer, F. The coelioscopic treatment of common bile duct stones: which results? Surg Endosc. 1993;7:117(A)
19. .Brodish, RJ, Fink AS. ERCP, cholangiography, and laparoscopic cholecystectomy. The Society of American Gastrointestinal Endoscopic Surgeons (SAGES) opinion survey. Surg Endosc. 1993;7:3.

Section VII
Transplantation of the liver

26
Liver transplantation: current status 1996

Y. BAYRAKTAR, A. GURAKAR, A. COLANTONI, N. DeMARIA and D. H. VAN THIEL

GENERAL CONSIDERATIONS

Liver transplantation (LTx) for desperately ill patients with end-stage liver disease has matured from an experimental operation performed at only a few centres to a well-accepted, lifesaving procedure performed at many centres worldwide. Although several different techniques for LTx exist (auxiliary, partial, orthotopic), the replacement of the native, diseased liver with a normal liver harvested from a brain-dead, heart-beating donor, placed in the orthotopic position is the preferred and most widely used approach[1].

One-year graft and patient survival rates have improved steadily over the past decade from values of 30% in the early 1980s to values of 85–90% currently[1,2]. These improvements in graft and patient survival are a result of improvements in operative technique, the selection of candidates, organ preservation, and immunosuppression. As a result, LTx has become the therapy of choice for patients with advanced end-stage liver disease and acute liver failure for whom no other medical or surgical therapy exists[1–4]. However, not all individuals with lethal liver disease are candidates for LTx.

Before beginning a discussion of clinical LTx it is necessary to define the terms used by transplant physicians and surgeons. An autograft is a transplant involving an individual's own organ or tissues. An isograft is a transplant performed using an organ obtained from a syngeneic individual or an identical twin. An allograft or homograft is a transplant between individuals having different genetic backgrounds. A xenograft is a transplant across species, such as the transplantation of other animal tissue or organs into humans.

TYPES OF LIVER TRANSPLANTS

1. Orthotopic LTx is the most frequently used procedure. It consists of the use of a cadaver donor liver to replace a diseased organ with the graft being placed in the normal anatomical location[1–4].

2. Reduced size (segmental) and split-liver transplants are modifications of orthotopic LTx wherein a part of a cadaveric organ (either the right or left lobe) is used and placed in the orthotopic position. Split-liver transplantation is a modification of reduced-size cadaveric transplantation wherein the two portions of a split cadaveric organ, usually the right lobe and left lateral segment, are used to replace the diseased liver in two different individuals, one of which is usually an infant or child[2,5–7].

3. Living donor LTx is a technique wherein a child receives a liver graft, usually the left lateral segment, from a living related donor. In living related cases the donor is usually a relative of the recipient. This procedure is usually reserved for individuals such as infants for whom a cadaveric liver is unlikely to be available or when the recipient resides in a country where cadaveric LTx is not permitted legally[2,6–8].

4. Auxiliary heterotopic transplantation is a technique wherein an individual with a potentially life-threatening but reversible liver disease, such as fulminant hepatic failure, receives a cadaveric graft placed in a non-anatomical site. With reversal of the underlying liver disease in the recipient the graft can either be removed, or the immunosuppression used can be discontinued and the graft will be rejected as the natural liver assumes all of the functions required of a normal liver[6].

HISTORY OF LTx

In 1955 Welch performed the first LTx in a dog[9]. Since then, clinical LTx has matured from an experimental procedure first performed in 1963 to an accepted lifesaving, widely performed procedure today. As noted earlier in this chapter, the current success with LTx is a consequence of improvements in surgical techniques, organ preservation, and immunosuppression occurring over the past three decades[1–4]. These include the use of steroids, cyclosporin, and, more recently, FK506 (tacrolimus); the use of the University of Wisconsin preservation fluid; and the use of different techniques for portal and hepatic vein and hepatic material vascular anastomoses[2].

GRAFT REJECTION

Graft rejection is an immunological reaction wherein the cellular and humoral immune systems of the host damage the graft as a consequence of specific immunological mechanisms[10,11]. Despite major advances in immunosuppression it remains a major problem affecting long-term graft survival. Acute cellular rejection is manifest by an infiltration of the graft (liver) with mononuclear cells consisting of T lymphocytes, eosinophils, and other mononuclear cells such as plasma cells and macrophages. These immunologically active cells usually accumulate in the portal areas, or along the vascular endothelium of the portal and hepatic venules and/or biliary epithelium[10–13].

Hyperacute rejection is a consequence of a humoral immune response wherein antibody deposition occurs along vascular endothelial surfaces followed by polymorphonuclear leucocyte adhesion leading to vascular thrombosis and ischaemic necrosis of the graft within hours (non-hepatic grafts) or several days (hepatic grafts) of the transplant procedure[10,11].

Chronic rejection is a consequence of a cellular immune response directed towards alloantigens with an activation of mononuclear cell cytokine cascades leading to organ damage, and ultimately loss of bile ducts and hepatic arterial occlusion as a consequence of an accumulation of subendothelial foam cells (histiocytes). This type of injury leads to a progressive portal fibrosis, loss of functioning bile ducts and progressive cholestatic liver disease[10–13].

ALLOGRAFT REJECTION MECHANISMS

The major histocompatibility complex (MHC or HLA) provides the antigens which provoke allograft rejection between members of the same species. The intensity of allograft-specific T lymphocyte reactivity can be established by limiting dilution analysis wherein a fixed number of irradiated allogeneic stimulator or target cells are cultured with serial dilutions of potential alloreactive lymphocytes. Individuals with a very high level of *alloreactive cells* are more likely to react with the allograft. Whereas merely a fraction of a per cent of an individual's T cell population are able to react to given alloantigens not characteristic of the individual, once transplanted, these alloantigen proteins become the signal for allograft rejection and specific host T cell proliferation directed at the allograft. Once activated, these alloantigen specific T cells produce cytokines and directly damage allograft cells, ultimately leading to graft injury and loss of graft function[11,14–16].

The specific antigens involved in graft rejection are under genetic control. Thus, uniovular twins who are genetically identical can be transplanted without the need for immunosuppression. The genes controlling these antigens have been identified and characterized by inbreeding experiments in animals, and serological and cellular antigenic studies performed in humans. Because inbred mice breed true within a given strain, and always accept grafts from animals of the identified strain, they are presumed to be homozygous for 'transplantation' or major histocompatibility (MHC) genes. Let us consider two such inbred strains, P and R, with MHC genes differing at only one locus as a result of inbreeding until the progeny have a common genetic constitution, either P/P or R/R respectively. Crossing animals of strains P and R yields a first generation (F1) of animals having a MHC constitution P/R. All of the F1 generation animals will accept a graft from either parent as they are tolerant to both P and R strains. By crossing pairs of the F1 generation, a F2 generation is produced, consisting of an average distribution of MHC genotypes as follows: P/P, P/R, P/R, and R/R. One in four of the F2 generations would have no P genes and would therefore reject a graft because of a lack of tolerance for P antigens. Similarly one in four would reject an R graft for the same reason, lack of R antigen tolerance. Conversely, two of four being PR would accept a graft from either parent, as they would be tolerant to both P and R antigens[11,17–21].

Although approximately 40 different antigenic loci have been established in the mouse, some are predominant in that they control the expression of 'strong' transplantation antigens which are capable of provoking intense allograft reactions. Other loci control minor transplantation antigens. The term 'minor' does not imply that these antigens do not give rise to serious rejection problems, rather they do so either more slowly or less frequently[17–23].

When transplant antigens (MHC in other animals and HLA in humans) are not compatible between a donor organ or tissue, the recipient T cells are stimulated to become blast cells and proliferate. Mixing lymphocytes having different MHC or HLA antigens together *in vitro* (mixed lymphocytic reaction) leads to the proliferation of lymphocytes reacting to MHC class II determinants on the surface of the other lymphocyte population. During this reaction, many different proteins (cytokines) are produced by the transformed activated lymphocytes. The mixed lymphocyte reaction is the *in-vitro* equivalent of an *in-vivo* rejection reaction. It is possible to make the cells in either situation unresponsive to each other with the addition of powerful immunosuppressive agents. Among various lymphocytes subpopulations, the CD4 T lymphocytes are the predominant responding cells, and are stimulated by the presence of different MHC or HLA class II determinants present on B lymphocytes, macrophages and particularly dendritic antigen-presenting cells (APC). It is also possible to inhibit the mixed lymphocyte reaction by the addition of antisera to class II determinants on the stimulator cells, or by treatment of responding cells with cellular toxins such as mitomycin C, irradiation and, as noted earlier, with the use of powerful immunosuppressive agents[11,17,24,25].

In addition to lymphocyte proliferation, a second consequence of MHC incompatibility is cell-mediated lympholysis (CML). The MHC class II antigens involved in the initiation of transplantation rejection manifested by CML can be used as a test for histocompatibility (or lack thereof) manifested by the presence of cytotoxic T cells directed at antigen determinants of potential donor cells[17,25,26].

The third consequence of MHC or HLA incompatibility is the graft-versus-host reaction. When competent T cells are transplanted from a donor (via the graft) to a recipient, who is not able to reject the transferred T cells, the graft T cells survive and react to host antigens. Subsequently they proliferate, and can attack the host or recipient. Instead of the normal transplantation reaction of host cells reacting to a transplanted tissue or organ, a reverse reaction, wherein the grafted donor T cells react to the recipient's cells, occurs as the graft-versus-host reaction[27]. In humans this phenomenon is manifested clinically as fever, splenomegaly, weight loss, diarrhoea, and anaemia[28]. During this reaction, as occurs also in allograft rejection reactions, cytokines (particularly tumour necrosis factor, TNF) are generated. In both allograft rejections and graft-versus-host disease, the stronger the transplantation antigen difference between host and graft, the more severe the resultant immunological reaction[27].

THE PREVENTION OF ALLOGRAFT REJECTION

The methods available for prevention of graft reaction are: (1) suppression of the immune system using powerful immunosuppressive drugs, or (2) selection of well-matched individuals as donors and recipients.

Knowledge about MHC or HLA antigens in humans has increased considerably. The following generalizations can be made:

1. Three classes of HLA gene products or antigens are encoded within the 4-kilobase region of the MHC locus. Class I antigens consist of a heavy and light chain polypeptide complexes which are expressed on virtually all cell surfaces. They are further subdivided as HLA-A and HLA-B antigens. Class II HLA antigens consist of two polypeptide chains of unequal length which are expressed on the surface of B lymphocytes, some monocytes, and activated T lymphocytes, and are encoded by closely linked genes, collectively termed HLA-D antigens. Class III HLA antigens consist of the C4, C2, and Bf components of complement[11].
2. Class I and II antigens are directed at self-versus-non-self discrimination, and are the effector phases of the immune response[11].

The clinical use of immunosuppressant drugs such as FK506 (tacrolimus) and cyclosporin A has remarkably reduced the untoward effects of mismatching HLA antigens in solid organ transplantations[11,29,30]. Matching donors and recipients for DR antigens (MHC class II antigens) is the most important factor responsible for long-term graft survival in the absence of immunosuppression. Its role is greater in kidney than in liver transplantation[30].

THE MECHANISMS OF LIVER GRAFT ACCEPTANCE AND TOLERANCE

The transplanted liver was the first allograft to be identified as having a chimeric composition. Recent experimental and clinical studies have shown that, within minutes of the transplant, normally sessile, but potentially migratory leucocytes that are part of the normal architecture of the graft leave the graft and migrate throughout the recipient. At the same time recipient cells migrate into and replace the donor cells that exit the graft without disturbing the highly specialized donor parenchymal cells. Graft tissue leucocytes, including Kupffer cells and sinusoidal endothelial cells in the recipient, manifest the recipient phenotype within 100 days of the transplant. In contrast, the hepatocytes continue to retain donor specificity[17,31].

The same process occurs in successfully transplanted small intestine. The epithelium of the transplanted bowel retains donor specificity while the lymphoid, dendritic, and other leucocytes within the lamina propria manifest host specificity[31,32].

This cell migration phenomenon makes comprehensible the unexpected inability of donor-recipient HLA matching to accurately predict the outcome of whole-organ transplantation. Neither the transplanted organ nor the recipient remains the same soon after the transplant procedure is concluded. Both become chimeras (e.g. have cells with donor and recipient HLA specificity). The role of chimerism in long-term graft acceptance or tolerance is currently highly controversial[31,32].

INDICATIONS FOR LTx

Candidates for LTx are individuals who have irreversible liver disease for which alternative medical or surgical treatments have been exhausted, or do not exist. Table 1 lists the hepatic diseases for which LTx can be utilized. The specific evaluation of a potential liver transplant candidate varies considerably, depending on specific disease indication for which the liver transplant is being considered. The first goals of a transplant evaluation are to identify a specific liver disease diagnosis, to stage the disease and finally to determine whether or not alternative therapies are available. If no other therapy is available, identifying the timing of the transplant procedure is critically important in determining the clinical outcome and cost of LTx.

Table 1a Indications for liver transplantation in adults

  I. *Parenchymal liver disease*
      Chronic viral liver disease
         Virus B (HBV-DNA negative)
         Virus C
         Virus D
      Chronic drug-induced liver disease
      Alcoholic liver disease
      Chronic autoimmune liver disease
      Cryptogenic liver cirrhosis

  II. *Cholestatic liver disease*
      Chronic drug reactions (rare)
      Chronic hepatic rejection
      Graft-versus-host disease
      Primary biliary cirrhosis
      Secondary biliary cirrhosis
      Primary sclerosing cholangitis

  III. *Vascular disease of the liver*
      Budd–Chiari syndrome
      Veno-occlusive disease

  IV. *Metabolic liver disease*
      Wilson's disease
      Haemochromatosis
      Alpha-1 antitrypsin deficiency

  V. *Malignant hepatic disease*
      Hepatocellular carcinoma
      Hepatoblastoma
      Metastatic neuroendocrine tumours

  VI. *Fulminant liver failure*
      Viral hepatitis: A, B, C, D, E and Epstein–Barr virus
      Acute alcoholic hepatitis
      Drug induced–acute toxic hepatitis
      Metabolic liver disease
         Organic aciduria
         Reye's syndrome
         Fulminant Wilson's disease
         Acute fatty liver of pregnancy

Table 1b   Indications for liver transplantation in children

I. *Inherited disorders of metabolism*
 Wilson's disease
 Tyrosinaemia
 Glycogen storage disease (types I and IV)
 Homozygous type IIA hypercholesterolaemia
 Lysosomal storage diseases
 Protoporphyria
 Crigler–Najjar disease (type I)
 Type A and B haemophilia
 Oxalosis
 Alpha-1 antitrypsin deficiency

II. *Cholestatic liver disease*
 Biliary atresia
 Neonatal hepatitis
 Alagille's syndrome
 Byler's disease

III. *Parenchymal liver disease*
 Hepatitis B and C
 Autoimmune liver disease
 Cryptogenic liver disease
 Congenital hepatic fibrosis

Improved timing and better patient selection procedures have contributed substantially to the increased success of LTx in the 1990s. Although the hepatic disease should be advanced, and any opportunity for spontaneous or medically induced disease stabilization or recovery should be allowed, transplantation should be performed at an early enough time in the terminal phase of the liver disease to give the surgical procedure a chance to succeed. The conventional criteria used to identify the ideal candidate and the optimal time for the transplantation are presented in Table 2. These procedures assess the synthetic, metabolic, and excretory function of the liver and the quality of life of the potential recipient with end-stage liver disease. Ideally, LTx should be considered only for liver disease patients who have experienced a life-threatening complication of their hepatic disease, or have a quality of life that has deteriorated to an unacceptable level. Moreover, the transplant should be performed early enough such that no contraindications or extrahepatic irreversible systemic deterioration has occurred.

CONTRAINDICATIONS FOR LTx

In evaluating an individual for LTx it is important to evaluate the candidate for the presence of any absolute or relative contraindications for LTx. Table 3 lists the absolute and relative contraindications for LTx. As a result of improvements in surgical technique and intraoperative and postoperative care, the number of contraindications for LTx has been reduced substantially over the past decade. Finally, all individuals being considered for LTx need to have their heart, lungs and kidney function assessed. Non-hepatic disease can adversely affect the

Table 2 Clinical and biochemical variables that determine the need for a liver graft

I. *Chronic liver disease*
    Parenchymal liver disease
        Albumin <2.5 g/dl
        Advanced hepatic encephalopathy
        Prothrombin time >5 s above the normal value
    Cholestatic liver disease
        Bilirubin >10 mg/dl
        Intractable pruritus
        Hepatic osteodystrophy
        Recurrent biliary sepsis

II. *Acute hepatic insufficiency*
    Bilirubin level >10 mg/dl
    Prothrombin time >10 s above normal

III. *Factors applicable for any type of liver disease*
    Hepatorenal syndrome
    Recurrent spontaneous bacterial peritonitis
    Intractable ascites
    Recurrent variceal bleeding

Table 3 Contraindications for liver transplantation

I. *Absolute contraindications*
    Life-threatening systemic disease
    Uncontrolled extrahepatic bacterial or fungal infection
    Advanced cardiovascular and pulmonary disease
    Acquired immunodeficiency syndrome
    Hepatobiliary malignancy with extrahepatic metastasis
    Active drug and/or alcohol abuse

II. *Relative contraindications*
    Advanced age >65 years
    Portal vein thrombosis
    Marked obesity
    Human immunodeficiency virus positivity without ARC or AIDS
    Prior major abdominal surgery
    Hepatitis B virus-related liver disease with HBV-DNA positivity
    Poor compliance
    Severe hypoxaemia resulting from right to left intrapulmonary shunts
    Cholangiocarcinoma

success of LTx. Renal function prior to LTx has been shown to be a major predictive factor for LTx survival, the presence of clinically advanced renal disease may necessitate combined renal and liver transplantation. Candidates with a confounding cardiomyopathy associated with haemochromatosis, alcoholism, or glycogen storage require specific cardiological assessments. Individuals with diabetes, hypertension, arterial vascular disease, or an age greater than 50 years may need to be assessed for the presence of coronary artery disease.

SPECIFIC DISEASE INDICATIONS FOR LTx

Chronic parenchymal liver disease

End-stage liver disease caused by HBV, HCV, HDV, or non-A–non-B–non-C viral liver disease is the most common indication for LTx throughout the world. Transplant candidates having liver disease related to any of these hepatitis viruses account for more than 30% of all adult transplants[33]. Prior to LTx the HBV or HCV replicative status of the patient needs to be assessed. If the individual is HBV-DNA and HBeAg-negative, the LTx is likely to be successful and the risk of disease recurrence is low[34–39]. On the other hand, if the individual is HBV-DNA and/or HbeAg-positive, disease recurrence is almost 100%. Recurrent HBV disease progresses much faster than HBV infection occurring in a native liver[34,36]. Thus, replicative HBV infection is considered a strong relative contraindication for LTx.

Individuals coinfected with the delta virus typically have low levels of viral replication, as do individuals with fulminant hepatic failure[35,40–42]. Disease recurrence rates in individuals with these types of HBV disease, when treated with hepatitis B immune globulin (HBIG) postoperatively, are greatly reduced post-LTx[34,43–48]. Without HBIG, HBV infection recurrence rates are unacceptably high in individuals with replicative HBV disease. Current HBIG regimens attempt to maintain Hbs antibody titres greater than 100 IU/ml and potentially as high as 500 IU/ml for an indefinite period of time. Even under these circumstances the recurrence rate of HBV infection is 30%[36–49]. HBIG treatment is expensive and may be associated with serious complications such as mercury poisoning. Clearance of HBV-DNA prior to transplantation should result in markedly enhanced graft and patient survival rates. Recent developments in antiviral nucleoside analogue therapy for HBV may make HBV clearance prior to transplantation possible. Lamivudine is a potent inhibitor of HBV-DNA replication in patients with chronic viral B hepatitis[50]. At doses of 100–300 mg orally daily, viral clearance can be achieved in patients after only 3 months of treatment. How long lamivudine therapy must be continued in transplant patients post-LTx remains to be determined[51]. Famciclovir has also been used successfully for this purpose in transplant cases[52]. If current ongoing trials of oral nucleoside analogues, used both before and after LTx, prove to be effective, prevention of recurrent hepatitis B infection may be possible and HBV-associated liver disease may become the major disease indication for LTx.

HCV recurrence rates are as high as, if not greater than, those experienced for HBV[53–55]. Disease recurrence, however, develops slower over 3–5 years rather than 1–3 years and, as a result, has only recently become recognized[56,57]. Unfortunately, unlike the situation with HBV, no oral nucleoside analogues or hepatitis C immunoglobulin preparations exist that are effective at reducing the rate of recurrent HCV disease in liver allografts.

Cholestatic liver disease

The indications for LTx for cholestatic liver disease include any of the complications of advanced cholestatic liver disease such as hepatic osteodystrophy, variceal bleeding, spontaneous bacterial peritonitis, the hepatic renal syndrome and/or intractable pruritus.

Disease recurrence can occur but is a minor, rather unusual, problem as opposed to what occurs with viral liver disease. As a result, the long-term post-transplant prognosis for individuals transplanted for cholestatic liver disease is excellent[58–60].

GENERAL PREPARATION OF THE POTENTIAL LTx CANDIDATE

The blood group, HLA, A, B, and DR antigens, the presence of antibodies to cytomegalovirus, EBV and hepatitis C virus and all of the markers of hepatitis B virus infection should be determined. In patients with malignant disease the presence of metastases must be sought out using all available means, including computerized tomography scans of the chest, abdomen, and brain, as well as bone scans. Obviously the presence of any and all possible complications of end-stage liver disease must be assessed, particularly the development of primary liver cancer.

EVALUATION OF THE DONOR

The donor should not have a transmissible disease, and should be free of liver injury occurring as a consequence of the donor's agonal state. Ideally, bio-chemical assays of hepatic injury should be within normal limits and the donor should not have experienced a period of prolonged hypotension or anoxia. Except for emergent transplants the donor should be blood group compatible with the recipient[2,61].

The remarkable success of LTx and the increasing size of LTx candidate lists, as well as the expanded indications for LTx, have created a marked increase in the demand for donor organs. Unfortunately the organ donation rate has remained constant. The actual donor pool has been expanded, however, as a result of the use of more liberal criteria for donor selection and improvements in organ preservation. Nonetheless, the median waiting time for LTx has increased substantially[62]. Donor and recipient matching for LTx is based solely on ABO blood group compatibility and estimated liver size, which correlates with the height, weight, and thoracic circumference of the donor and recipient.

MATCHING OF HLA ANTIGENS

In contrast to kidney transplantation, HLA matching has either had no effect on LTx survival rates, or has a paradoxical negative impact on liver graft survival[30]. There is some evidence to suggest that class II (HLA-DR) mismatching may be advantageous in reducing the intensity of recurrent viral hepatitis and reducing the frequency of the vanishing bile duct syndrome[63].

VIRAL INFECTIONS IN THE DONOR

Cytomegalovirus (CMV)

One of the more important viral infections in clinical LTx is CMV infection. The mortality of CMV infection in immunosuppressed individuals has been reduced remarkably as a result of the use of ganciclovir. Livers harvested from CMV-seropositive donors are associated with an increased risk for clinically severe CMV infection in the graft recipient[64].

Hepatitis B

Contrary to CMV, it is very difficult to justify the use of a liver harvested from a donor with evidence of a prior viral hepatitis due to HBV. If the potential donor is positive for either HBsAg, anti-HBc IgM or HBV-DNA, the liver should not be used for transplantation. If the donor is positive only for anti-HBc (IgG) and all other markers of HBV infection are negative, and the liver has a normal histology, the organ can be used for a recipient who is HBV-DNA positive or has detectable anti-HBsAg.

Hepatitis C

The use of a liver obtained from a donor who is anti-HCV positive is associated with a near-universal rate of post-transplant HCV infection. In a study of 105 confirmed HCV seropositive donors for whom liver biopsy was available, 21% had persistent chronic hepatitis, 45% had chronic active hepatitis, and 7% had active cirrhosis. Moreover, in all studies to date, the use of a donor liver from a donor who is anti-HCV positive has led to HCV infection in the recipient. Thus, the use of a liver obtained from a seropositive donor should be avoided except under very unusual circumstances or recipient need, and should then be limited to those recipients who are anti-HCV positive themselves[65,66].

THE ALCOHOL ABUSER AS A DONOR

Grafts obtained from donors with a history of alcohol abuse and elevated blood alcohol levels are acceptable for transplantation if the hepatic histology is normal and liver function is good. No correlation between an elevated blood alcohol level in the donor and subsequent initial graft function or short-term survival has been demonstrated[61].

LIVER GRAFT ASSESSMENTS

In order to assess donor organ quality or viability, multiple testing procedures have been utilized. The monoethylglycinexylide (MEGX) test is a simple, practical and inexpensive test that has been used for this purpose. It quantifies the conversion of lidocaine to MEGX by the liver and correlates well with conventional liver function tests[67,68]. Unfortunately, the sensitivity of the MEGX test at selecting donor organs with good post-transplant function has been reported to be only 65%. Whenever the MEGX test value is less than 50 ng/ml the potential donor liver should be considered at high risk for poor post-transplant function. The most valuable criterion used to reject donor livers with poor post-transplant function has been the histological demonstration of hepatic steatosis involving more than 30% of the hepatic parenchymal cells. Donor livers with high-grade steatosis, hydropic degeneration of hepatocytes, or perivenular hepatocyte necrosis are at increased risk of poor post-transplant graft function. An important factor in determining post-transplant function is the duration of time the donor was in the intensive care unit before organ procurement. Longer stays in the ICU are associated with depletion of hepatic glycogen and an increased risk of poor post-transplant graft function[67].

FOLLOW-UP OF LIVER ALLOGRAFT RECIPIENTS

Obviously, a major problem of concern to physicians following liver allograft recipients is the recognition and treatment of allograft rejection, the recognition of recurrent hepatic disease, and the recognition and specific identification of new confounding liver disease. In addition to these obvious hepatic problems the recognition of, and specific treatment of, opportunistic infections due to viral or parasitic organisms is a second major challenge for physicians and surgeons following liver allograft recipients. These problems often occur following an episode of treated allograft rejection as they represent untoward consequences of 'excessive' immunosuppression. A third important responsibility of physicians caring for allograft recipients is to recognize and treat neoplasms that occur at increased rates in individuals, who are immunosuppressed for long periods, potentially lifelong. These include skin cancer; breast cancer; cervical and vulvar cancer; renal cancer; colonic, prostatic and gastric cancer as well as post-transplant lymphoproliferative diseases or neoplasms. These lesions should be identified early by prophylactic screening procedures and knowledge of an increased awareness of these cancers in transplant recipients. A fourth responsibility of the transplant physician is to monitor the immunosuppression utilized by the allograft recipient. This includes increasing it for episodes of rejection, reducing it during opportunistic infections or with increasing periods of rejection-free time post-transplant. This also includes a continuing monitoring of all of the medications that the allograft recipient takes, that might either enhance or inhibit the metabolism of cyclosporin or tacrolimus. A fifth and critical, often-ignored, responsibility of the physicians caring for allograft recipients is to manage the medical problems associated with the use of lifelong immunosuppression. These problems include obesity, hypertension, renal failure, marrow hypocellularity or failure, diabetes mellitus, atherosclerosis and coronary artery disease.

CONCLUSIONS

Currently, LTx is a common, readily available procedure for individuals with end-stage liver disease. The requirement for LTx has exceeded the availability of donor organs. Current approaches to resolve this problem of greater numbers of potential recipients as compared to donors include the use of reduced size, split-liver and lung-related donor organs. With the increasing success of antiviral therapies the demand for donor organs is likely to increase to levels much greater than those currently experienced. It would appear that the only realistic resolution of this disparity of donor organs will be the use of xenotransplants. Considerable research is ongoing to enable clinical xenotransplantation to become a reality.

References

1. Maddrey WC, Van Thiel DH. Liver transplantation: an overview. Hepatology. 1988;8:948–59.
2. Wood RP, Ozaki CF, Katz SM *et al.* Liver transplantation. The last ten years. Surg Clin N Am. 1994;74:1133–54.
3. Starzl TE, Demetris AJ, Van Thiel DH. Medical progress: liver transplantation (part I). N Engl J Med. 1989;321:1014–22.
4. Starzl TE, Demetris AJ, Van Thiel DH. Medical progress: liver transplantation (part II). N Engl J Med. 1989;321:1092–9.
5. Malago M, Rogiers X, Broelsch CE. Reduced-size hepatic allografts. Annu Rev Med. 1995;46:507–12.
6. Pappas SC, Rouch DA, Stevens LH. New techniques for liver transplantation: reduced-size, split liver, living-related and auxiliary liver transplantation. Scand J Gastroenterol. 1995;208:97–100.
7. Sloof MJ. Reduced size liver transplantation, split liver transplantation and living-related liver transplantation in relation to the donor organ shortage. Transpl Int. 1995;8:69–73.
8. Bhatnagar V, Rela M, Heaton ND, Tan KC. Liver transplantation from living related donors: review of world experience and its implications for India. Ind J Pediatr. 1994;61:387–93.
9. Welch CS. A note on transplantation of the whole liver in dogs. Transplant Bull. 1955;2:54.
10. Anonymous. Terminology for hepatic allograft rejection. International Working Party. Hepatology. 1995;22:648–54.
11. Vierling JM. Immunologic mechanisms of hepatic allograft rejection. Sem Liv Dis. 1992;12:16–27.
12. Hubscher SG. Pathology of liver allograft rejection. Transplant Immunol. 1994;2:118–23.
13. Hubscher SG. Histological findings in liver allograft rejection – new insight into the pathogenesis of hepatocellular damage in liver allografts. Histopathology. 1991;18:377–83.
14. Perkins JD, Rakela J, Sterioff S *et al.* Results of treatment in hepatic allograft rejection depend on the immunohistologic pattern of the portal T lymphocyte infiltrate. Transplant Proc. 1988;20:223–5.
15. Fung JJ, Zeevi A, Starzl TE *et al.* Functional characterization of infiltrating T lymphocytes in human hepatic allografts. Hum Immunol. 1986;16:182–99.
16. Markus BH, Demetris AJ, Saidman S *et al.* Alloreactive T lymphocytes cultured from liver transplant biopsies: association of HLA specificity with clinicopathological findings. Clin Transplant. 1988;2:70–75.
17. Kamada N. Animal models of hepatic allograft rejection. Sem Liv Dis. 1992;12:1–15.
18. Kamada N. The immunology of experimental liver transplantation in the rat. Immunology. 1985;55:369–76.
19. Zimmermann FA, Davies HFFS, Knoll PP *et al.* Orthotopic liver allografts in the rat. The influence of strain combination in the fate of the graft. Transplantation. 1984;37:406–10.
20. Kamada N, Brons G, Davies HFFS. Fully allogeneic liver grafting in rats induces a state of systemic nonreactivity to donor transplantation antigens. Transplantation. 1980;29:429–31.
21. Kamada N, Davies HFFS, Roser BJ. Fully allogeneic liver grafting and the induction of donor-specific unreactivity. Transplant Proc. 1981;13:837–41.
22. Howard JC. The major histocompatibility complex of the rat: a partial review. Metabolism. 1983;32 (Suppl. 1):41–50.
23. Cortese Hassett AL, Misra DN, Kunz HW, Gill TJ III. The major histocompatibility complex in the rat. In: Srivastava R, Ram BP, Tyle , (editors). Immunogenetics of the major histocompatibility complex. New York: VCH; 1991:236–44.

24. Gunther E, Stark O. At least two loci of the major histocompatibility complex can determine mixed lymphocyte stimulation in rat. Tissue Ant. 1978;11:465–70.
25. Peters M, Vierling JM, Gershwin ME *et al.* Immunology and the liver. Hepatology. 1991;13:977–94.
26. Davis MM, Bjorkman PJ. T-cell receptor genes and T-cell recognition. Nature. 1988;334:395–402.
27. Burakoff SJ, Deeg HJ, Ferrara J, Atkinson K (editors). Graft vs host disease: immunology, pathophysiology and treatment. New York: Marcel Dekker; 1990.
28. Roberts JP, Ascher NL, Lake J *et al.* GVHD after liver transplantation in humans: a report of 4 cases. Hepatology. 1991;14:274–81.
29. Starzl TE, Todo S, Fung J *et al.* FK-506 for liver, kidney and pancreas transplantation. Lancet. 1989;2:1000–4.
30. Gunson BK, Hathaway M, Buckels JA *et al.* HLA matching in liver transplantation: a retrospective analysis. Transplant Proc. 1992;24:2434–5.
31. Starzl TE, Demetris AJ, Murase N *et al.* Cell migration, chimerism and graft acceptance. Lancet. 1992;339:1579–82.
32. Steininan KM, Inaba K, Austin JM. Donor derived chimerism in recipients of organ transplants. Hepatology. 1993;17:1153–6.
33. Fagiuoli S, Shah G, Wright HI, Van Thiel DH. Types, causes and therapies of hepatitis occurring in a liver allograft. Dig Dis Sci. 1993;38:1–8.
34. Lake J. Should liver transplantation be performed for patients with chronic hepatitis B? Liver Transplant Surg. 1995;1:260–5.
35. Samuel D, Muller R, Alexander G *et al.* Liver transplantation in European patients with the hepatitis B surface antigen. N Engl J Med. 1993;329:1842–7.
36. Van Thiel DH, Wright HI, Fagiuoli S. Liver transplantation for hepatitis B virus associated cirrhosis. Hepatology. 1994;20:20–3S.
37. Konig V, Hopf U, Neuhaus P *et al.* Long-term follow-up of hepatitis B virus infected recipients after orthotopic liver transplantation. Transplantation. 1994;58:553–9.
38. O'Grady JG, Smith JM, Davies SE *et al.* Hepatitis B virus reinfection after liver transplantation: serological and clinical implications. J Hepatol. 1992;14:104–11.
39. Todo S, Demetris AJ, Van Thiel DH *et al.* Orthotopic liver transplantation for patients with hepatitis B virus-related liver diseases. Hepatology. 1991;13:619–26.
40. Ottobrelli A, Marzano S, Smedile A *et al.* Patterns of hepatitis delta virus reinfection and disease in liver transplantation. Gastroenterology. 1991;101:1649–55.
41. Villamil FG, Vierling JM. Recurrence of viral hepatitis after liver transplantation: insight into management. Liver Transplant Surg. 1995;1:89–99.
42. Williams R, Wendon J. Indications for orthotopic liver transplantation in fulminant liver failure. Hepatology.1994;20:5–10S.
43. Lauchart W, Muller R, Pichlmayer R. Long-term immunoprophylaxis of hepatitis B virus reinfection in recipients of human allografts. Transplant Proc. 1987;19:4051–3.
44. Pruett TL. HBIg immunoprophylaxis in the United States: IV. Studies. Presentation at American Association for the Study of Liver Diseases, Single topic Symposium, Liver transplantation for chronic viral hepatitis, Reston, Virginia, March 1995.
45. Mora NP, Klintmalm GB, Poplawski SS *et al.* Recurrence of hepatitis B after liver transplantation: does hepatitis B immunoglobulin modify the recurrent disease? Transplant Proc. 1990;22:1549–50.
46. Muller R, Gubernatis G, Farle M *et al.* Liver transplantation in HBs antigen (HBsAg) carriers. Prevention of hepatitis B virus (HBV) recurrence by passive immunization. J Hepatol. 1991;13:90–6.
47. Samuel D, Bismuth A, Mathieu D *et al.* Passive immunoprophylaxis after liver transplantation in HBsAg positive patients. Lancet. 1991;337:813–15.
48. Samuel D, Bismuth A, Serres C *et al.* HBV infection after liver transplantation in HBsAg positive patients: experience with long-term immunoprophylaxis. Transplant Proc. 1991;23:1492–4.
49. Marcellin B, Samuel D, Arias J *et al.* Pretransplantation treatment and recurrence of hepatitis B virus infection after liver transplantation for hepatitis-B related end stage liver disease. Hepatology. 1994;19:6–12.
50. Tyrrel DLJ, Mitchell MC, DeMan RA *et al.* Phase II trial with lamivudine for chronic hepatitis B. Hepatology. 1993;18:112A.

51. Benhamou Y, Dohin E, Lunel-Fabiani F *et al.* Efficacy of lamivudine on replication of hepatitis B virus in HIV-infected patients (letter). Lancet. 1995;345:396–7.
52. Schalm SW, DeMan RA, Heijtink RA, Niesters HG. New nucleoside analogues for chronic hepatitis B. J Hepatol. 1995;22:52–6.
53. Pons JA. Role of liver transplantation in viral hepatitis. J Hepatol. 1995;22:146–53.
54. Wright TL, Donegan E, Hsu HH *et al.* Recurrent and acquired hepatitis C viral infection in liver transplant recipients. Gastroenterology. 1992;103:317–22.
55. Poterucha JJ, Rakela J, Lumeng L *et al.* Diagnosis of chronic hepatitis C after liver transplantation by the detection of viral sequences with polymerase chain reaction. Hepatology. 1992;15:42–5.
56. Shah G, Demetris AJ, Gavaler JS *et al.* Incidence, prevalence and clinical course of hepatitis C following liver transplantation. Gastroenterology. 1992;103:323–9.
57. Ferrcl LD, Wright TL, Roberts J *et al.* Hepatitis C viral infection in liver transplant recipients. Hepatology. 1992;16:865–76.
58. Harrison J, McMaster P. The role of orthotopic liver transplantation in the management of sclerosing cholangitis. Hepatology. 1994;20:14–19S.
59. Benhamou W. Indications for liver transplantation in primary biliary cirrhosis. Hepatology. 1994;11–13S.
60. Wiesner RH, Porayko MK, Dickson ER *et al.* Selection and timing of liver transplantation in primary biliary cirrhosis and primary sclerosing cholangitis. Hepatology. 1992;16:1290–9.
61. Strasberg SM, Howard TK, Molmenti EP, Herti M. Selecting the donor liver: risk factors for poor function after orthotopic liver transplantation. Hepatology. 1994;20:829–38.
62. UNOS 1995 annual report of the U.S. scientific registry of transplant recipients and the organ procurement and transplantation network. International Standard Book N. 1–886651–10–8.
63. Demetris AJ, Murase N, Delaney CP *et al.* The liver allograft, chronic (ductopenic) rejection, and microchimerism: what can they teach us? Transplant Proc. 1995;27:67–70.
64. Stratta RJ, Shaeffer MS, Markin RS *et al.* Cytomegalovirus infection and disease after liver transplantation. An overview. Dig Dis Sci. 1992;37:673–88.
65. Aswad S, Obispo E, Mendez RG, Mendez R. HCV + donors: should they be used for organ transplantation? Transplant Proc. 1993;25:3072–4.
66. Shah G, Demetris AJ, Irish W *et al.* Frequency and severity of HCV infection following orthotopic liver transplantation. Effect of donor and recipient serology for HCV using a second generation ELISA test. J Hepatol. 1993;18:279–83.
67. Potter JM, Balderson GA, Hickman PE *et al.* The value of the donor MEGX test in predicting liver allograft recipient outcome. Transplantation. 1994;58:524–6.
68. Potter JM, Hickman PE, Lynch SV *et al.* Use of MEGX test as a liver function test in the liver transplant recipient. Transplantation. 1993;56:1385–8.

27
Surgical complications after liver transplantation

J. J. FUNG and A. PINNA

INTRODUCTION

Orthotopic liver transplantation (OLTx) has become an accepted means for the treatment of end-stage liver disease. Although the technique of OLTx has been refined to a relatively standardized approach, the operation remains a formidable surgical challenge. As such, OLTx can have numerous technical complications, to which pretransplant conditions, donor, iatrogenic and immunological factors may all contribute. The purpose of this discussion is to identify the technical complications during the hepatectomy, anhepatic phase and reimplantation of the allograft in OLTx. In addition, means of prevention, diagnosis and management of complications are discussed.

HEPATECTOMY

The 'standard incision' for OLTx has historically been a bilateral subcostal incision with an upper midline extension to the xiphoid (sometimes called an inverted Y or Mercedes incision). Other incisions have been used; however, the principle in determining the type of incision is to gain adequate exposure to the liver and to other intra-abdominal structures, such as the infrarenal aorta, should the need arise. The type of incision is of paramount importance and choosing the wrong incision can make the operation difficult. The presence of previous incisions may require modifications to the planned incision, in order to avoid flap necrosis from devascularization. The incision should be made with electrocautery, due to the presence of portal hypertension and coagulopathy in the patient with end-stage liver disease. Even so, the blood loss from an incision can be significant. Thus, all the larger subcutaneous venous collaterals should be ligated.

In the case of pre-existing surgery, particular attention must be paid upon entering the abdominal cavity, as the presence of vascular adhesions can lead to both significant blood loss and/or violation of the gastrointestinal tract. With inadvertent injuries to the bowel, the area should be reinforced, as tissue breakdown is common during the postoperative period, when the patients are in a catabolic state and malnourished, as well as receiving high doses of corticosteroids.

Usually the hepatectomy is the most difficult part of the liver transplant operation. Consequently, technical misadventures during this phase of the operation may result in significant complications. This is particularly true during the hepatectomy in patients with previous upper abdominal surgery. Excessive bleeding is the most common complication. This can be the result of carelessness, massive portal hypertension, presence of unusual collaterals (especially in the presence of portal vein thrombosis), and/or adhesions. The dissection of adhesions (often vascularized) must be undertaken using a combination of electrocautery and ligation. A relatively slow, methodical and bloodless dissection translates in a much smoother operation and, ironically, a considerably shorter total case time. Haemostatic sutures must be applied with great care, especially when there are extensive collaterals, since they are thin-walled and apt to be torn with improperly placed haemostatic sutures. Early portal decompression with the veno-venous bypass (see below) may aid in avoiding massive bleeding. It is particularly difficult to perform surgical haemostasis once the allograft is already in, especially if there is any degree of post-reperfusion coagulopathy.

A potentially serious complication during hepatectomy is injury to the right adrenal gland, which results in severe bleeding that is difficult to control, and may require adrenalectomy. This can be avoided by staying on the liver surface during the dissection of the right lobe. Some surgeons have advocated a subcapsular approach to the hepatectomy, which minimizes the possibility of adrenal injury. Another feared complication is injury to the right renal vein during mobilization of the infrahepatic vena cava. Dissection of the vena cava at too low a level must be avoided. If the renal vein is injured this has to be recognized immediately, and the vessel repaired. If necessary, a segment of donor iliac vein can be used for the repair. In some cases a right nephrectomy may be lifesaving if the renal vein injury cannot be controlled. One method of avoiding the necessity of encircling the infrahepatic vena cava is to place a vascular clamp in an anterior/posterior fashion, and to dissect the posterior aspect of the vena cava only after the liver is removed.

Injury of the wall of the suprahepatic vena cava is an uncommon but potentially disastrous complication. Rarely, the insertion of the right hepatic vein is at a higher level than that of the left and middle hepatic veins. An attempt to create a common cloaca with the hepatic veins and suprahepatic vena cava may result in a posterior wall that is unable to hold sutures. In such cases, as well as in injury of the suprahepatic cava with a resulting cuff that is too short, the diaphragm may have to be opened and the vena cava isolated within the pericardium, to allow placement of the vascular clamp close to or at the level of the right heart atrium. If necessary, the suprahepatic vena cava may need to have the sutures closed, and venous outflow of the hepatic allograft may require a caval–atrial anastomosis.

Another potential complication is injury to the right phrenic nerve. This occurs when an excessive amount of diaphragm is included in the suprahepatic vascular clamp, particularly in the paediatric patient. This injury is usually self-reversible, but on occasion it can lead to permanent paralysis of the right hemidiaphragm.

Finally, injury to the retrohepatic venous collaterals can lead to persistent and occasionally severe bleeding. As in avoidance of right adrenal injuries (see above), dissection close to the liver, or under Glisson's capsule, will avoid this problem. Bleeding that has already occurred can be controlled with running Prolene sutures, and pledgeted sutures may allow secure haemostasis, even when tissues are friable.

Additionally, a better understanding of the anatomy of the diseased liver has allowed novel approaches to the hepatectomy. This is especially true in patients with extensive previous perihepatic surgery, who have difficult dense and vascular adhesions. In the case of previous operations involving the hepatic hilum, the usual approach to the hilar dissection may not be possible, and an approach from either side of the hilum may be safer. An approach from the left side, dividing the hepatogastric ligament, identifying the caudate process and cautiously moving laterally until the hepatic artery is identified, is usually the safest approach. This method permits early division of the hepatic artery and cannulation of the portal vein for veno-venous bypass decompression. An alternative method involves the cannulation of the portal vein via the inferior mesenteric vein at the very beginning of the operation, thus assuring portal decompression before initiation of the hilar dissection.

At times it may not be possible to dissect a completely 'frozen' hilum from either an anterior or lateral approach. In such cases the suprahepatic vena cava can be approached and divided first. Subsequently, the liver can be removed from 'above' and the hilum approached from a posterior direction, after the infrahepatic vena cava has been transected. Conversely, a completely frozen suprahepatic vena cava can be approached from behind, after the hilum has been completely transected and the liver mobilized from behind and below.

ANHEPATIC PHASE

The introduction of the veno-venous bypass has been an important factor in the improvement of liver transplantation results during the past decade. The early portal and caval decompression afforded by veno-venous bypass has manifested favourably on both the morbidity and mortality previously noted with total crossclamping during the anhepatic phase. However, the veno-venous bypass can cause complications; some of them fatal.

The most frequent complication is the wound lymphocele, both in the inguinal and axillary incisions. These can be avoided by careful dissection and ligation of all lympathics. Lymphoceles are usually self-limiting and self-healing, but occasionally chronic lymphorrhoea can be quite disabling and require surgical correction. Newer approaches to percutaneous cannulation of the femoral vein and internal jugular vein may obviate the wound complications associated with cutdowns; however, the risk of haematoma formation or venous perforation exists with these techniques.

Damage to the axillary, femoral and/or portal vein is also possible. There are several mechanisms of portal vein injury: (a) improper placement of the portal vein cannulae, with inadequate decompression; (b) injury of the wall of a mesenteric vein with resultant perforation; and (c) torsion of the portal vein which can result in avulsion of small tributaries, with resultant massive and perhaps uncontrollable bleeding in patients with portal hypertension. The injury to the axillary or subclavian vein can result in either thrombosis or massive haematoma. Perforation of the subclavian vein with an improperly placed axillary vein cannula can result in haemothorax or massive haematoma. Care should be taken in patients with previous indwelling central venous catheters, and particularly those with peritoneal–venous shunts, since central venous thrombosis may lead to life-threatening superior vena caval syndromes during veno-venous bypass.

Damage to the brachial plexus or isolated nerve trunks has been described, and can be extremely disabling and frequently permanent. This can be avoided only by identification and protection of the nerves during dissection of the axillary vein. Appropriate positioning of the arm should be accomplished, to avoid hyperextension, with resultant brachial plexus injury.

Clot or air embolization can occur during the use of the veno-venous bypass. Blood clots originate during periods of low flow and thus can be avoided by achieving a flow of at least 1 L/min. Attempts to correct bleeding, either surgical or medical, by use of exogenous coagulation factor administration, during veno-venous bypass, should be avoided, since the risk of fatal pulmonary embolism is markedly increased due to creation of a hypercoagulable state. Air embolism is rare, but can occur if there is a tear in the portal vein, or if the portal cannula is not secured, through which air may be sucked in. Occasionally, a patent right-to-left intracardiac shunt (e.g. patent foramen ovale) may lead to systemic embolization, and has been associated with post-transplant strokes.

Recently, some controversy has arisen concerning the use of veno-venous bypass, with an increasing number of transplant surgeons questioning its need. This is due in part to the improved intraoperative haemodynamic management of the patient by the anaesthesiology team, and in part to the improved technical skills of the surgeons. The preservation of the entire retrohepatic vena cava and anastomosis of the new liver to a cuff formed from one or more of the main suprahepatic veins, has been advocated as a method of avoiding veno-venous bypass. The advantages of preserving the vena cava can be significant, but this technique (also known as the 'piggy-back technique') requires high skills and complete knowledge of, and confidence with, the standard OLTx with veno-venous bypass. Essentially, the technique consists of dissection of the caudate process and right lobe of the liver from the retrohepatic vena cava, until only the suprahepatic veins remain. Subsequently, the suprahepatic veins are clamped and interconnected, thus forming a cuff that can then be anastomosed to the suprahepatic vena cava of the donor liver, in an end-to-side fashion. After flushing the liver to clear the preservation solution, the infrahepatic cava of the allograft can be simply ligated. The new liver will finish by lying on top of the recipient's vena cava, but this can result in compression of the recipient's vena cava, with development of thrombosis.

There are several potential advantages of this technique, including less bleeding, less chance of adrenal gland and renal vein injury, shortening the anhepatic phase by eliminating the lower caval anastomosis, and potentially less haemodynamic instability. In this situation, if portal crossclamping in the patient with existing portal hypertension is well tolerated, it may be appropriate not to utilize veno-venous bypass. In cases without pre-existing portal hypertension (e.g. fulminant hepatitis), a temporary portacaval shunt can be fashioned during the initiation of the anhepatic phase, to achieve mesenteric vein decompression without veno-venous bypass.

REIMPLANTATION

Numerous complications can occur during, or as a result of, vascular anastomoses. The most common complication is a stenosis of the vascular anastomoses. In end-to-end arterial anastomoses, strictures can be avoided by the use of a Carrel patch or by allowing a slight redundancy in the continuous vascular suture to allow for expansion of the suture line upon reperfusion (also known as a 'growth factor'). The 'growth factor' is used routinely in portal vein anastomosis, and occasionally for caval anastomoses. When, despite all measures, a stricture does occur, percutaneous balloon dilatation can be attempted, with fairly good success. Failure to dilate the stricture by angioplasty may require operative correction of the problem, which can be difficult.

Complete thrombosis of the hepatic artery (HAT) is usually quite a dramatic complication. It can lead to acute, massive necrosis, formation of a central biloma secondary to intrahepatic duct necrosis, multiple biliary structures, or intermittent bacteraemia. Occasionally, rarely in adults but more often in children, HAT can be asymptomatic. The factors which determine whether a liver fails or survives in the face of complete HAT are not known; however, the presence of collateral circulation (e.g. from the phrenic artery via vascularized adhesions to the liver) is usually associated with a more benign course after HAT. Segmental or lobar HAT has also been described. Left HAT (usually associated with an injury to an unrecognized anomalous left hepatic artery arising from the left gastric artery) is generally benign. However, right HAT (usually associated with an injury to an unrecognized anomalous right hepatic artery arising from the superior mesenteric artery, or from technically imperfect reconstruction of the anomalous right hepatic artery at the backtable) is associated with development of biliary strictures, due to the dependence of biliary viability on the right hepatic artery.

One must recognize that patients with anomalous hepatic arterial anatomy may not have a sufficiently large common hepatic artery to use as inflow. Patients with coeliac axis stenosis may also have inadequate inflow. The median arcuate ligament syndrome has been described as affecting arterial inflow in liver transplantation. In these circumstances the use of a donor iliac arterial conduit from the infrarenal (or occasionally supracoeliac) aorta to the allograft, may be necessary. The availability of iliac or carotid arteries from the donor allows one to utilize alternative inflow sites. Artificial conduits, e.g. PTFE (Gortex) grafts, should be avoided, due to the risk of thrombosis and infection.

Kinking of the anastomosis is another potential problem that can easily be avoided by correct orientation of the vessels to be attached together. When kinking of the suprahepatic vena cava anastomosis occurs, particularly if a large native liver is replaced with a much smaller organ, a Budd–Chiari-like syndrome may be seen, with ascites, congested liver and elevated liver function tests. This can best be avoided in this situation by using a size-matched liver or by reattaching the suspensory ligaments of the liver if there is significant play in the transplanted liver in the right upper quadrant. The differential causes of this syndrome include: suprahepatic vena caval stenosis or thrombosis, right heart failure, or veno-occlusive disease associated with rejection. Redundancy of the vessels can also cause kinking. This is avoided by trimming the vessels until they look almost too short, since the vessels are apt to elongate after flow is re-established. For the hepatic artery, where the site of the anastomosis is also dictated by the diameter of the vessels and the presence of patches, a long artery can be bolstered with an omental pedicle, which prevents kinking.

Intimal dissection of the artery can result from too vigorous manipulation of the vessels, either in the donor or the recipient. If not recognized early, intimal flaps will lead to arterial thrombosis.

Finally, imperfect haemostasis or slippage of a tie may result in postoperative bleeding, requiring re-exploration. Even if easily controlled, postoperative bleeding leads to increased cost, morbidity and mortality.

The biliary anastomosis has been referred to as the 'Achilles tendon' of the liver transplant operation. Because of the insensitivity of nuclear medicine scans and ultrasonography in detecting biliary complications, use of T-tube cholangiograms (TTC), percutaneous transphepatic cholangiograms (PTC), or endoscopic retrograde cholangiopancreatograms (ERCP) usually allows early and positive diagnosis of biliary complications.

There are two currently practised biliary reconstructions after OLTx. The most common is the choledochocholedochostomy (duct-to-duct anastomosis), and the other is the choledochojejunostomy (to a Roux-en-Y defunctionalized intestinal loop). Other 'historic' types of biliary reconstructions include the choledochoduodenostomy and the now-defunct cholecystoduodenostomy (the 'Wadell–Calne' biliary reconstruction). While there are variations of all of these biliary reconstructions, there are similar patterns of complications regardless of the type of reconstruction. The most common biliary complication is biliary stenosis. This is the result of either imperfect anastomotic technique or ischaemia of the bile duct, which appears as a stenotic area in the common bile duct, either at or slightly proximal to the biliary anastomosis, with proximal biliary dilatation. Recurrent bouts of cholangitis or persistent abnormal liver function tests may indicate an obstruction to bile outflow. Percutaneous balloon dilatation can be successful, but surgical revision has historically been employed. In the case of choledochocholedochostomy, the revision consists in a conversion to an end-to-side choledochojejunostomy with a Roux-en-Y loop.

It has been hypothesized that the papilla of Vater is innervated by fibres coursing through the hepatic branch of the vagus, and that hepatectomy can result in a syndrome known as 'ampullary dysfunction'. Radiological examination of the biliary tree reveals dilatation of both the donor and recipient bile ducts, with or without intrahepatic biliary dilatation. Treatment consists of conversion to a choledochojejunostomy. The alternative treatment, which utilizes endoscopic papillotomy, has been attempted with some success.

Multiple intrahepatic strictures of the biliary tree have been described by various groups. The causes and pathophysiology of these intrahepatic strictures have not been clearly elucidated. In many cases the strictures seem to be associated with a hepatic artery thrombosis or stenosis, and ischaemia of the biliary tree is probably the aetiology. Preservation damage of the allograft may result in multiple intrahepatic biliary strictures, with or without biliary sludge and casts. An immunological association to a positive lymphocytotoxic positive cross-match has also been hypothesized. In some patients who were originally transplanted for primary sclerosing cholangitis, recurrence of the disease seems a possibility. Finally, an association of intrahepatic bile duct strictures with cytomegalovirus infection has also been reported. While some patients with multiple intrahepatic strictures eventually need to be retransplanted, others can live for years with minimal difficulties, especially if they receive chronic antibiotic prophylaxis.

The most feared complication of the biliary anastomosis is the bile leak. Technically speaking, this is usually the result of an imperfect anastomosis, but it may also be impacted by preservation injuries to the allograft. This complication is particularly lethal in the choledochojejunostomies, since the bile collection is rapidly infected with enteric organisms, resulting in an inflamed and friable operative site during attempted repair. In the choledochocholedochostomies, the leaks usually occur at the exit site of the T-tube. In order to avoid this, a purse-string suture should be placed around the exit site. Leakage at the T-tube exit site is usually self-containing, and no treatment is necessary as long as the distal bile duct empties well. Some surgeons have advocated not using any stenting following choledochocholedochostomy, in an attempt to avoid the risk of T-tube site leakage.

When a Roux-en-Y loop is used, bleeding can occur at the jejunojejunostomy. In about half of the cases this is a self-limiting problem; in the other half exploration for haemostasis may be necessary. This can be avoided by using a haemostatic running suture to approximate the mucosa and submucosa.

Finally, internal hernias through the mesentery at the jejunojejunostomy can occur, often with disastrous consequences due to small-bowel volvulus and necrosis. Careful closure of the defect in the mesentery prevents this complication.

CONCLUSIONS

While the results of OLTx have improved dramatically over the past 20 years, many of the same technical considerations have plagued the procedure since its inception, over 30 years ago. With the increasing complexity of candidate undergoing OLTx, an improved understanding of the pathophysiology of donor organ preservation, reperfusion injury, improved immunosuppression, more effective diagnostic tools, and new anti-infective agents, have all contributed to a smoother post-transplant course. Nevertheless, none of these advances can negate a poorly performed technical procedure.

28
New trends in liver transplantation

C. E. BROELSCH, M. HERTL, M. MALAGO, X. ROGIERS and
M. BURDELSKI

INTRODUCTION

The field of liver transplantation (LTx) has been in continuous development since its beginning three decades ago. It has its roots in the late 1950s and early 1960s. The first human LTx was performed by Starzl in 1963[1–4]. The first successful transplantation was carried out in 1967 by the same surgeon[5]. In the 1960s and 1970s the technique of homotransplantation was developed, but the long-term success rate remained poor, mainly due to inefficient immunosuppression. The 1-year survival rate in the late 1970s was approximately 30%[6]. This changed dramatically with the introduction of the more potent immunosuppressive drugs, namely cyclosporin A (CyA). The survival rate after 1 year rose to 75% in the Pittsburgh group[6]. The 1980s also brought further refinements in surgical technique, and in 1987 the introduction of the UW solution (see below). What added to the much-improved outcome was the fact that LTx was no longer being reserved for critically ill patients as a last rescue therapy.

As the technique proved to be successful, indications and timing of transplantation changed, and the operation was performed on a more elective basis. As a result the number of LTx rose steadily. In 1980 a total of 182 LTx were performed in the United States; in 1989 there were 2192; and this number increased to 3056 by 1992. The limit for further expansion of numbers now became the lack of suitable organ donors, while the number of patients dying on the waiting list was increasing[6]. In 1990 24.3% of the 2200 potential LTx candidates in the United States died while awaiting transplantation[7]. This distressing observation led to the increased use and further refinement of reduced-size transplantation, split-liver transplantation and living-donor-liver transplantation. The goal of the 1990s and of the turn of the century will be improving organ utilization by increased donor pool and routine application of the above-mentioned techniques and the further improvement in immunosuppression, making preservation of the donor liver even more effective. New avenues such as xenotransplantation, hepatocyte transplantation and artificial liver support need further investigation and study[8–10].

"

LTx has emerged during the past two decades from a desperate and often unsuccessful treatment to the standard therapy for end-stage liver disease. The 1-year survival rate for some indications such as primary biliary cirrhosis is now around 90%; the 5-year survival rate up to 80%. This has become reality through important innovations in the area of liver preservation; surgical technique and growing experience; pre-, peri- and postoperative care; treatment and avoidance of rejection; dealing with infectious complications and prevention of disease recurrence. The following sections will focus on current developments in these areas and describe the newest 'trends'.

INDICATIONS FOR LTx

The indications for LTx have not changed much in recent years[11–19]. However, improvements in outcome have led to wider acceptance of LTx for a greater number of patients. This has also led to decreasing restrictions according to age (in both directions), and the willingness to perform even multiple retransplantation. The majority of the patients is still being transplanted for end-stage cirrhosis, which untreated would be fatal. Indications for LTx for malignant disease have been restricted because of poor long-term survival[20–22]. On the other hand, transplantation for abstinent alcoholic liver disease has become more widely accepted[17] and, as pointed out earlier[23], there is no real reason why it should not.

Portal vein thrombosis occurs in up to 10% of cirrhotic patients and is a relative contraindication for LTx. If only partial obstruction is present a thrombectomy or dilatation may be possible. If the obstruction reaches the bifurcation of splenic and mesenteric veins a reconstruction with a donor graft vein may be possible. However, if the thrombus reaches the branches of the mesenteric vein, LTx is not a viable option[24].

The situation in the paediatric transplant group has very much improved. While in former years about 20% of such children were dying on the waiting list[25,26], at our institution there has been no recent death due to organ shortage. This has become possible not only through improved availability of whole livers, but mainly through the consequent use of split-livers and living-donor-liver transplantation.

PRESERVATION

The liver is explanted after extensive systemic and topic cooling with crushed ice. The pioneers in the field of preservation are Collins with the EuroCollins solution, and Belzer and Southard from the University of Wisconsin. In 1987 the latter came forward with a newly designed solution, the so-called UW solution[27–29]. Using this solution preservation time could be increased from up to 8 h in the EuroCollins era to up to 24–30 h[30–33]. However, recent studies have cautioned against exceeding long cold storage[34]. The Achilles heel of preservation is the bile ducts, and it could be shown that preservation times over 12 h increase the risk of bile duct complications. The diffuse intra–extrahepatic stricture rate increases from 2% when organs are stored for less than 12 h to up to

35% for livers stored for longer periods[35]. The reason for the susceptibility of the bile ducts probably lies in lack of contact with the preservation solution, which is only perfused through the blood vessels of the porta hepatis and lack of peri-bile duct capillary diffusion. A back-flush with preservation solution up the common bile duct or via the gallbladder is highly recommended, and it was shown that sludge formation in the biliary tract is suppressed using that technique. It was found in clinical and experimental studies that it is very important to keep storage temperature low. It is not sufficient for the liver to be stored at refrigerator temperature, which is commonly around 4°C. Storage on crushed ice at 0–1°C is superior[36]. The mode of flush-out is also a topic of recent research. Some centres flush only through the hepatic artery via the abdominal aorta; most others also flush through the portal vein. The superiority of one method over the other has not yet been conclusively proven, but there are data which indicate that aortic flush alone is at least as good[37]. Perfusion pressure is usually not determined scientifically, but it should be noted that a portal perfusate pressure exceeding the normal portal venous pressure is unphysiological and should be avoided. The widely applied technique of perfusing artery and vein at the same pressure is probably not the best technique. Again, more studies are needed before one can make concise statements. At the end of preservation the liver is usually taken out of the cold solution and implanted in the right upper abdomen. At this stage it is important to keep the organ as cold as possible and the warm ischaemic time as short as possible. A close association with length of sewing-in and rate of initial poor function and non-function was demonstrated[38,39]. The solutions used to flush out the potassium-rich UW solution prior to reperfusion differ from centre to centre. In most centres an albumin or albumin–glucose solution is used, usually at room temperature[30]. The Carolina Rinse solution, developed by the North Carolina group at Chapel Hill[40–42], and used by some centres, contains adenosine and antioxidants, and has been shown in a rat transplant model to be beneficial in reducing reperfusion damage[41,42]. Controlled clinical trials are still necessary.

SURGICAL TECHNIQUE

The experience of transplant centres is another important factor. The technical quality and speed of implantation, and its duration, are related to the postoperative function of the liver[43–46] and obviously related to the rate of complications.

As an important point when discussing the feasibility, usefulness and ethical applicability of new techniques, one has also to consider death on the waiting list while waiting for a transplant. At the University of Chicago the mortality of children on the waiting list was only 1% compared to 10–25% at other centres at the same time[47]. This mortality rate also has to be taken into account when comparing post-transplant survival among individual groups. Any patient who dies while waiting for an organ can be seen as an 'unsuccessful transplant'. The shortage of donors, especially of paediatric donors, has led to three attempts to improve current resources, legal and social measures, in an attempt to increase the availability of grafts for adults and children. These new surgical techniques are based on the reduction of a full liver to a smaller functional size by means of an anatomical hepatectomy. The reduced size transplantation allograft techniques available today are Reduced-Size Cadaveric Liver Transplantation (RLT), Split Liver Transplantation (SLT) and Living Related Liver Transplantation (LRLT). The first two utilize livers from cadaveric donors, while in LRLT an in vivo hepatectomy is performed.

Reduced-size liver transplantation

One method to reduce organ shortage is reduced-size hepatic transplantation[48,49]. Its evolution in animal studies dates back to the 1950s[50]. Even in 1955 hepatic auxiliary transplantation was considered the only viable option to replace liver function, because with that technique the difficult part of clamping the portal vein and interrupting the venous flow could be omitted. This technique does not increase the organ pool in general, but redistributes the livers from larger adult recipients to children, who show more deaths on the waiting list because their donor pool is much smaller[25,51–53]. Technically a right lobe graft (segments 5–8, achieving a donor–recipient size reduction of 1:2) is prepared by dissection in the principal fissure, staying on the left side of the inferior vena cava and tying off the left hepatic duct, the left branch of the hepatic artery and the left portal vein. The left branches of the hepatic vein are also tied. For preparing a left lobe graft (segment 2–4, 1:4 reduction[54]) one has to stay on the right side of the inferior vena cava, tying off the right portal vein, the right branch of the hepatic artery and the right hepatic duct. The middle and left hepatic veins remain intact[53]. If one wants to prepare only the left lateral segments (segments 2 and 3, 1:10 reduction[54]), the procedure is very much the same as for retrieving the left lobe, but the bile duct is cut much shorter in order to ensure an adequate blood supply and to prevent bile duct necrosis. The reconnection of the hepatic vein of the left lateral segment is performed retaining the donor inferior vena cava, which has to be reduced in circumference. Nowadays, the recipient vena cava is preserved and an end-to-side anastomosis, directly to the vena cava (piggyback), is made.

Split-liver transplantation

SLT means transplanting to separate grafts obtained from a single cadaveric liver in two different recipients. The shortage of organs soon led to a search for other sources. In 1988 Pichlmayr *et al.* were the first to report a case of transplanting one donor liver in two recipients[55]. The basic difference compared to reduced-size liver transplantation is that both parts of the split liver are used for transplantation[25,50]. As the inferior vena cava can be used for only one of the grafts, usually the right side of the liver, the remaining part of the donor liver has therefore to be revascularized directly to the recipient's vena cava. The common hepatic artery and portal vein can also remain only with one graft, so that vascular structures on the remaining side have to be reconstructed. The results of split-liver transplantation grafts have initially not been as good as for reduced-size liver transplantation[25]. The reasons for this were long ischaemic times due to longer dissection of the liver, often necrosis of the left median segment (segment 4), thrombosis of hepatic artery, biliary tract complications and outflow block to the inferior vena cava[52,56]. To address these problems the extensive use of interposition grafts, the splitting into right lobe (segments 4–8) and left lateral segment and not left lobe have been recommended[56]. Discarding segment 4 when preparing the left lateral lobe also has the advantage of obtaining more length on artery and portal vein[25]. Shortening of the bile duct to ensure good blood supply and a long venotomy on the inferior vena cava, rather than an anastomosis of the left hepatic vein to the stump of the left hepatic vein of the recipient, have been advocated in selected cases. It should be kept in mind that only excellent livers should be used for splitting. In cases of fatty infiltration or long preservation time one should be aware that two recipients are potentially put in danger by transplanting these grafts.

The results presented by the European Workshop[56] on split-liver transplantation showed that the rate of primary non-function and dysfunction was low (4%). Vascular thrombosis occurred in 7% of cases, biliary complications in 14.3% of right grafts and 23.4% of left grafts; this is no higher than in other publications[35]. Overall graft and patient survival was not statistically different between this group and the group of transplants performed conventionally during the same time period. However, the rate of retransplantation in the adult group was higher (22% vs 10%), but the 6-month survival rate was also better (89% vs 80%). At this point it is safe to say that split-liver transplantation has, in experienced hands, no disadvantage compared to conventional LTx, and should be considered as a routine procedure.

In-situ splitting of the liver

In 1995 a first report concerning *in-situ* splitting of the liver was published by our group[57]. This technique in preliminary reports proves to have several advantages over the *ex-situ* splitting procedure. First, by taking only the left lateral segments (segments 2 and 3) the right lobe of the liver and its vascular supply is left untouched, the transplantation of the right liver resembles a whole-liver transplantation. Since the operation is done in the heart-beating donor, perfusion of segment 4 can be checked before implantation. Another advantage is complete haemostasis on the cutting surface before harvesting of the liver. Since one problem of *ex-situ* splitting was the longer cold ischaemic time, compared to conventional LTx, with *in-situ* splitting this can be kept short.

Disadvantages are the longer duration of the explant procedure, the more technically demanding operation and the more difficult implantation of the left segment, which resembles a living-donor procedure. Overall, however, the advantages of the operation, if performed by an experienced team, outweigh its drawbacks; it could become a powerful tool in fighting donor shortage in young children as well as in small-size adults for whom, up to now, often only a reduced-size liver could be used.

Living-donor-liver transplantation

The lack of size-matched organs for the paediatric population is the most limiting problem in paediatric LTx. While split-liver transplantation may alleviate that problem, at this point in time it cannot be the solution for all transplant candidates[58]. With the splitting technique, however, it could be proved that dividing the liver into two viable organs can be done safely. So the next logical step was, in analogy to living-donor-kidney transplantation, the introduction of living-donor-liver transplantation[59]. While split-liver grafts probably demand the highest surgical skills, the use of living-donor-liver grafts involves a wealth of ethical problems. The first to address these issues was the team at the University of Chicago[25,26,52,60]. The possibly beneficial effects of having a live donor include a decreased rate of non-function and dysfunction (probably due to the lack of trauma and ischaemia to the graft before retrieval), the ability to schedule the operation electively and, additionally, the psychological benefit for the family, which is relieved of the pressure of having to wait for an uncertain time for the transplantation. On the other hand, of course, there is risk for the donor and, in case of living non-related liver donation, the potential economic background.

The classic operation is a left lateral segmentectomy without vascular exclusion. While the left lobe can be removed without endangering the blood supply to the remainder of the liver, removal of the entire left lobe has proved to be burdened with too many complications[47]. In most cases, therefore, removal of the left lateral segments is performed. This has several advantages: first, the left lateral segments are the smallest part of the liver one can easily explant (donor–recipient size 1:10). This makes LTx possible in even the smallest children. Secondly, the anatomy and vascular structures of segments 2 and 3 are well defined, which makes surgical isolation easier. It could be shown that the portal venous blood supply to segment 4 can be impaired without inducing necrosis. Thirdly, the cut surface of the liver left of the falciforme ligament is very small, minimizing blood loss and the chance of leaking bile ducts. The dissection of the segments is carried out without interruption of blood flow to the liver, and blood transfusions are usually not required[26,61].

A total of more than 600 cases have been performed world-wide with 1-year graft survival of 83% (Living Donor Registry, Hamburg). The results are very encouraging, and survival rates for living-donor-liver transplantation are as good as, if not better than, those for cadaveric transplantation[34,62,63].

Piggyback (PB)/side-to-side cavocavostomy transplantation

The technique of this procedure is to preserve the recipient vena cava and to perform an end-to-side (piggyback) or a side-to-side[64] cavocavostomy and to oversew the distal stump of the donor inferior vena cava. The main advantage of these techniques lies in the possibility of anastomosing vessels even if there is a major discrepancy between donor and recipient organ size. The disadvantage is the danger of outflow obstruction through kinking, in the PB transplantation, and pressure by the liver upon the vena cava. This technique should therefore be reserved for cases with a large discrepancy between donor and recipient size[24]. This technique can avoid the use of veno-veno bypass by partial side clamping of the vena cava or very short vena cava clamping time. A temporary portocaval shunt can be used if splanchnic decompression is needed.

Auxiliary liver transplantation

This is another option in cases of metabolic disorders or fulminant hepatic failure. Only a small portion of functional liver or only temporary support is needed to compensate for the impairment of liver function of the native liver[12,25,50], even though both right and left grafts can be used (most commonly a left lateral graft). The graft is usually implanted in the right upper abdomen after resection of the left lobe of the recipient's liver. In heterotopic transplantation the graft is implanted in a non-anatomical position and the recipient liver is left intact. This procedure has been less successful because of difficult haemo-dynamics and abdominal volume scarcity, leading to pressure ischaemia. These problems can be avoided by placing the venous outflow as proximal and close to the diaphragm as possible[50]. The strategy in auxiliary transplantation is to give the native liver a chance to recuperate, and eventually to discontinue immunosuppression[24]. The transplanted liver will then be rejected and become atrophic, or it must be removed surgically[51]. The group at King's College Hospital in London[65], and the one at Villejuif, France[66], have set up guidelines for the correct timing of LTx.

Xenotransplantation

A completely new avenue in organ transplantation is the transplantation of organs from another species into humans. The first xenotransplants were done in the 1960s, all of them unsuccessful. The first liver xenotransplantation pro-gramme was initiated by the University of Pittsburgh group in 1992. They trans-planted two baboon livers into two human recipients. The second recipient died soon after surgery from peritonitis without ever regaining consciousness after the operation. The first patient died 70 days after the operation from dissemi-nated fungal infection. The baboon liver, which initially was much smaller than the original organ, had reached nearly the appropriate size within only a few weeks, indicating the immense regenerative potency of the liver[67–69]. It is thought that the patient, to whom cyclophosphamide was also administered, to prevent the humoral component of rejection, actually died from a too-aggressive immunosuppressive regimen.

Xenotransplantation is not yet a clinical reality because of major problems such as infections, hyperacute rejection and complement cascade-related prob-lems as well as the need for high immunosuppressive regimens.

GENERAL PROBLEMS OCCURRING IN LIVER TRANSPLANTATION

Reperfusion

This is begun after performing the suprahepatic and infrahepatic venous anasto-moses, then portal vein anastomosis and finally arterial anastomosis. Most centres reperfuse after portal vein anastomosis is accomplished, without having completed arterial anastomosis. The advantage is that, in cases in which a veno-venous bypass has not been used, the period of intestinal congestion is short-ened. The disadvantage is the uneven initial perfusion of the graft, and the danger is further reperfusion injury while finishing the arterial anastomosis. For that reason it is recommended to perform simultaneous arterial and portal reper-fusion, when a venovenous bypass is employed. Using UW it is mandatory to flush out this potassium-rich perfusate. This can be accomplished by perfusion with colloid or crystalloid solutions (albumin solution, Ringer's solution or

Carolina Rinse solution). Another method is using a blood-flush, using the recipient's own blood. It has not yet been determined in large randomized trials which flush solution, at what temperature, is optimal to minimize reperfusion injury.

Biliary anastomosis

To date biliary anastomosis remains a challenge in the otherwise fairly standardized field of liver transplantation[35,70–72]. Most centres use the end-to-end-technique, which carries a complication rate of 10–50%. In cases of sclerosing cholangitis a choledochocholedochostomy is not advisable, so a Roux-en-Y reconstruction should be performed. A side-to-side-reconstruction has been shown to carry the lowest complication rate of all techniques (2.3% surgical-related complications[24]). The rate of complications between reduced-size and full-size LTx is comparable[73].

Immunosuppression

The use of CyA in 1979 brought a tremendous change in the field of clinical liver transplantation[74]. The substitution of azathioprine for CyA increased the 1-year survival rate from 30% to 75%. The early 1990s saw the introduction of FK506, a macrolide antibiotic produced by the soil fungus *Streptomyces tsukubaensis*[75,76]. This acts in a way similar to CyA, but it is 100 times more effective. It is also of use as a rescue drug in patients with acute rejection under CyA therapy[77]. In several double-blind studies of FK506 versus CyA the superiority of FK506 was proved[6,78]. Another drug used in CyA-resistant rejection is OKT3[79] or FK506 switch.

Chimaerism

Chimaerism means that in the organ recipient donor-derived lymphatic cells become engrafted and functionally active. The significance of this finding could become profound in the near future. It is possible that patients with a high grade of chimaerism may need less immunosuppression, and in some cases may not need any at all. To date chimaerism has not been shown to have real clinical importance. At any rate, a more thorough understanding of chimaerism may lead to a more sophisticated drug regimen.

RECURRENCE OF PRE-EXISTING DISEASE

Hepatitis B

LTx in patients with chronic hepatitis B lead to almost universal disease recurrence if untreated after surgery[80]. Patients who are HBV DNA-positive show disease recurrence in more than 90%, even with postoperative administration of hepatitis B immunoglobulin[15,81]. Patients who are HBV DNA-negative have a better outcome with concomitant IgG administration; disease recurrence is around 40%. Fulminant hepatitis, HBV delta and HBV DNA-positive patients have scaling rates of recurrence[53]. Pretreatment with interferon and lamivudine in HBV DNA-positive patients seems a possible strategy to rescue these cases, who today are considered poor indications for LTx[82,83].

If the disease recurs, disease exacerbation is much faster than before transplantation. To slow down the disease process, interferon, or antiviral drugs such as lamivudine, have been used with some success[15,84]. However, in patients who are unsuccessfully treated, retransplantation has to be considered, keeping in mind that the time until recurrence is usually 50% of the one after the first transplantation.

Hepatitis C

Hepatitis C-related LTx carries a much better prognosis than hepatitis B. The actuarial survival rates in 97 liver transplant recipients 1, 2 and 3 years after transplantation were 94%, 89% and 87%, respectively[16]. Of 11 deaths in this group only two were directly related to disease recurrence. The University of Pittsburgh group investigated the use of interferon for recurrent disease, and results were not promising. Interferon–ribavirin seems to be the most effective regimen in controlling aggressive recurrent hepatitis C[82,85].

References

1. Starzl TE, Marchiori TL, Von Kaulla KN, Hermann G, Brittain RS, Waddell WR. Homotransplantation of the liver in humans. Surg Gynecol Obstet. 1963;117:659–76.
2. Starzl TE, Demetris AJ. Liver transplantation: a 31-year perspective. Part I. Curr Probl Surg. 1990;17:55–116.
3. Starzl TE, Demetris AJ. Liver transplantation: a 31-year perspective. Part II. Curr Probl Surg. 1990;17:129–36.
4. Starzl TE, Demetris AJ. Liver transplantation: a 31-year perspective. Part III. Curr Probl Surg. 1990;17:187–240.
5. Starzl TE, Demetris AJ, van Thiel D. Liver transplantation. N Engl J Med. 1989;321:1014–22.
6. Wood RP, Ozaki CF, Katz SM, Monsour HP, Dyer CH, Johnston TD. Liver transplantation. Surg Clin N Am. 1994;74:1133–54.
7. Alexander JW, Vaughin WK. The use of 'marginal' donors for organ transplantation. Transplantation. 1991;51:135–41.
8. Yarmush ML, Dunn JCY, Tompkins RG. Assessment of artificial liver support technology. Cell Transplant. 1992;1:323–41.
9. Neuzil DF, Rozga I, Moscioni AD, Ro MS, Hakim R, Demetriou AA. Use of a xenograft liver support system to treat a patient with acute liver failure. Hepatology. 1991;14:246A.
10. Ricordi C, Starzl TE. Cellular transplantation. Transplant Proc. 1991;23:73–6.
11. Calne R. Contraindications to liver transplantation. Hepatology. 1994;20:3–4S.
12. Williams R, Wendon J. Indications for orthotopic liver transplantation in fulminant liver failure. Hepatology. 1994;20:5–10S.
13. Benhamou J-P. Indications for liver transplantation in primary biliary cirrhosis. Hepatology. 1994;20:11–13S.
14. Harrison J, McMaster P. The role of orthotopic liver transplantation in the management of sclerosing cholangitis. Hepatology. 1994;20:14–19S.
15. Van Thiel DH, Wright HI, Fagiuoli S. Liver transplantation for hepatitis B virus-associated cirrhosis: a progress report. Hepatology. 1994;20:20–23S.
16. Ascher NL, Lake JR, Emond J, Roberts J. Liver transplantation for hepatitis C virus-related cirrhosis. Hepatology. 1994;20:24–27S.
17. Krom RAF. Liver transplantation and alcohol: who should get transplants? Hepatology. 1994;20:28–32S.
18. Otte J-B, de Ville de Goyet J, Reding R et al. Sequential treatment of biliary atresia with Kasai portoenterostomy and liver transplantation: a review. Hepatology. 1994;20:41–48S.

19. Lidofsky SD. Liver transplantation for fulminant hepatic failure. Gastroenterol Clin N Am. 1993;22:257–69.
20. Pichlmayr R, Weimann A, Ringe B. Indications for liver transplantation in hepatobiliary malignancy. Hepatology. 1994;20:33–40S.
21. Pichlmayr R, Weimann A, Steinhoff G, Ringe B. Liver transplantation for hepatocellular carcinoma: clinical results and future aspects. Cancer Chemother Pharmacol. 1992;31 (Suppl. I):S157–61.
22. Keeffe EB, Esquivel CO. Controversies in patient selection for liver transplantation. West J Med. 1993;159:586–93.
23. Hertl M, Broelsch CE, Stand der Lebertransplantation. In: Nilius R, Paquet K-J, editors. Prävention, Progressionshemmung und Rehabilitation von Lebererkrankungen. Freiburg: Karger GmbH;1995:192–203.
24. Neuhaus P, Platz K-P. Liver transplantation: newer surgical approaches. Bailliere's Clin Gastroenterol. 1994;8:481–93.
25. Broelsch CE, Emond JC, Whitington PF, Thistlethwaite JR, Baker AL, Lichtor JL. Application of reduced-size liver transplants as split grafts, auxiliary orthotopic grafts, and living related segmental transplants. Ann Surg. 1990;212:368–77.
26. Broelsch CE, Lloyd DM. Living related donors for liver transplants. Adv Surg. 1993;26:209–31.
27. Wahlberg JA, Love R, Landegaard L, Southard JH, Belzer FO. 72-hour preservation of the canine pancreas. Transplantation. 1987;43:5–8.
28. Belzer FO, Southard JH. Principles of solid organ preservation by cold storage. Transplantation. 1988;45:673–6.
29. Belzer FO. Clinical organ preservation with UW solution. Transplantation. 1989;47:1097.
30. Belzer FO, Southard JH, D'Alessandro AM, Knechtle SJ, Sollinger HW, Kalayoglu M. Update on preservation of liver grafts. Transplant Proc. 1993;25:2010–11.
31. Todo S, Nevy J, Yanaga K, Podesta L, Gordon RD, Starzl TE. Extended preservation of human liver grafts with UW solution. J Am Med Assoc. 1989;261:711–14.
32. Kocoshis SA, Tzakis A, Todo S, Reyes J, Nour B. Pediatric liver transplantation. Clin Pediatr. 1993;32:386–92.
33. Vogelbach P, Emond JC, Thistlethwaite JR, Broelsch CE. Die Konservierung von Spenderlebern mit University of Wisconsin-Lösung. Helv Chirurg Acta. 1991;58:159–61.
34. Bismuth H, Azoulay D, Dennison A. Recent developments in liver transplantation. Transplant Proc. 1993;25:2191–4.
35. Krom RAF. The biliary tree – the Achilles tendon of liver transplantation. Transplantation. 1992;53:1167.
36. Hertl M, Chartrand PB, West DD, Harvey PRC, Strasberg SM. The effects of hepatic preservation at 0°C compared to 5°C. Cryobiology. 1994;31:434–40.
37. De Ville de Goyet J, Hausleithner V, Malaise J, et al. Liver procurement without in situ portal perfusion. Transplantation. 1994;57:1328–32.
38. Furukawa H, Todo S, Inventarza O et al. Cold ischemia time versus outcome of human liver transplantation using UW solution. Transplant Proc. 1991;23:1550–1.
39. Furukawa H, Todo S, Inventarza O, et al. Effect of cold ischemia time on the early outcome of human hepatic allografts preserved with UW solution. Transplantation. 1991;51:1000–4.
40. Currin RT, Thurman RG, Lemasters JJ. Carolina Rinse solution protects adenosine triphosphate-depleted hepatocytes against lethal cell injury. Transplant Proc. 1991;23:645–7.
41. Gao W, Takei Y, Marzi I et al. Carolina Rinse solution – a new strategy to increase survival time after orthotopic liver transplantation in the rat. Transplantation. 1991;52:417–24.
42. Gao W, Hijioka T, Linder KA, Caldwell-Kenkel JC, Lemasters JJ, Thurman RG. Evidence that adenosine is a key component in Carolina Rinse responsible for reducing graft failure after orthotopic liver transplantation in the rat. Transplantation. 1991;52:992–8.
43. Cisneros C, Guillén F, Gomez R et al. Analysis of warm ischemia time for prediction of primary nonfunction of the hepatic graft. Transplant Proc. 1991;23:1976.
44. Cywes R, Clavien P-A, Sanabria JR, Greig PD, Harvey PRC, Strasberg SM. Glycogen repletion and metabolism during porcine hepatic allograft retrieval and preservation. Hepatology. 1991;14:57 (abstract).
45. Kamiike W, Burdelski M, Steinhoff G, Ringe B, Lauchart W, Pichlmayr R. Adenine nucleotide metabolism and its relation to organ viability in human liver transplantation. Transplantation. 1988;45:138–43.

46. Kanematsu T, Higashi H, Takenaka K, Matsumata T, Maehara Y, Sugimachi K. Bioenergy status of human liver during and after warm ischemia. Hepato-Gastroenterology. 1990;37 (Suppl.):160–2.

47. Thistlethwaite JR, Emond JC, Heffron TG, Whitington PF, Black DD, Broelsch CE. Innovative use of organs for liver transplantation. Transplant Proc. 1991;23:2147–51.

48. Bismuth H, Houssin D. Reduced size orthotopic liver graft in hepatic transplantation in children. Surgery. 1984;95:367–72.

49. Broelsch CE, Emond JC, Thistlethwaite JR, Withington PF. Orthotopic transplantation of hepatic segments in infants with biliary atresia. Langenbecks Chirurg Arch. 1984 (Suppl.):105–9.

50. Broelsch CE, Whitington PF, Emond JC. Evolution and future perspectives for reduced-size hepatic transplantation. Surg Gynecol Obstet. 1990;171:353–60.

51. Pappas SC, Rouch DA, Stevens LH. New techniques for liver transplantation: reduced-size, split-liver, living-related and auxiliary liver transplantation. Scand J Gastroenterol. 1995;30(Suppl.):97–100.

52. Broelsch CE, Emond JC, Thistlethwaite JR *et al.* Liver transplantation, including the concept of reduced-size liver transplants in children. Ann Surg. 1988;208:410–20.

53. Emond JC, Heffron TG, Whitington PF, Broelsch CE. Reconstruction of the hepatic vein in reduced size hepatic transplantation. Surg Gynecol Obstet. 1993;176:11–17.

54. Malago M, Rogiers X, Broelsch CE. Reduced-size hepatic allografts. Annu Rev Med. 1995;46:507–12.

55. Pichlmayr R, Ringe B, Gubernatis G. Transplantation einer Spenderleber auf zwei Empfänger: eine neue Methode in der Weiterentwicklung der lebersegment Transplantation. Langenbecks Arch Chirurg. 1989;373:127–30.

56. De Ville de Goyet J. Split liver transplantation in Europe – 1988 to 1993. Transplantation. 1995;59:1371–6.

57. Rogiers X, Malago M, Habib N *et al. In situ* splitting of the liver in the heart-beating cadaveric donor for transplantation in two recipients. Transplantation. 1995;59:1081–3.

58. Otte JB. Is it right to develop living related liver transplantation? Do reduced and split livers not suffice to cover the needs? Transplant Int. 1995;8:69–73.

59. Slooff MJH. Reduced size liver transplantation, split liver transplantation, and living related liver transplantation in relation to the donor organ shortage. Transplant Int. 1995;8:65–8.

60. Broelsch CE, Whitington PF, Emond JC *et al.* Liver transplantation in children from living related donors. Ann Surg. 1991;214:428–39.

61. Broelsch CE, Burdelski M, Rogiers X *et al.* Living donor for liver transplantation. Hepatology. 1994;20:49–55S.

62. Rogiers X, Burdelski M, Broelsch CE. Liver transplantation from living donors. Br J Surg. 1994;81:1251–3.

63. Ota K, Teraoka S, Kawai T. Transplantation in Asia: organ transplantation in Japan. Transplant Proc. 1995;27:1463–5.

64. Lerut J, de Ville de Goyet J, Donataccio M, Reding R, Otte JB. Piggyback transplantation with side-to-side cavocavostomy is an ideal technique for right split liver allograft implantation. J Am Coll Surg. 1994;179:573–6.

65. O'Grady JG, Alexander GJM, Hayllar KM. Early indicators of prognosis in fulminant hepatic failure. Gastroenterology. 1989;97:439.

66. Bernuau J, Goudeau A, Poynard T *et al.* Multivariate analysis of prognostic factors in fulminant hepatitis B. Hepatology. 1986;6:648–51.

67. Starzl TE. Liver allo- and xenotransplantation. Transplant Proc. 1993;25:15–17.

68. Starzl TE, Fung J, Tzakis A, Van Thiel D. Baboon-to-human liver transplantation. Lancet. 1993;341:65–71.

69. Fox IJ, Sindhi R, Shaw BW. Xenografts: do they have a role? Bailliere's Clin Gastroenterol. 1994;8:441–54.

70. Kadmon M, Bleyl J, Kueppers B, Otto G, Herfarth C. Biliary complications after prolonged University of Wisconsin preservation of liver allografts. Transplant Proc. 1993;25:1651–2.

71. Donovan J. Nonsurgical management of biliary tract disease after liver transplantation. Gastroenterol Clin N Am. 1993;22:317–35.

72. Van Thiel DH, Fagiuoli S, Wright HI, Rodriguez-Rilo H, Silverman W. Biliary complications of liver transplantation. Gastrointest Endosc. 1993;39:455–60.

73. Heffron TG, Emond JC, Whitington PF *et al.* Biliary complications in pediatric liver transplantation. Transplantation. 1992;53:391–5.
74. Calne RY, Rolles K, White DJ *et al.* Cyclosporin A initially as the only immunosuppressant in 34 recipients of cadaveric organs: 32 kidneys, 2 pancreases, 2 livers. Lancet. 1979;2:1033–6.
75. Hooks MA. Tacrolimus, a new immunosuppressant – a review of the literature. Ann Pharmacother. 1994;28:501–10.
76. Fung JJ, Todo S, Tzakis A *et al.* Conversion of liver allograft recipients from cyclosporine to FK 506-based immunosuppression: benefits and pitfalls. Transplant Proc. 1991;23:14–21.
77. Platz K-P, Mueller Z, Bechstein W-O, Blumhardt G, Lobeck H, Neuhaus P. OKT3 versus FK 506 rescue management of acute steroid-resistant and chronic rejection. Transplant Proc. 1995;27:1111–13.
78. Woodle ES, Perdrizet GA, So SKS, White HM, Marsh JW. FK506 rescue therapy for hepatic allograft rejection: experience with an aggressive approach. Clin Transplant. 1995;9:45–52.
79. Höckerstedt K. Treatment and prevention of liver allograft rejection with OKT3. Clin Transplant. 1993;7:403–13.
80. Holt CD, Millis JM, Busuttil RW. Role of liver transplantation in patients with hepatitis B infection. Clin Transplant. 1995;9:269–76.
81. Langrehr JM, Lemmens HP, Keck H *et al.* Liver transplantation in hepatitis B surface antigen positive patients with postoperative long-term immunoprophylaxis. Transplant Proc. 1995;27:1215–16.
82. Bizollon T, Ducerf C, Trepo C. New approaches to the treatment of hepatitis C virus infection after liver transplantation using ribavirin. J Hepatol. 1995;23:22–5.
83. Marcellin P, Benhamou J-P. Treatment of chronic viral hepatitis. Bailliere's Clin Gastroenterol. 1994;8:233–53.
84. Fung JJ, Eghtesad B, Todo S, Rakela J, Magnone M, Starzl TE. Hepatitis B virus (HBV) re-infection following liver transplantation: theory and practice. Clin Transplant. 1995;9:262–8.
85. Gane EJ, Tibbs CJ, Ramage JK, Portmann BC, Williams R. Ribavirin therapy for hepatitis C infection following liver transplantation. Transplant Int. 1994;8:61–4.

Index

cholestasis 40
  mechanisms 125–6
  neonatal *see* neonatal cholestasis
cholic acid 139
cimetidine 130
cis-diaminodichloroplatinum 231
clometacin 95
clonidine 156
colchicine 78, 136, 193–4
collagen 72, 74
contraceptives 87
copper
  deficiency 104
  hepatic concentration 116
  radiocopper 117
  urinary excretion 116
Cpd-861 198 (table), 199–208
  liver fibrosis, treatment 199–208
    chronic liver disease 207–8
cryoglobulinaemia, mixed 33
cyclosporin 130
cyclosporin A 136, 277, 295
cysteine 72
cytochrome P450
  antigen 95
  supergene family 9
cytochrome P450 2E1 92
cytokine-mediated antiviral mechanisms
  46–8
cytokines 22
cytomegalovirus, donor liver transplant 283
cytoskeletal proteins 180

decorin 195
dehydralazine 96
dexamethasone 196
α-dihydroxy bile acids 139
diphtheria toxin A 44, 48
diuretics 156
DNA-based prophylactic vaccination 48–9
drug susceptibility factors 93–4
drug-associated hepatitis 85–97
  diagnosis of drug reactions 87–9
  drug reactions 90–1
  drugs causing 85, 88 (table)
  epidemiology of drug reactions 85–7
  patterns 89–90

elastosis perforans serpiginosa 120
enfurane 70
epirubicin 231
Erk-1 179
Erk-2 179
erythromycin 130
ethanol *see* alcohol
extracorporeal shockwave lithotripsy, for
  gallstones 247–9
extrahepatic biliary atresia 130

famciclovir 29, 55, 59–60, 62
fatty liver 75–6
fenobrate 95
ferritin 102–3
FK506 (tacrolimus) 277
flucloxacillin 130
flu-like syndrome 34, 57
flumazenil 190
5-fluorouracil 230–1

gallstones
  cholesterol 241–2
  extracorporeal shockwave lithotripsy
    247–9
  laparoscopic cholecystectomy *see*
    laparoscopic cholecystectomy
  non-surgical management 244–50
    expectant 244–5
  oral bile acid dissolution 246–7
  pigment 242
  surgical treatment 252–60
  therapeutic intervention 245–6
    treatment options 246 (table)
ganciclovir 55, 62
glucocorticoids 136
γ-glutamyl-transpeptidase 39–40
glutathione (GSH) 72–3, 125
graft rejection 274–5
granulocyte-macrophage-colony-stimulating
  factor (GM-CSF) 29

haemochromatosis 100–6
  biochemical defect 102–4
  diagnosis 100–1
  genetics 104–6
  hepatocyte membrane transport 103–4
  inheritance 100
  intestinal mucosal cell 102–3
  liver 103
  non-transferrin bound iron 103–4
  parenchymal cell defect 104
  pathology 101
  prognosis 106
  reticuloendothelial system 104
  treatment 106
haemophiliacs 33
halothane 87, 95
HbsAg-positive chronic hepatitis 17
hepatectomy 288–90
hepatic cirrhosis 17, 79–80
  metabolic alkalosis 185
  pathobiochemistry 185 (fig.)
hepatic encephalopathy 78, 176–90
  astrocyte swelling 177–80
  hepatic ammonia detoxication 181–6
  liver transplantation 190
  precipitating factors 182 (fig.), 187
  treatment 187–90

interferon α 27–8, 44, 55–8
  action in HbsAg carriers   54
  adverse effects   57–8
  liver fibrosis   194–5
  lymphoblastoid   30
  oriental HbsAg carriers vs. caucasian HbsAg
    carriers   56–7
  recombinant   38
  steroid therapy preceding   56
interferon β 44
interferon γ, liver fibrosis   194–5
interleukin-2   29
interleukin-6   22
intravenous drug users   33
iron   100
  absorption   102
    defective control   102
  binding proteins   102
isoniazid   70, 96–7
isosorbide dinitrate   156
isosorbide-5-mononitrate   156

K^+ canrenoate   169
ketanserin   156
kidney
  cystic degeneration   130
  grafts   33
Kupffer cells   104

lactilol   188
lactulose   188
lamivudine   29, 55, 60–2, 63
laparoscopic cholecystectomy
  complicated   255–7
    acute cholangitis   257
    acute cholecystitis   255–6
    gallstone pancreatitis   256–7
  complications   257–60
    biliary injuries   257–60
    bowel injury   260
    cardiopulmonary   260
    discharge of stones   260
    hernias   260
    intra-abdominal abscess   260
    spillage of stones   260
    subcutaneous abscess   260
    vascular injury   260
    would infection   260
  in:
    children   255
    cirrhosis   255
    diabetics   255
    pregnancy   255
  indications/contraindications   252–7
    asymptomatic cholelithiasis   252–4
    symptomatic cholelithiasis   254, 258
      (fig.)
lecithin   77
lipoidal   228

lipogranulomas   75
liposomes   48
liver disease
  autoimmune   9
  drug induced   9
  viral   9
liver fibrosis   193–208
  treatment
    antisense DNA   197
    colchicine   193–4
    Cpd-861   199–208
    D-penicillamine   196
    interferon α 195
    interferon γ 194–5
    lufironil   195
    lysyl oxidase inhibitor   195–6
    PDGF blocking agents   197
    pentoxifylline   197
    polyunsaturated lecitine   194
    prostaglandins E2   196
    retinoids   195
    steroids   196
    TGF β 197
    traditional Chinese medicine   197–202
    zinc   196
liver glutaminase   183–5
liver transplantation   273–303
  acceptance/tolerance   277
  alcohol abuser as a donor   283
  allograft rejection mechanisms   275–6
    prevention   276–7
  anhepatic phase   290–2
  anomalous hepatic artery anatomy   292
  ascites   173
  assessments of graft   283–4
  auxiliary liver   300–1
  biliary anastomosis   301–2
  chimaerism   302
  coeliac axis stenosis   292
  contraindications   279–80
  donor evaluation   282
  follow-up of allograft recipient   284
  graft rejection   274–5
  hepatectomy   288–90
  hepatic artery thrombosis   292
  hepatic encephalopathy   190
  hepatitis B, recurrence   302
  hepatitis C, recurrence   303
  history   274
  HLA antigens matching   282
  immunosuppression   302
  in situ splitting   299
  indications   278–9, 281–2, 296
    cholestatic liver disease   281–2
    chronic parenchymal liver disease   281
  living donor   299–300
  patient preparation   282
  piggyback   291, 300
  preservation   296–7

Falk Symposium Series

43. Reutter W, Popper H, Arias IM, Heinrich PC, Keppler D, Landmann L, eds.: *Modulation of Liver Cell Expression*. Falk Symposium No. 43. 1987   ISBN: 0-85200-677-2*

44. Boyer JL, Bianchi L, eds.: *Liver Cirrhosis*. Falk Symposium No. 44. 1987
    ISBN: 0-85200-993-3*

45. Paumgartner G, Stiehl A, Gerok W, eds.: *Bile Acids and the Liver*. Falk Symposium No. 45. 1987   ISBN: 0-85200-675-6*

46. Goebell H, Peskar BM, Malchow H, eds.: *Inflammatory Bowel Diseases – Basic Research & Clinical Implications*. Falk Symposium No. 46. 1988   ISBN: 0-7462-0067-6*

47. Bianchi L, Holt P, James OFW, Butler RN, eds.: *Aging in Liver and Gastrointestinal Tract*. Falk Symposium No. 47. 1988   ISBN: 0-7462-0066-8*

48. Heilmann C, ed.: *Calcium-Dependent Processes in the Liver*. Falk Symposium No. 48. 1988   ISBN: 0-7462-0075-7*

50. Singer MV, Goebell H, eds.: *Nerves and the Gastrointestinal Tract*. Falk Symposium No. 50. 1989   ISBN: 0-7462-0114-1

51. Bannasch P, Keppler D, Weber G, eds.: *Liver Cell Carcinoma*. Falk Symposium No. 51. 1989   ISBN: 0-7462-0111-7

52. Paumgartner G, Stiehl A, Gerok W, eds.: *Trends in Bile Acid Research*. Falk Symposium No. 52. 1989   ISBN: 0-7462-0112-5

53. Paumgartner G, Stiehl A, Barbara L, Roda E, eds.: *Strategies for the Treatment of Hepatobiliary Diseases*. Falk Symposium No. 53. 1990   ISBN: 0-7923-8903-4

54. Bianchi L, Gerok W, Maier K-P, Deinhardt F, eds.: *Infectious Diseases of the Liver*. Falk Symposium No. 54. 1990   ISBN: 0-7923-8902-6

55. Falk Symposium No. 55 not published

55B. Hadziselimovic F, Herzog B, Bürgin-Wolff A, eds.: *Inflammatory Bowel Disease and Coeliac Disease in Children*. International Falk Symposium. 1990 ISBN 0-7462-0125-7

56. Williams CN, eds.: *Trends in Inflammatory Bowel Disease Therapy*. Falk Symposium No. 56. 1990   ISBN: 0-7923-8952-2

57. Bock KW, Gerok W, Matern S, Schmid R, eds.: *Hepatic Metabolism and Disposition of Endo- and Xenobiotics*. Falk Symposium No. 57. 1991   ISBN: 0-7923-8953-0

58. Paumgartner G, Stiehl A, Gerok W, eds.: *Bile Acids as Therapeutic Agents: From Basic Science to Clinical Practice*. Falk Symposium No. 58. 1991   ISBN: 0-7923-8954-9

59. Halter F, Garner A, Tytgat GNJ, eds.: *Mechanisms of Peptic Ulcer Healing*. Falk Symposium No. 59. 1991   ISBN: 0-7923-8955-7

60. Goebell H, Ewe K, Malchow H, Koelbel Ch, eds.: *Inflammatory Bowel Diseases – Progress in Basic Research and Clinical Implications*. Falk Symposium No. 60. 1991
    ISBN: 0-7923-8956-5

61. Falk Symposium No. 61 not published

62. Dowling RH, Folsch UR, Löser Ch, eds.: *Polyamines in the Gastrointestinal Tract*. Falk Symposium No. 62. 1992   ISBN: 0-7923-8976-X

63. Lentze MJ, Reichen J, eds.: *Paediatric Cholestasis: Novel Approaches to Treatment*. Falk Symposium No. 63. 1992   ISBN: 0-7923-8977-8

64. Demling L, Frühmorgen P, eds.: *Non-Neoplastic Diseases of the Anorectum*. Falk Symposium No. 64. 1992   ISBN: 0-7923-8979-4

64B. Gressner AM, Ramadori G, eds.: *Molecular and Cell Biology of Liver Fibrogenesis*. International Falk Symposium. 1992   ISBN: 0-7923-8980-8

*These titles were published under the MTP Press imprint.

Falk Symposium Series

65. Hadziselimovic F, Herzog B, eds.: *Inflammatory Bowel Diseases and Morbus Hirschprung*. Falk Symposium No. 65. 1992   ISBN: 0-7923-8995-6

66. Martin F, McLeod RS, Sutherland LR, Williams CN, eds.: *Trends in Inflammatory Bowel Disease Therapy*. Falk Symposium No. 66. 1993   ISBN: 0-7923-8827-5

67. Schölmerich J, Kruis W, Goebell H, Hohenberger W, Gross V, eds.: *Inflammatory Bowel Diseases – Pathophysiology as Basis of Treatment*. Falk Symposium No. 67. 1993   ISBN: 0-7923-8996-4

68. Paumgartner G, Stiehl A, Gerok W, eds.: *Bile Acids and The Hepatobiliary System: From Basic Science to Clinical Practice*. Falk Symposium No. 68. 1993   ISBN: 0-7923-8829-1

69. Schmid R, Bianchi L, Gerok W, Maier K-P, eds.: *Extrahepatic Manifestations in Liver Diseases*. Falk Symposium No. 69. 1993   ISBN: 0-7923-8821-6

70. Meyer zum Büschenfelde K-H, Hoofnagle J, Manns M, eds.: *Immunology and Liver*. Falk Symposium No. 70. 1993   ISBN: 0-7923-8830-5

71. Surrenti C, Casini A, Milani S, Pinzani M , eds.: *Fat-Storing Cells and Liver Fibrosis*. Falk Symposium No. 71. 1994   ISBN: 0-7923-8842-9

72. Rachmilewitz D, ed.: *Inflammatory Bowel Diseases – 1994*. Falk Symposium No. 72. 1994   ISBN: 0-7923-8845-3

73. Binder HJ, Cummings J, Soergel KH, eds.: *Short Chain Fatty Acids*. Falk Symposium No. 73. 1994   ISBN: 0-7923-8849-6

73B. Möllmann HW, May B, eds.: *Glucocorticoid Therapy in Chronic Inflammatory Bowel Disease: from basic principles to rational therapy*. International Falk Workshop. 1996   ISBN 0-7923-8708-2

74. Keppler D, Jungermann K, eds.: *Transport in the Liver*. Falk Symposium No. 74. 1994   ISBN: 0-7923-8858-5

74B. Stange EF, ed.: *Chronic Inflammatory Bowel Disease*. Falk Symposium. 1995   ISBN: 0-7923-8876-3

75. van Berge Henegouwen GP, van Hoek B, De Groote J, Matern S, Stockbrügger RW, eds.: *Cholestatic Liver Diseases: New Strategies for Prevention and Treatment of Hepatobiliary and Cholestatic Liver Diseases*. Falk Symposium 75. 1994.   ISBN: 0-7923-8867-4

76. Monteiro E, Tavarela Veloso F, eds.: *Inflammatory Bowel Diseases: New Insights into Mechanisms of Inflammation and Challenges in Diagnosis and Treatment*. Falk Symposium 76. 1995.   ISBN 0-7923-8884-4

77. Singer MV, Ziegler R, Rohr G, eds.: *Gastrointestinal Tract and Endocrine System*. Falk Symposium 77. 1995.   ISBN 0-7923-8877-1

78. Decker K, Gerok W, Andus T, Gross V, eds.: *Cytokines and the Liver*. Falk Symposium 78. 1995.   ISBN 0-7923-8878-X

79. Holstege A, Schölmerich J, Hahn EG, eds.: *Portal Hypertension*. Falk Symposium 79. 1995.   ISBN 0-7923-8879-8

80. Hofmann AF, Paumgartner G, Stiehl A, eds.: *Bile Acids in Gastroenterology: Basic and Clinical Aspects*. Falk Symposium 80. 1995   ISBN 0-7923-8880-1

81. Riecken EO, Stallmach A, Zeitz M, Heise W, eds.: *Malignancy and Chronic Inflammation in the Gastrointestinal Tract – New Concepts*. Falk Symposium 81. 1995   ISBN 0-7923-8889-5

82. Fleig WE, ed.: *Inflammatory Bowel Diseases: New Developments and Standards*. Falk Symposium 82. 1995   ISBN 0-7923-8890-6

Falk Symposium Series

82B. Paumgartner G, Beuers U, eds.: *Bile Acids in Liver Diseases.* International Falk Workshop. 1995   ISBN 0-7923-8891-7

83. Dobrilla G, Felder M, de Pretis G, eds.: *Advances in Hepatobiliary and Pancreatic Diseases: Special Clinical Topics.* Falk Symposium 83. 1995.   ISBN 0-7923-8892-5

84. Fromm H, Leuschner U, eds.: *Bile Acids – Cholestasis – Gallstones: Advances in Basic and Clinical Bile Acid Research.* Falk Symposium 84. 1995   ISBN 0-7923-8893-3

85. Tytgat GNJ, Bartelsman JFWM, van Deventer SJH, eds.: *Inflammatory Bowel Diseases.* Falk Symposium 85. 1995   ISBN 0-7923-8894-1

86. Berg PA, Leuschner U, eds.: *Bile Acids and Immunology.* Falk Symposium 86. 1996   ISBN 0-7923-8700-7

87. Schmid R, Bianchi L, Blum HE, Gerok W, Maier KP, Stalder GA, eds.: *Acute and Chronic Liver Diseases: Molecular Biology and Clinics.* Falk Symposium 87. 1996   ISBN 0-7923-8701-5

88. Blum HE, Wu GY, Wu CH, eds.: *Molecular Diagnosis and Gene Therapy.* Falk Symposium 88. 1996   ISBN 0-7923-8702-3

88B. Poupon RE, Reichen J, eds.: *Surrogate Markers to Assess Efficacy of TReatment in Chronic Liver Diseases.* International Falk Workshop. 1996   ISBN 0-7923-8705-8

89. Reyes HB, Leuschner U, Arias IM, eds.: *Pregnancy, Sex Hormones and the Liver.* Falk Symposium 89. 1996   ISBN 0-7923-8704-X

89B. Broelsch CE, Burdelski M, Rogiers X, eds.: *Cholestatic Liver Diseases in Children and Adults.* International Falk Workshop. 1996   ISBN 0-7923-8710-4

90. Lam S-K, Paumgartner P, Wang B, eds.: *Update on Hepatobiliary Diseases 1996.* Falk Symposium 90. 1996   ISBN 0-7923-8715-5